COGNITIVE REHABILITATION IN OLD AGE

COGNITIVE REHABILITATION IN OLD AGE

ROBERT D. HILL

LARS BÄCKMAN

ANNA STIGSDOTTER NEELY

New York   Oxford
OXFORD UNIVERSITY PRESS
2000

Oxford University Press

Oxford   New York

Athens   Auckland   Bangkok   Bogota   Bogotá   Bombay   Buenos Aires   Calcutta
Cape Town   Chennai   Dar es Salaam   Delhi   Florence   Hong Kong   Istanbul
Karachi   Kuala Lumpur   Madrid   Melbourne   Mexico City   Mumbai
Nairobi   Paris   São Paulo   Singapore   Taipei   Tokyo   Toronto   Warsaw

and associated companies in
Berlin   Ibadan

Published by Oxford University Press, Inc.
198 Madison Avenue, New York, New York 10016

Oxford is a registered trademark of Oxford University Press

Library of Congress Cataloging-in-Publication Data

Cognitive rehabilitation in old age / edited by Robert D. Hill, Lars
Bäckman, Anna Stigsdotter Neely.
p.   cm.
Includes bibliographical references and index.
ISBN 0-19-511985-1
1. Cognition disorders in old age—Patients—Rehabilitation.
2. Geriatric psychiatry.   I. Hill, Robert D.   II. Bäckman, Lars.
III. Neely, Anna Stigsdotter.
[DNLM: 1. Aging—psychology.   2. Cognition—in old age.
3. Cognition Disorders—rehabilitation.   WT 145 C6765 2000]
RC524.C645   2000
618.97′689—dc21   99-11189
DNLM/DLC for Library of Congress

1 3 5 7 9 8 6 4 2

Printed in the United States of America
on acid-free paper

Preface

Cognitive deficits are part of the normal aging process and are exacerbated in various diseases that affect adults in old and very old age, such as dementia, depression, and stroke. A significant scientific and social effort has been expended to evaluate whether cognitive deficits can be remediated through systematic interventions. Thus, the editors, as well as the chapter authors, represent a variety of viewpoints that span theory, as well as practice. One of the goals of this book is to extend what is apparent in the theoretical literature on cognitive aging to normative issues facing older adults, as well as to nonnormative conditions reflective of diseases such as dementia, depression, and stroke. The principal purpose of this volume is to provide meaningful coverage of cognitive intervention research on normal and pathological aging, with a specific focus on the application of cognitive training strategies in natural settings. An important feature of this book is that it is grounded in contemporary theory about cognitive aging that should be applicable to both the practicing clinician and the researcher. Thus, it is important to note that this book was designed to be relevant to scholars studying basic issues in cognitive aging and to professionals working with older adults in preventive or remedial settings.

In this text, rehabilitation is broadly defined as encompassing not only the outcomes that may occur when a particular function is fully restored to its premorbid level, but also the outcomes that may result in mitigating the slope of decline in everyday functional ability (as is seen in dementia). Thus, the concept of rehabilitation may produce a diversity of expectations, from full restoration of function through improvement within a restricted ability range to preserving essential abilities that are necessary for function in an assisted-living or other caregiving context. It is our belief that the term *rehabilitation* best captures this variability in subject capability that is often used to gauge intervention programs that will best address cognitive changes that are inherent in both normal and pathological aging.

This text is organized into four parts that systematically move from theory-driven principles to the provision of practical techniques and ideas that can be used in a number of contexts. Part I highlights prominent theoretical principles that are important in conceptualizing and planning rehabilitation programming. In this section, chapters focus on plasticity in intellectual functioning, theoretical issues to consider in memory training, and factors that may influence the extent to which transfer and generalization are possible. These concepts provide essential background for Part II, which examines cognitive rehabilitation strategies in normal aging, with a specific focus on remediating memory deficits that are considered normative in old and very old age. The first chapter in this section is a general overview of the kinds of memory-training strategies that have been used with older adults and the extent to which they can be applied as rehabilitation aids. The two following chapters highlight innovative ideas and adjunctive techniques that can be used to augment rehabilitation strategies. In general, Part II explores the extent to which memory training can promote a sense of self-control over cognitive capabilities in everyday living.

Part III examines the interplay between cognitive function and lifestyle patterns that include physical exercise and cigarette smoking. In addition to lifestyle choices, Part III also addresses the role of selected psychological processes such as executive function and depression on cognitive capabilities in old and very old age. The fourth and final part focuses on rehabilitation strategies that address issues in pathological (or diseased) aging (dementia, depression, and stroke). Although this section deals with the domain that is often stereotypically viewed as the subject matter of rehabilitation, we have included this section last to encourage the reader to think of cognitive rehabilitation as a collection of strategies and procedures that are applicable to both normal aging and disease processes in old and very old age. In short, we believe that aging as a developmental process should be viewed as a continuum from optimal to maladaptive conditions. Thus, this book suggests that intervention strategies that are applicable to normal aging may also have some benefit when adapted to those who are experiencing age-related disease.

We appreciate the hard work of our chapter authors who assisted in helping us develop the concepts and ideas that form the foundation and organization of the book. This book is dedicated to our spouses and children; namely, Debra Hill, Darren and Justin; Agnenta Herlitz, Daniel, Hannes, Elias, and Miriam; Greg Neely, Tor and Ruyna.

Contents

Contributors

EDITORS

Lars Bäckman, Ph.D.
Stockholm Gerontology Research Center
Dalagatan 9-11, S-11382
Stockholm, Sweden

Robert D. Hill, Ph.D.
Counseling Psychology Program
Department of Educational Psychology,
  327 MBH
University of Utah
Salt Lake City, UT 84112

Anna Stigsdotter Neely, Ph.D.
Department of Psychology
University of Umea
S-90187
Umea, Sweden

CONTRIBUTORS

Michael J. Bird, Ph.D.
Department of Psychology
National Health and Medical Research
  Council
Social Psychiatry Research Unit
The Australian National University
Canberra, ACT, 0200
Australia

Cameron J. Camp, Ph.D.
Myers Research Institute
Menorah Park Center for the Aging
27100 Cedar Road FL 1
Beachwood, OH 44122

Katie E. Cherry
Department of Psychology
236 Audubon Hall
Louisiana State University
Baton Rouge, LA 70803

Jeffrey W. Elias, Ph.D.
Sanford Center on Aging
University of Nevada, Reno
Reno, NV 89557-0133

Charles F. Emery, Ph.D
Department of Psychology
Ohio State University
Columbus, OH 43210

Michael K. Gardner, Ph.D.
Department of Educational Psychology,
  327 MBH
University of Utah
Salt Lake City, UT 84112

Margie E. Lachman, Ph.D.
Department of Psychology
Brandeis University
Psychology Department MS#062
Waltham, MA 02254-9110

Bernice A. Marcopulos, Ph.D., ABPP.Cn.
Department of Psychiatric Medicine
University of Virginia
Charlottesville, VA 22908
and
Western State University
Staunton, VA 24401

Patrick J. Miller, Ph.D.
Psychology Service, 116B
VA Medical Center
Salt Lake City, UT 84112

Nancy A. Pachana, Ph.D.
School of Psychology
Massey University
Private Bag 11 222
Palmerston North
New Zealand

Thomas Schenkenberg, Ph.D.
Department of Neurology
School of Medicine
50 North Medical Drive
Salt Lake City, UT 84132

Karen Rothballer Seelert, M.A.
University of Utah
1705 East Campus Center Drive
Room 327
Salt Lake City, UT 84112

Clive Skilbeck, Ph.D.
Doctoral Program in Clinical Psychology
School of Health
University of Teeside
Middlesbrough TS1 3BA
United Kingdom

David L. Strayer
Department of Psychology
University of Utah
380 S. 1530 E., Rm. 502
Salt Lake City, UT 84112

Kellie A. Takagi, Ph.D.
Veterans Affairs Palo Alto Healthcare
  System
Stanford University School of Medicine
Stanford, CA 94304

Julia E. Treland, Ph.D.
Private Practice
14265 Domingo Ct.
Reno, NV 89511-6617

Paul Verhaeghen, Ph.D.
Department of Psychology
430 Huntington Hall
Syracuse University
Syracuse, NY 13244-2340

Duana C. Welch, Ph.D.
California State University, Fullerton
P.O. Box 6846
Fullerton, CA 92831-6846

Robin L. West, Ph.D.
Box 112250
Department of Psychology
University of Florida
Gainesville, FL 32611-2250

Dan J. Woltz
Department of Educational Psychology
University of Utah
1705 E. Campus Center Drive
Rm. 327
Salt Lake City, UT 84112-9255

Monica S. Yassuda
University of Florida
Department of Psychology
P.O. Box 112250
Gainesville, FL 32611-2250

PART I

THEORY-DRIVEN GUIDELINES FOR COGNITIVE REHABILITATION STRATEGIES IN OLDER ADULTS

I

The Interplay of Growth and Decline

Theoretical and Empirical Aspects of Plasticity of Intellectual and Memory Performance in Normal Old Age

PAUL VERHAEGHEN

Research on Plasticity in Old Age: A Short History

As cognitive aging researchers, we care for our subjects. Most scientists and practitioners do, of course, but there seems to be a quite inordinate amount of sympathiz-
ing in cognitive aging circles. I usually look very much forward to testing people
from our older adult research panel—they are so much different from the typical
undergraduate student, who breezes into the lab and seems to want nothing more than
to breeze out as quickly as possible. We get acquainted over a cup of coffee, and I
usually get to hear some pretty interesting stories (thanks to my research subjects,
I know more about nuclear waste management than is good for my sense of security,
I have an inkling of the usefulness of Bach sonatas for the beginning piano player,
and I will never consider a career switch to operating high-rise cranes). It is always
quite distressing to see how these interesting, highly motivated, and articulate human
beings then struggle with the cognitive tasks set before them—they certainly do not
breeze through. This contrast between high performance in daily life and less than
optimal performance in the laboratory has not been lost on most researchers in the
field. Our laboratory data and our theories about basic effects of aging on cognition
say one thing (decline, growing inflexibility, powerlessness); our hearts, and also our
eyes, say another (accumulated experience, openness to life, potential).

In fact, a major impetus for the initiation of plasticity research in the 1970s was
precisely the "general theoretical scenario of gerontological work" (Baltes & Lindenberger, 1988, p. 284) then prevalent: Cognitive aging was considered a process of
universal, cumulative, and gradual decline. The growing dissatisfaction with this limited view on aging resulted in conceptualizations of cognitive aging as a multidimen-

sional, multidirectional process with much individual variety in developmental trajectories (e.g., Baltes, Dittmann-Kohli, & Dixon, 1984). One of the cornerstones of such conceptions was the performance-potential distinction, which led researchers to look for modifiability-toward-potential as a function of the experiences accumulated by the individual rather than just to focus on scores on standard tests of cognitive performance (e.g., Baltes & Labouvie, 1973; Baltes & Schaie, 1976; Baltes & Willis, 1982; Labouvie-Vief, 1976). This modifiability within individuals was subsequently labeled *plasticity,* and intervention studies were started in the domain of psychometric intelligence by researchers at Penn State (the ADEPT [Adult Development and Enrichment] program), and later at the Max Planck Institute for Human Development and Education in Berlin (the PRO-ALT [Projekt Altersintelligenz, Intelligence in Old Age Project]).

Soon, the concept of plasticity became synonymous with the type of modifiability tapped by these and similar (though less ambitious) programs. Whereas Baltes and Willis (1982) defined plasticity in a generic sense as "the range of functioning at the individual level, whether ontogenetic (how variable is the individual course of development?) or concurrent (how variable is the performance at a given point in ontogenetic time?)" (pp. 355–356), in practice, the term has been narrowed down to mean "the range of intellectual aging under conditions not normally existent in either the living ecology of older persons or in the standard assessment situation provided by classical tests of psychometric intelligence," restricted "for ethical reasons, . . . to conditions assumed to be performance enhancing" (Baltes & Willis, 1982, p. 356). After first and largely unsuccessful attempts to modify performance on paper-and-pencil intelligence tests by increasing response speed (Hoyer, Hoyer, Treat, & Baltes, 1979; Hoyer, Labouvie, & Baltes, 1973; speed was indeed found to have increased after practice, but this did not have a large impact on intelligence test performance), plasticity researchers turned to the investigation of the effects of instruction and practice on performance on specific subtests of intelligence tests.

It is important to note here that these programs tapping plasticity in intellectual functioning have been developed explicitly for theoretical reasons, and not for the remediation of problems encountered in the day-to-day living ecology of the participants. The theories, moreover, were rather vague. Merely demonstrating the existence of plasticity was considered more important (at least at first) than a thorough investigation of plasticity as a phenomenon. In this, as Salthouse (1985) pointed out, 1970s accounts of plasticity often attacked a straw man position, as if any true psychologist could earnestly state that older people have no capacity to benefit from experience. Theory was not the only thing that was on researchers' minds—direct links to social policy issues were involved, in a sort of vicarious emancipatory reflex, as exemplified in the following quote from Baltes and Willis (1982):

> Research on plasticity is inherently aimed at providing a knowledge base apt to suggest procedures for optimization . . . and redistribution of education resources according to a life-span perspective. . . . In this sense, research on plasticity contributes to a foundation of social policy that is inherently preventive, corrective, and equity-oriented rather than discriminatory or defeatist. (p. 357)

Since those early days, things have changed. More recently, much emphasis has been placed on the fact that the demonstration of the existence of plasticity is not enough, and that plasticity in its turn needs to be explained (e.g., Baltes & Kliegl, 1986; Baltes, Kliegl, & Dittmann-Kohli, 1988; Baltes & Lindenberger, 1988; Kliegl & Baltes, 1987; Willis, 1989, 1990). Some of the controversial issues that surround plasticity as a phenomenon (rather than a concept) are the nature and directionality of the effects of treatment. With regard to the *nature of training effects*, there is some controversy over whether the training really attains the level of the ability trained (as was the explicit goal of the ADEPT program; Willis, 1989) or rather remains at the level of the specific skill taught (Willis called this "teaching the test," 1989, p. 554). Likewise, *directionality of the effects* is an issue under debate. The abilities trained are known to decline with age, and it may be tempting to assume that training remediates at least part of the decline that individuals experience, by activating skills that have gone lost or rusty through disuse. However, given the large individual differences in the timing of decline and the exact abilities that show decline, Willis (1989) suggested that "training effects may reflect remediation, incrementation, or compensation, depending on a given individual's prior performance history on a specific ability" (p. 557).

Another interesting development is that plasticity research has moved out of the tradition of psychometric intelligence (and out of the laboratory) and into the domain of episodic memory functioning. Unlike the ADEPT or PRO-ALT studies, memory-training studies were often constructed with the explicitly pragmatic goal of boosting memory performance in the real world. Maybe because the explicit goals of these two research traditions were so diverse, the experimental design and procedures for the two types of research have been quite different, so that a direct comparison of results is difficult. For instance, research into plasticity in psychometric intelligence has used different types of control groups and control measures; control procedures are the exception rather than the rule in memory-training research. Another difference is that the psychometric intelligence tradition has not used age-comparative designs, whereas quite a number of memory-training studies exist in which the treatment gains of older adults are compared to the treatment gains of young adults. The new line of findings has led researchers to focus on other issues of interest to plasticity theory, such as (age-related) *limits to plasticity* (Baltes & Kliegl, 1986; Lerner, 1990) and individual differences associated with *individual differences in plasticity* (Willis, 1990).

In the remainder of this chapter, I will briefly summarize some key results from these two main lines of plasticity research, paying special attention to the controversies and questions mentioned above: the nature and directionality of training effects, the age-related limits of plasticity, and individual differences in training responsiveness.

Plasticity in Psychometric Test Performance

Plasticity in Psychometric Test Performance: Study Design

As stated above, the studies devised to tap plasticity in psychometric intelligence performance have been designed with the initial goal of demonstrating the existence of plasticity, rather than offering direct theoretical insights into its nature and anteced-

ents. In order to demonstrate plasticity, a number of carefully planned control procedures have been included in the design of the studies. One simple control procedure
is to compare treatment gain in trained subjects with the gain obtained when subjects
are merely retested. This control group is used to estimate the baseline for plasticity
due to testing experience alone. Some of the later studies (Baltes et al., 1988; Baltes,
Sowarka, & Kliegl, 1989) also included a group receiving extensive practice; that is,
participants were repeatedly retested under the standardized instructions for the test,
and without receiving any feedback. This type of intervention serves as an estimate
for the amount of performance gain subjects can achieve on the basis of cognitive
skills already in their repertoire or by applying new but entirely self-taught skills.
Two studies (Hayslip, 1989; Labouvie-Vief & Gonda, 1976) included stress inoculation treatment as a placebo group.

All of these types of control treatments are contrasted to explicit training in ability-
specific problem-solving skills. The exact content of the skills trained is determined
through task analysis of the marker tests for these abilities. For instance, for a training
in figural relations, standard tests for this ability would be analyzed, relational rules
would be identified that should be applied to the material, and these rules would then
be taught in the training program. Items used for training were always similar to, but
not identical to the items of the standardized test. Results obtained from such training
groups yield an estimate of the amount of plasticity that can be reached when optimal
strategies are applied to the task.

Another type of control procedure used in psychometric intelligence plasticity involves measuring the effects of the training on a number of transfer tests. First and
foremost, tests of the ability trained are used as indicators of near-near transfer, that
is, transfer from the specific items taught to the items of a test measuring the same
ability. Second, tests for related abilities are used as indicators of near transfer. All
training programs involve fluid abilities, and consequently tests for other fluid abilities
are used as near transfer measures (in the one study on attention, memory span was
used as a near transfer measure). Third, tests for abilities unrelated to the trained
ability (e.g., tests for crystallized abilities) are used as indicators of far transfer. If the
effect is ability-specific, as opposed to being a general reactivation effect, one should
expect performance gain on near-near transfer tasks to exceed performance gain on
the other transfer tasks. It might even be expected that transfer on near transfer tasks
would be larger than transfer on far transfer tests.

Plasticity in Psychometric Test Performance: Some Key Findings

An overview of the results of the different training studies can be found in Table 1.1.
In this table, pre-to-posttest treatment gains are expressed in terms of mean standardized differences. Thus, the numbers indicate by how many standard deviations performance was shifted from a test prior to training or the relevant control procedure to a
test after the training or control treatment. A meta-analysis of these findings is presented in Table 1.2 (for an introduction to meta-analysis, see Bangert-Drowns, 1986,
or Mullen, 1989; a quick tutorial can be found in Verhaeghen, Marcoen, & Goossens,
1992). Note that the subjects in Baltes, Dittmann-Kohli, and Kliegl (1986) and Baltes
et al. (1988) were trained in both figural relations and inductive reasoning, so that

Table 1.1 Studies Included in the Meta-Analysis on Pre-to-Posttest Differences in Control, Placebo, and Treatment Groups for Psychometric Intelligence Research

Study	Type	n	d	Lower	Upper
				95% confidence limits for d	
Control groups					
Baltes, Dittmann-Kohli, and Kliegl (1986)	FR	68	0.75	0.40	1.10
Baltes, Kliegl, and Dittmann-Kohli (1988)	FR	29	0.36	−0.15	0.88
Baltes, Sowarka, and Kliegl (1989)	FR	24	0.39	−0.18	0.96
Plemons, Willis, and Baltes (1978)	FR	15	1.55	0.73	2.37
Baltes et al. (1986)	IR	68	0.90	0.54	1.25
Baltes et al. (1988)	IR	29	0.23	−0.29	0.75
Hayslip (1989)	IR	88	1.21	0.89	1.54
Willis, Cornelius, Blow, and Baltes (1983)	AT	24	0.64	0.06	1.22
Extended practice					
Baltes et al. (1986)	FR	29	0.88	0.34	1.42
Baltes et al. (1988)	FR	24	0.87	0.27	1.46
Baltes et al. (1988)	IR	29	0.82	0.28	1.35
Stress inoculation					
Hayslip (1989)	IR	92	1.51	1.18	1.84
Ability training					
Baltes et al. (1986)	FR	136	1.36	1.09	1.62
Baltes et al. (1988)	FR	29	0.67	0.15	1.20
Baltes et al. (1989)	fR	24	0.74	0.15	1.32
Plemons et al. (1978)	fR	15	2.08	1.19	2.97
Baltes et al. (1986)	IR	136	1.34	1.07	1.60
Baltes et al. (1988)	IR	29	0.80	0.27	1.34
Hayslip (1989)	IR	76	1.81	1.44	2.19
Willis and Schaie (1986)	SO	118	0.45	0.19	0.70
Willis et al. (1983)	AT	24	1.04	0.44	1.64
Near transfer					
Baltes et al. (1986)	FR	136	0.66	0.42	0.90
Baltes et al. (1988)	FR	29	0.41	−0.11	0.93
Baltes et al. (1989)	FR	24	0.38	−0.19	0.95
Plemons et al. (1978)	FR	15	0.70	−0.04	1.44
Baltes et al. (1986)	IR	136	0.66	0.42	0.90
Baltes et al. (1988)	IR	29	0.41	−0.11	0.93
Willis et al. (1983)	AT	24	0.37	−0.20	0.94
Far transfer					
Baltes et al. (1986)	FR	136	0.36	0.12	0.60
Baltes et al. (1988)	FR	29	0.07	−0.44	0.59
Baltes et al. (1989)	FR	24	0.25	−0.32	0.81
Baltes et al. (1986)	IR	136	0.36	0.12	0.60
Baltes et al. (1988)	IR	29	0.07	−0.44	0.59
Willis and Schaie (1986)	IR	110	0.20	−0.07	0.46
Willis et al. (1983)	SO	24	0.19	−0.06	0.45

Note. FR = figural relations; IR = inductive reasoning; SO = spatial orientation; AT = attention; d = point estimate of means standardized difference between pretest and posttest. The comparisons between Figural Relations and Inductive Reasoning by Baltes et al. (1986) and Baltes et al. (1988) are within-subject. Transfer effects versus training effects in all relevant studies are measured within-subject; effects of training versus control, extended practice or stress inoculation in all studies are measured between-subject.

Table 1.2 Summary of Effect Size Statistics (Effects of Skill Training on Intelligence Performance as Compared With the Effects of Various Control Procedures)

Measure	k	d_+	95% Confidence limits for d_+ Lower	Upper	Q_W
Figural relations					
Ability training	4	1.21	0.99	1.41	11.30[a]
Near transfer	4	0.59	0.39	0.79	1.34
Far transfer	3	0.30	0.10	0.50	1.01
Control	4	0.67	0.42	0.91	6.93
Extended practice	2	0.87	0.48	1.27	0.00
Inductive reasoning					
Ability training	4	1.08	0.92	1.24	35.74[a]
Near transfer	2	0.62	0.39	0.84	0.71
Far transfer	3	0.26	0.10	0.43	1.37
Control	3	0.92	0.71	1.14	10.12[a]
Extended practice	1	0.82	0.28	1.35	
Stress inoculation	1	1.51	1.18	1.84	
Spatial orientation					
Ability training	1	0.45	0.19	0.70	
Far transfer	1	0.19	−0.06	0.45	
Attention					
Ability training	1	1.04	0.44	1.64	
Near transfer	1	0.37	−0.20	0.94	
Control	1	0.64	0.06	1.22	

Note. k = number of studies; d_+ = mean weighted effect size (mean standardized difference); Q_W = chi-square statistic for homogeneity within groups.

[a]Significant nonhomogeneity at $p < .05$, according to chi-square test.

effect sizes for these measures (within the control, extended-practice, and ability-training treatment groups) are not independent; also note that treatment gains could not be calculated because of design problems or insufficient data in four other relevant studies (Blackburn, Papalia-Finlay, Foye, & Serlin, 1988; Blieszner, Willis, & Baltes, 1981; Labouvie-Vief & Gonda, 1976; Willis, Blieszner, & Baltes, 1981).

A number of results from the meta-analysis seem noteworthy. First, training in ability-specific problem-solving skills generally results in larger performance gains than retesting. This finding indicates that the training has an effect above and beyond the effect of mere retesting. However, these differences are reliable only for the ability of figural relations ($Q_B = 10.53$; $p < .05$), and not for inductive reasoning or attention ($Q_B = 1.37$ and 0.86, respectively; *ns*). In fact, a more striking result is that for both skill training and retesting, effect sizes are fairly large. This finding indicates that retesting itself is a quite potent elicitor of plasticity in intellectual performance, improving performance by two thirds of a standard deviation or more.

Second, extended-practice groups show no reliably smaller treatment gain than skill-training groups ($Q_B = 2.08$ and 0.88 for figural relations and inductive reasoning, respectively; *ns*; and note that in the three studies that included both conditions, the effect size for extended practice was actually larger than that for skill training). This finding strongly suggests that the crucial factor in the difference between the outcome of retesting and skill-training treatments is not the experimenter-guided instruction. Rather, as Baltes et al. (1988) formulated it, this difference seems an indication that "the performance gains obtained in past cognitive training research with psychometric measures of intelligence in the elderly were possible . . . because of the activation and practice of existing cognitive skills" (p. 399). This interpretation of the data is further supported by the fact that in the Baltes et al. (1988) study, ability-trained subjects did not solve more difficult items than the subjects having received extensive practice. Further support for the skill activation/practice hypothesis comes from the result that stress inoculation treatment resulted in reliably larger treatment gain than skill training in the one study investigating both (Hayslip, 1989)—maybe reducing stress helped subjects activate metacognitive operations and thus allowed them access to efficient skills. Skill reactivation appears to be a fairly rapid process, in that it already seems to operate when people are given a power assessment of the test (e.g., giving them more time and fewer items to solve; Baltes et al., 1988) rather than the usual speeded assessment.

With regard to transfer, tests for near-near transfer do indeed show a trend toward larger performance gains than either near transfer or far transfer tasks, with the latter showing the least amount of pre-to-posttest treatment gain. Inspection of the 95% confidence intervals indicates that for the abilities of figural reasoning and inductive reasoning, performance gains in ability tests are larger than those for near transfer and far transfer tests, with no reliable difference between the latter two. This finding, then, suggests that the effects of training remain largely confined to the ability trained.

Effects of cognitive skill training have also proven to be reasonably durable. Maintenance of training effects for fluid abilities have been examined over a 6-month period by Baltes et al. (1986), Willis et al. (1981), and Willis, Cornelius, Blow, and Baltes (1983), with posttest-to-follow-up-test mean standardized differences of 0.42, −0.06, and −0.14, respectively, showing either gain over this period or a decline that was relatively modest compared with the pre-to-posttest gain.

Plasticity in Psychometric Test Performance: Controversial Issues

What do these results teach us about the *nature of observed plasticity* in psychometric intelligence? As Willis stated in 1989: "The primary concern in training research is not a change in performance on a letter-series test or the 20-questions task per se, but rather change in the latent construct the test is said to represent" (p. 554). Unfortunately, the available evidence is largely inconclusive. The design of the studies, while ingenious, is not well suited for distinguishing between a change due to teaching-the-test and change at the latent construct level. For instance, in order to conclude that a change in ability has indeed occurred, one needs to demonstrate that long-term effects are present—but long-term effects could also be present if one merely has learned the skills to do well on the particular test and these skills are retained over the follow-up period, as we shall see in the review of memory plasticity studies.

A finding that at first sight seems like hard evidence for ability change is the fact that in the Willis and Schaie (1986) study, where training outcome was assessed at the factorial (i.e., presumably ability) level, performance was boosted more for the trained than for an untrained ability. However, this again is a necessary but not a sufficient condition for demonstrating that training has reached the ability level. In this study, subjects were trained in spatial orientation, and most tests for this ability require a common skill, namely, mental rotation. If subjects master this skill well—for instance, because they have learned to "focus on two or more features of the figure during rotation" (Willis & Schaie, 1986, p. 241)—they might apply this skill to all kinds of rotation tests, including those that look quite different from the test on which they were trained.

The most stringent test for demonstrating effects at the ability level would be to assess changes in performances on tasks relying on the ability, both in a laboratory context and in the living ecology. For instance, if one claims to have raised the spatial intelligence of students and spatial intelligence is correlated with certain types of study results (say, in geometry), then one should expect an increase in study results on the specified tasks after training. To my knowledge, no explicit tests for this type of generalization of ability training to other tasks requiring the ability have been conducted. However, it is interesting to observe that training in perceptual speed through extended practice does not result in a sizable increase in fluid intelligence scores (Hoyer et al., 1979; Hoyer et al., 1973), even though perceptual speed appears to be a major determinant of fluid intelligence (Horn, 1982; Salthouse, 1996; Verhaeghen & Salthouse, 1997).

In sum, while the results are consistent with the possibility that training reached the ability level, they are equally consistent with the hypothesis that effects remained at the level of the specific skill.

Another controversial issue concerns the *direction of training improvement*. Does training truly provide rehabilitation, in that it installs not only levels of performance previously available, but reinstalls lost skills? Schaie and Willis (1986) investigated this question by training 229 older adults from the Seattle Longitudinal Study on either Inductive Reasoning or Spatial Orientation. These subjects had taken standardized intelligence tests 7 and 14 years prior to training, and training improvement could thus be compared to their prior level of functioning. It was found that people whose performance had declined reliably (i.e., by one standard error or more in the course of 14 years) showed larger treatment gain at the level of the test taught than stable subjects; both groups showed equal gain when performance was measured at the factorial level. For 40% of the declining subjects, performance was equal to or larger than their performance 14 years earlier. Schaie and Willis (1986) concluded that what their "intervention procedures seem to accomplish is to reactivate behaviors and skills that have remained in the subjects' behavioral repertoire but have not been actively employed" and that "at least a portion of the previously observed decline may be attributable to disuse" (p. 230). Unfortunately, one can make this assertion with full confidence only if information about the 1970 skills (rather than just the 1970 performance) is available—which is not the case. The question also remains: What, then, is altered in the stable subjects, who also performed better at pretest than decliners, and thus presumably deployed superior skills or used them more efficiently already at pretest? It is quite possible that the stable subjects also had the trained skills unused in their repertoire, which would imply that performance decrements of decliners over the 14-year period are not necessarily due to disuse of these skills. In fact, it remains entirely possible that young adults also have the same skills dormant in their repertoire. Before firm conclusions regarding the role of disuse in adult age differences in intelligence can be reached, it is absolutely necessary to include groups of young adults in the designs (Salthouse, 1991). If disuse is indeed a major determinant of adult age differences and reactivation a potent elicitor of treatment gain, young adults should show less training gain than the old (Light, 1991; Salthouse, 1991). Salthouse (1991, p. 166) reviewed seven relevant studies on extended practice in intelligence or short-term memory performance and found that in none of these studies did the young show smaller treatment gain than the old.

Plasticity in Psychometric Test Performance: Conclusions

Results from plasticity research in psychometric intelligence shows that considerable malleability of performance is indeed present in old age. The locus of these changes appears to lie largely in the older adults themselves: Given enough practice with the task, they seem perfectly able to reach the level of performance reached by their age peers who have been subjected to explicit training in the relevant skills. In fact, this research shows that a procedure for fair assessment of older adults' performance on traditional intelligence tests should include either practice with the task or power rather than speeded assessment. There seems to be no conclusive evidence yet as to the nature or directionality of the plasticity effect. Thus, it remains possible that training or self-taught improvement does not reach the ability level and is not truly reactivation, but fast learning of a new skill or increased efficiency in executing an existing skill.

Plasticity in Memory Performance

Plasticity in Memory Performance: Mnemonics, Skills, or Ability?

Interestingly, some of the controversial issues surrounding plasticity in the domain of psychometric intelligence do not apply to the domain of memory plasticity. Memory plasticity research is almost exclusively concerned with teaching particular skills or strategies that might help boost memory performance, and boosting performance is the goal—the goal is not a change in memory ability. This is already evident from definitions of memory skills or strategies such as the one offered by Bellezza (1983): A memory strategy is "a particular procedure that an individual can use to memorize a particular set of materials under a specific set of conditions" (p. 53). One can make a loose distinction between memory *skills,* such as rehearsal, semantic elaboration, or the use of imagery or organization, which have broad applicability to subclasses of memory tasks, and more specific *strategies,* such as the method of loci or the pegword mnemonic or other formal systems for encoding and retrieving information, which can be applied to only a narrow range of tasks and materials. Memory skills are often applied spontaneously by many research subjects, because they are usually part of the behavioral repertoire of most adults, being relatively standard ways of operating on to-be-remembered materials. Formal techniques are rarely used spontaneously; they need to be learned explicitly and typically need conscious control for their initiation and execution (Cavanaugh, Grady, & Perlmutter, 1983; Harris, 1980; Intons-Peterson & Fournier, 1986; Park et al., 1990).

Two strategies that have been used extensively in research with older adults are the method of loci and the name-face mnemonic (for more details on these and other strategies, see Bellezza, 1983). In the method of loci, subjects learn, in a first step, a sequence of locations, such as landmarks in a city or places around their home. When a list of words has to be learned, each word is linked through interactive imagery to one of the locations. Retrieval occurs by taking a mental walk along the sequence of locations, retrieving the mental image at each location, and decoding the original word from it. In the face-name mnemonic (see Lorayne, 1976, for an extensive description), subjects select a prominent feature of the face to be learned, make a concrete, high-imagery transformation of the person's name, and then form an interactive image of the facial feature and the name transformation.

From these brief descriptions, it is clear that the effects of training in these mnemonics will probably result in highly specific effects. Training in the method of loci should be of little help to subjects learning to associate names and faces. Likewise, training in the name-face mnemonic would be of little avail when one is confronted with a list of words that have to be learned in sequence. The training effects are thus tied to performance, not to a change in an underlying ability. Kliegl and Baltes (1987) illustrated this by offering an analogy with high jumping. Trained athletes do high jumping by twisting the body after pushing off, so that they go back down, head first over the bar, a technique called the *Fosbury flop* after the person who used it first at the 1968 Olympic games. This technique has to be learned, and the locus of change is clearly not the trainee's intrinsic ability to high-jump, but merely her or his performance. Note that the technique can be applied only under certain circumstances; for instance, it presupposes a shock-absorbent surface at landing—it's clearly not recommended for jumping the garden wall. Performance increments always occur in a specific context and make sense only within that particular context. Note that the assumed specificity of training effects also means that from a clinical point of view, it may be worthwhile to teach the metaskill of deciding what technique to use when one is faced with a particular task and a particular set of materials under specified conditions (Wong, 1989). To my knowledge, no research on the effects of training such metacognitive skills, though potentially useful, has been conducted.

Likewise, when a mnemonic strategy is taught, the *directionality* of effects is usually clear: Reactivation is highly improbable, because most people never had these mnemonic strategies in their behavioral repertoire (and, interestingly, even people who know these techniques and understand their effectiveness, such as professional memory researchers, do not tend to use them; Park et al., 1990). Rather, memory strategy training entails the learning and honing of a completely new skill.

Another difference between training in the use of memory skills or strategies and training in psychometric intelligence concerns individual differences. Whereas training in psychometric intelligence is always (that is, if the task analysis has been done carefully) training in the optimal technique for the test (there is only one good way to perform well on an intelligence test), this is not the case for mnemonic training. There is more than one effective way to learn, for instance, a list of words in sequence. One could apply the method of loci, the pegword mnemonic, or one could make up a story using the words in sequence or make a phrase of the first few letters of each word. Certain individuals may prefer one technique over the other, and this preference may have to do with particular abilities these individuals are strong in, or with their preferred cognitive style.

Plasticity in Memory Performance: Some Key Findings

The key results of plasticity in the domain of episodic memory functioning were summarized in a meta-analysis of 32 studies by Verhaeghen et al. (1992). Here, I wish to highlight four results from that analysis.

First, the effects of memory training appeared to be larger than the effects of mere retesting or placebo treatment (placebo treatment consisted of all interventions that did not consist of teaching memory skills or strategies; it included giving feedback, teaching relaxation techniques, or having group discussions of memory problems). Memory training boosted performance by 0.73 standard deviations; mere retesting enhanced performance by 0.38 standard deviations; and placebo treatment resulted in a gain of 0.37 standard deviations. Consequently, the locus of treatment effects appears to have been primarily the training itself. It can also be concluded that the effects of relaxation techniques, group discussions, and the like on memory performance probably entailed no more than a retesting effect. The reader may note that the specific effect of the instruction (0.73 − 0.38 = 0.35) was somewhat larger than the specific effect of the instruction in psychometric intelligence (which had a weighted average of 0.20, all types of abilities combined). On the other hand, the retest effect for memory tests was only about half the size of the retest effect for intelligence tests. Taken together, these results suggest that no dramatic self-initiated change in skill or strategy or optimization of skills or strategies occurred in retested subjects, but that the net effects of memory training were quite large indeed.

Second, there was indeed a differential effect of training on memory tasks tailored to measure progress after training in the specific technique (e.g., a list of words to be recalled in sequential order for training in the method of loci; Verhaeghen et al. called this a "target task") and measures that consisted of near transfer tasks (for training in the method of loci, a near transfer task could be recall for the association between faces and names). This result indicates that the effects of training in a memory technique were quite specific indeed. This is a clear indication that the locus of the training effect is the technique taught, and not reactivation of general memory skills.

Third, no differential treatment gain was observed for the different types of skills or strategies taught. This was true regardless of whether the specific skills or strategies were directly compared with each other, or whether verbal techniques were contrasted with imagery techniques, or whether skills were contrasted with strategies. Thus, when the effect is measured on target tasks, there does not seem to be any technique that is clearly superior to any other.

Fourth, a regression analysis was conducted to determine some of the characteristics of the studies that were reliably associated with treatment gain. It was found that treatment gains were largest when the subjects were younger, when pretraining (usually involving training in imagery) was provided, when training was carried out in groups, when some form of memory-related intervention (such as attention training, providing information about memory and aging, and group discussion) was included in the program, and when sessions were relatively short. Part of these effects have to do with optimizing the learning environment. For instance, with regard to session duration, it should be mentioned that mean session duration in these studies was 90 minutes—an inordinate amount of time when one wishes to hold someone's attention. Thus, it makes sense that shorter sessions should be more fruitful. The enhancement of effect when other interventions are combined with the training proper may be due to increased motivation, or such interventions may simply provide a break in the sessions, thus reducing the need for sustained attention. The positive effects of conducting the training in a group environment may have to do with peer learning, or again, they may be due to enhanced motivation. The effect of pretraining could be explained in similar terms, or it may be a real effect of learning a new skill in the pretraining phase that can be applied to the memory technique in the training phase. Or the effect of pretraining might be artifactual, in that more testing occasions were provided in these programs, and increased familiarity with the material may have played a role. The age-relatedness of plasticity, within a group of older adults, is a finding that will be expanded upon in the next section.

Like the effects of training in psychometric intelligence, the effects of memory training appear to be reasonably durable. A small number of studies have investigated follow-up effects over either a 6-month interval (Stigsdotter Neely & Bäckman, 1993a, 1993b) or a 3-year interval (Anschutz, Camp, Markley, & Kramer, 1987; Scogin & Bienias, 1988; Stigsdotter Neely & Bäckman, 1993a). A meta-analysis on these studies shows that the net maintenance effect of training (i.e., pre-to-follow-up-test effect size minus pre-to-posttest effect size) was quite large. Over a 6-month interval, performance increased by 0.40 standard deviations (as compared to a 0.28 increase in retest groups); over 3 years, performance went down slightly, by 0.11 standard deviations (as compared to a 0.06 decrease in retest groups). Thus, the effects of memory training appear to be as durable as those of training in psychometric intelligence. The reader may note that since the nature of the treatment effect here is the skill or strategy rather than the ability, these results indicate that even skill or strategy training can clearly lead to durable effects.

Plasticity in Memory Performance: Testing-the-Limits and Individual Differences

A first text on the limits of plasticity in old age appeared in 1986 (Baltes & Kliegl). These authors apparently took their inspiration from theories about biopsychological adaptation in old age (Coper, Jänicke, & Schulze, 1985), which state that aging brings about increased vulnerability and a reduction in system adaptability. These problems should be most easily noticeable at limits of performance. Baltes and Kliegl trained their subjects in the method of loci, using a presentation time manipulation as a way of getting at the limits of the system. It was found (and this finding has been replicated since; Kliegl, Smith, & Baltes, 1990) that at posttest, differences between subjects, including age differences, were magnified. Moreover, 20 subsequent sessions of practice and testing did not at all reduce the age difference obtained at posttest (Baltes & Kliegl, 1992). Thus, this study points at clear limits to plasticity and found these limits to be age-related. Other studies have confirmed this finding as well: When the effects of memory training in a group of young and older subjects are compared, training effects are usually larger for young than for older adults (for details and a meta-analysis on seven such studies, see Verhaeghen & Marcoen, 1996). In the previous section, we saw that this effect also holds within the group of older adults: On the average, studies that have younger old participants yield larger effects than studies than have examined older old participants. And it has been found that even the effects of lifelong expertise do not totally counter the negative effects of age on plasticity, as research concerning the trainability of graphic designers in the method of loci demonstrates (Lindenberger, Kliegl, & Baltes, 1992).

An obvious hypothesis might be that age is negatively associated with plasticity in memory performance because the same variables that are associated with pretest performance are also associated with posttest performance, treatment gain, or both. Consider again the high-jump analogy. While the Fosbury flop is a very effective technique if one wants to engage in high-level high jumping, it does not necessarily offer opportunities for compensation. At least some of the same abilities or strengths associated with pre-Fosbury techniques will be associated with the flop: Muscle strength, sheer speed, joint flexibility, precision of kinesthetic sensations, and motor control will probably all be important, whatever technique one uses for high jumping. To carry the analogy to the domain of memory functioning, posttest performance is still memory performance, and some of the variables associated with pretest scores will probably also affect posttest scores. Inasmuch as these variables are negatively associated with age, treatment gain may well be a negative function of adult age. Indeed, a number of variables found to be correlated with plasticity are also negatively affected by age: speed of mental operations (Kliegl et al., 1990; Kliegl & Thompson, 1991), working memory (Kliegl & Thompson, 1991), and mental status (Hill, Yesavage, Sheikh, & Friedman, 1989; Yesavage, Sheikh, Friedman, & Tanke,1990; a nonsignificant trend in the same direction was found by Stigsdotter Neely & Bäckman, 1995; an overview of other variables can be found in Verhaeghen & Marcoen, 1996).

Verhaeghen and Marcoen (1996) tested this hypothesis directly by training a group of young and older adults in the method of loci and measuring a number of basic variables usually associated with age-related differences in cognition (speed, visual and auditory working memory, and associative memory), while also tapping strategy use through a questionnaire filled out immediately after the recalling of each list. One difference between the two age groups emerging from this study was that older adults were less susceptible to complying with instructions and truly applying the method of loci at posttest. All of the young adults stated that they did use the method at posttest; about one in four older adults stated they did not use the method at all at posttest. Noncomplying older adults were generally older than complying older adults, performed less well at pretest, and had lower scores on a measure of associative memory. Thus, interestingly, those subjects that presumably needed the mnemonic boost most were less willing or maybe less able to actually use it. It was also found that fewer older adults applied the method correctly: About two thirds of the older adults who did apply the method of loci at posttest mixed it with other strategies, such as making up a story and forming connections between words—only 40% of the young did not apply the method correctly. It was found that incorrect application of the technique in older adults was a perseverance effect: The subjects not inclined to use the method correctly were those who, at pretest, used efficient strategies with a higher frequency than subjects using the method incorrectly. This finding suggests that memory training needs to be concerned not only with learning the new technique, but also with helping older people to discontinue the use of old (and usually inefficient) techniques.

With regard to individual differences in plasticity, Verhaeghen and Marcoen (1996) found that the same mechanism appears to govern plasticity in young and old adults. In both groups, speed of mental operations influences the capability of forming and retaining associations, and this capability influences pretest directly and posttest both directly and indirectly through limiting the number of times the subject can go over the list of words. For young adults, but not older adults, visual working memory appeared to be a secondary resource that correlated with pretest performance. Paradoxically, it is precisely the similarity of the mechanisms of plasticity in young and older adults that drives the magnification of age differences, because the basic variable of the plasticity system, speed of mental operations, is negatively correlated with old age. Speed of mental operations is also one of the basic variables that are associated with the age-related decline in fluid cognition (including episodic memory performance); therefore, training adults in the method of loci will result in an amplification effect: Group or individual differences that exist at pretest will be amplified at posttest.

It may be important to note here that the limiting effect of speed appears to be internal rather than external; that is, mental slowing has consequences in the efficiency of cognitive operations that go beyond a mere need for longer study times. For instance, Verhaeghen and Marcoen (1996) found that even older adults who claimed they had had the time to study all the words twice when study time was 6 minutes recalled only one word more than young adults who claimed they had had just enough time to study the list once when study time was 2 minutes (18.8 items vs. 17.8 items, out of a total of 25).

Reanalysis of the data from Baltes and Kliegl (1992) by Verhaeghen and Kliegl (1998), focusing on the relation between performance and study time, sheds additional light on the amplification of age differences. In this study, training in the method of loci was found to have mainly two immediate effects: It raised the maximum level of performance (i.e., the level that could be attained if no time pressure was present), and it slowed subjects down (i.e., at posttest, subjects needed more time to reach their maximum level of performance than at pretest). After subjects had more practice with the method, the maximum level of performance did not change much, but the speed of forming associations increased. Age differences were found at three levels: (a) Older adults needed one session more than young adults in order to reach their maximum level of performance; (b) their maximum performance was lower; and (c) they were slower at forming associations between words and places. In sum, this study showed that the effects of aging on plasticity were tied both to the maximum level of accuracy and to mental speed.

Plasticity in Memory Performance: Conclusions

As in the domain of psychometric intelligence, there appears to be sizable malleability in memory performance in old age. In contrast with plasticity in intelligence, the effects appear to be tied to teaching of the mnemonic: The effect of retesting is much smaller, and the net effect of training larger. The effects of training remain restricted to materials to which the specific skill or strategy taught can be applied, but they appear to be quite durable. One consistent result is that there are age-related limits to plasticity tied to basic characteristics of the aging mind: Speed goes down, as does maximum accuracy.

Plasticity Beyond the Laboratory

The research and the theoretical positions reviewed above are aimed at a better understanding of cognitive aging. Many of the research efforts aimed at uncovering plasticity do not have remediation as a primary goal. Still, some lessons that can be drawn from the literature presented here should have an impact on clinical work.

First, one way to look at the data from the ADEPT and PRO-ALT programs and the meta-analytic data gathered by Verhaeghen et al. (1992) is that training programs accomplish what they are designed to do: Programs designed to boost scores on standard intelligence tests do boost those scores, and programs teaching a particular mnemonic technique can enhance memory performance. The same was found in a meta-analysis on subjective memory functioning (Floyd & Scogin, 1997): Programs designed to improve subjective memory functioning indeed do so. However, in all these cases, the gains are restricted to those tasks that are in the focus of the program. Thus, in intelligence test training, treatment gain in scores on near transfer tests are much lower than treatment gains in tests narrowly connected to the skills taught; in memory training, treatment gain is limited to tasks to which the mnemonic can be applied; expectancy modification programs work better than actual memory training in producing treatment gain in changing scores on tests tapping subjective memory functioning. If improvement in a specific aspect of a person's functioning (regardless of that person's age) is the goal, it is important to target the intervention as closely as possible to the behavior to be changed. And it may be worthwhile to consider what precisely that target is before we rush to the training room: It seems to me that changing how older persons look at their own memory functioning may be even more important for their general well-being than their ability in recalling lists of words in the correct sequence. In that case, an intervention should probably not entail much instruction in mnemonics but should focus on a person's feelings and perceptions of memory functioning.

Second, effects of training are very much limited to specific target tasks. Most memory problems associated with old age, however, extend beyond single tasks. One then has basically two options for training. One option is to teach broader skills rather than specific techniques, at the same time focusing on the applicability of these skills in different contexts. The other option is to teach a number of different specific techniques, again paying careful attention on when and where to apply what technique. In my opinion, training for strategy selection is as important for boosting performance in the daily life ecology as training specific techniques. Memory monitoring and on-line control thus appear essential ingredients for any real-life cognitive training in the old.

Third, the finding of contextualization of plasticity (plasticity is always about teaching a *specific* person a *specific* technique that can be used in *specific* circumstances) has clear consequences for treatment. Training effectiveness will probably be a function of the interaction between technique, task, and individual. If a person has a visualization impairment or is not inclined to engage in imagery, teaching imagery-based mnemonics is maybe not such a good idea. Strategies and skills taught should rely on the individual's strong points, and not on the individual's weaknesses.

Fourth, the perseverance effect needs to be taken into account. Older people who have a good repertoire of effective skills tend not to trade in these skills too easily for other techniques, even if these are much more powerful. It is important to realize that such apparent lack of behavioral flexibility probably results from a lifetime of selective optimization of behavior (Baltes & Willis, 1982), resulting in self-initiated compensation (Bäckman, 1989). It is quite understandable that people want to hang on to these adaptive operations. Thus, cognitive or memory trainers should make certain that they can convince older persons that the new technique is more effective than the self-taught techniques, for instance by providing extensive practice with feedback on performance, so that older persons can judge for themselves whether they want to adopt the new skills as their own.

Fifth, there is no such thing as easy and effortless remediation of age-related performance differences. Even in a laboratory setting, subjects often seem to expect a miracle worker rather than a trainer, and to strongly hope for total recall with zero effort. Both subjects and trainers should be aware that progress will be relative and that much effort is required to achieve it. This may seem self-evident, but even in the context of an experimental training (and with participants who are well aware that this is research and not therapy), people can be mightily disappointed—even when their performance is boosted by 200%—if they do not get everything correct.

Sixth, because general factors such as basic speed of mental operations influence treatment gain and will presumably do so in every form of training in mental skills or strategies, subjects ranking low on such basic abilities will derive little or no benefit from such training. This is most clearly the case with patients suffering from (even mild) dementia. Training demented patients appears to result in very small treatment gains (Bäckman, Josephsson, Herlitz, Stigsdotter, & Viitanen, 1991; Yesavage, 1982), and sometimes even in a decrease in performance (Zarit, Zarit, & Reever, 1982), or else it demands a quite extensive training program for relatively meager results (Diesfeldt & Smits, 1991). In this case, it seems more worthwhile to resort to the principles of behavior modification, or to train external rather than internal techniques (Camp et al., 1993; Moffat, 1989; Wilson & Watson, 1996). It may also be important to restrain our therapeutic furor from time to time. There is nothing wrong with teaching older adults correct use of an agenda or helping them in the subtle art of note taking, rather than teaching them a battery of memory tricks that even schooled memory researchers refrain from using. External aids can be very powerful, and they may take away some of the daily strains of a memory that is not working perfectly: Better to go to the supermarket with a shopping list than to return home without the bathroom tissue. For those who are interested in some expert advise on how to construe one's living ecology so that the daily hassles of sensory and cognitive aging are minimized, there is the excellent Skinner and Vaughan (1983) how-to book.

By way of a final comment, I wish to stress that even though the news about plasticity has not been so good lately (we have evidence of age-related limits that seem hardwired), there are doubts about the nature of the effect (limits on growth and even shallow effects do, after all, indicate tangible growth and real effect). Some of the effects seem to reside within the individuals themselves, who thus prove to be more resilient that psychologists generally think: They do not really need the training; they can boost their performance all by themselves. Depending on the focal point of the viewer (growth or decline), both an optimistic and a pessimistic view on cognitive aging can be held. I propose that we try to transcend these positions dialectically and move to what I assume is a realistic view of cognitive aging. Realism, without denial of the possibilities that still lie before the older person, but certainly without fear of looking at age-related constraints on functioning, may provide a key to a richer understanding of the complex phenomenon of cognitive aging.

Acknowledgments—I would like to thank Alfons Marcoen, Paul De Boeck, and Reinhold Kliegl for helpful discussions on earlier versions of this text. This text is partly based on my dissertation, defended at the University of Leuven, Belgium, with Alfons Marcoen advising.

Address correspondence to Paul Verhaeghen, Department of Psychology, 430 Huntington Hall, Syracuse, NY 13244-2340. Electronic mail can be sent to PVerhaeg@psych.syr.edu.

References

Anschutz, L., Camp, C. J., Markley, R. P., & Kramer, J. J. (1987). Remembering mnemonics: A three-year follow-up on the effects of mnemonics training in elderly adults. *Experimental Aging Research, 13,* 141–143.

Bäckman, L. (1989). Varieties of memory compensation by older adults in episodic remembering. In L. W. Poon, D. C. Rubin, & B. A. Wilson (Eds.), *Everyday cognition in adulthood and late life* (pp. 509–544). Cambridge: Cambridge University Press.

Bäckman, L., Josephsson, S., Herlitz, A., Stigsdotter, A., & Viitanen, M. (1991). The generalizability of training gains in dementia: Effects of an imagery-based mnemonic on face-name retention duration. *Psychology and Aging, 6,* 489–492.

Baltes, P. B., Dittmann-Kohli, F., & Dixon, R. A. (1984). New perspectives on the development of intelligence in adulthood: Toward a dual-process conception and a model of selective optimization with compensation. In P. B. Baltes & O. G. Brim (Eds.), *Life-span development and behavior* (Vol. 6, pp. 33–76). New York: Academic Press.

Baltes, P. B., Dittmann-Kohli, F., & Kliegl, R. (1986). Reserve capacity of the elderly in aging-sensitive tests of fluid intelligence: Replication and extension. *Psychology and Aging, 1,* 172–177.

Baltes, P. B., & Kliegl, R. (1986). On the dynamics between growth and decline in the aging of intelligence and memory. In K. Poeck, H. J. Freund, & H. Gänshirt (Eds.), *Neurology* (pp. 1–17). Berlin: Springer-Verlag.

Baltes, P. B., & Kliegl, R. (1992). Further testing of limits of cognitive plasticity: Negative age differences in a mnemonic skill are robust. *Developmental Psychology, 28,* 121–125.

Baltes, P. B., Kliegl, R., & Dittmann-Kohli, F. (1988). On the locus of training gains in research on the plasticity of fluid intelligence in old age. *Journal of Educational Psychology, 80,* 392–400.

Baltes, P. B., & Labouvie, G. V. (1973). Adult development of intellectual performance: Description, explanation, and modification. In C. Eisdorfer & M. P. Lawton (Eds.), *The psychology of adult development and aging* (pp. 157–219). Washington, DC: American Psychological Association.

Baltes, P. B., & Lindenberger, U. (1988). On the range of cognitive plasticity in old age as a function of experience: 15 years of intervention research. *Behavior Therapy, 19,* 283–300.

Baltes, P. B., & Schaie, K. W. (1976). On the plasticity of intelligence in adulthood and old age. *American Psychologist, 31,* 720–725.

Baltes, P. B., Sowarka, D., & Kliegl, R. (1989). Cognitive training research on fluid intelligence in old age: What can older adults achieve by themselves? *Psychology and Aging, 4,* 217–221.

Baltes, P. B., & Willis, S. L. (1982). Plasticity and enhancement of intellectual functioning in old age: Penn State's Adult Development and Enrichment Project (ADEPT). In F. I. M. Craik & E. E. Trehub (Eds.), *Aging and cognitive processes* (pp. 353–389). New York: Plenum Press.

Bangert-Drowns, R. L. (1986). Review of recent developments in meta-analytic method. *Psychological Bulletin, 99,* 388–399.

Bellezza, F. S. (1983). Mnemonic-device instruction with adults. In M. Pressley & J. R. Levin (Eds.), *Cognitive strategy research: Psychological foundations* (pp. 51–73). New York: Springer-Verlag.

Blackburn, J. A., Papalia-Finlay, D., Foye, B. F., & Serlin, R. C. (1988). Modifiability of figural relations performance among elderly adults. *Journals of Gerontology: Psychological Sciences, 43,* P87–P89.

Blieszner, R., Willis, S., & Baltes, P. B. (1981). Training research in aging on the fluid ability of inductive reasoning. *Journal of Applied Developmental Psychology, 2,* 247–265.

Camp, C. J., Foss, J. W., Stevens, A. B., Reichard, C. C., McKitrick, L. A., & O'Hanlon, A. M. (1993). Memory training in normal and demented elderly populations: The E-I-E-I-O model. *Experimental Aging Research, 19,* 277–290.

Cavanaugh, J. C., Grady, J. G., & Perlmutter, M. (1983). Forgetting and use of memory aids in 20 to 70 year olds' everyday life. *International Journal of Aging and Human Development, 17,* 113–122.

Coper, H., Jänicke, B., & Schulze, G. (1985). Biopsychological research on adaptivity across the life span of animals. In P. B. Baltes, D. L. Featherman, & R. M. Lerner (Eds.), *Lifespan development and behavior* (Vol.7, pp. 207–232). Hillsdale, NJ: Erlbaum.

Diesfeldt, H. F. A., & Smits, J. C. W. A. (1991). Gezichten krijgen namen: Een cognitieve training voor psychogeriatrische patiënten voor het onthouden van namen en gezichten [Faces getting names: Cognitive training in remembering names and faces for psychogeriatric patients]. *Tijdschrift voor Gerontologie en Geriatrie, 22,* 221–227.

Floyd, M., & Scogin, F. (1997). Effects of memory training on the subjective memory functioning and mental health of older adults: A meta-analysis. *Psychology and Aging, 12,* 150–161.

Harris, J. E. (1980). Memory aids people use: Two interview studies. *Memory and Cognition, 8,* 31–38.

Hayslip, B. (1989). Alternative mechanisms for improvements in fluid ability performance among older adults. *Psychology and Aging, 4,* 122–124.

Hill, R. D., Yesavage, J. A., Sheikh, J., & Friedman, L. (1989). Mental status as a predictor of response to memory training in older adults. *Educational Gerontology, 15,* 633–639.

Horn, J. L. (1982). The aging of human abilities. In B. B. Wolman (Ed.), *Handbook of developmental psychology* (pp. 847–870). Englewood Cliffs, NJ: Prentice Hall.

Hoyer, F. W., Hoyer, W. J., Treat, N. J., & Baltes, P. B. (1979). Training response speed in young and elderly women. *International Journal of Aging and Human Development, 9,* 247–253.

Hoyer, W. J., Labouvie, G. V., & Baltes, P. B. (1973). Modification of response speed deficits and intellectual performance in the elderly. *Human Development, 16,* 233–242.

Intons-Peterson, M. J., & Fournier, J. (1986). External and internal memory aids: When and how often do we use them? *Journal of Experimental Psychology: General, 115,* 267–280.

Kliegl, R., & Baltes, P. B. (1987). Theory-guided analysis of mechanisms of development and aging through testing-the-limits and research on expertise. In C. Schooler & K. W. Schaie (Eds.), *Cognitive functioning and social structures over the life course* (pp. 95–119). Norwood, NJ: Ablex.

Kliegl, R., Smith, J., & Baltes, P. B. (1990). On the locus and process of magnification of age differences during mnemonic training. *Developmental Psychology, 26,* 894–904.

Kliegl, R., & Thompson, L. (1991, July). *Cognitive abilities and adult age-differential training gains in mnemonic skill.* Paper presented at the 11th Biennial meetings of the International Society for the Study of Behavioural Development, Minneapolis.

Labouvie-Vief, G. (1976). Toward optimizing cognitive competence in later life. *Educational Gerontology, 1,* 75–92.

Labouvie-Vief, G., & Gonda, J. N. (1976). Cognitive strategy training and intellectual performance in the elderly. *Journal of Gerontology, 31,* 327–332.

Lerner, R. M. (1990). Plasticity, person-context relations, and cognitive training in the aged years: A developmental contextual perspective. *Developmental Psychology, 26,* 911–915.

Light, L. L. (1991). Memory and aging: Four hypotheses in search of data. *Annual Review of Psychology, 42,* 333–376.

Lindenberger, U., Kliegl, R., & Baltes, P. B. (1992). Professional expertise does not eliminate age differences in imagery-based memory performance during adulthood. *Psychology and Aging, 7,* 585–593.

Lorayne, H. (1976). *Remembering people.* London: Allen.

Moffat, N. J. (1989). Home-based cognitive rehabilitation with the elderly. In L. W. Poon, D. C. Rubin, & B. A. Wilson (Eds.), *Everyday cognition in adulthood and late life* (pp. 659–680). Cambridge: Cambridge University Press.

Mullen, B. (1989). *Advanced BASIC meta-analysis.* Hillsdale, NJ: Erlbaum.

Park, D. C., Smith, A. D., & Cavanaugh, J. C. (1990). Metamemories of memory researchers. *Memory and Cognition, 18,* 321–327.

Plemens, J. K., Willis, S. L., & Baltes P. B. (1978). Modifiability of fluid intelligence in aging: A short term longitudinal training approach. *Journal of Geronotology, 33,* 224–231.

Salthouse, T. A. (1985). *A theory of cognitive aging.* Amsterdam: North-Holland.

Salthouse, T. A. (1991). *Theoretical perspectives on cognitive aging.* Hillsdale, NJ: Erlbaum.

Salthouse, T. A. (1996). General and specific speed mediation of adults age differences in memory. *Journal of Gerontology: Psychological Sciences, 51B,* P30–42.

Schaie, K. W., & Willis, S. L. (1986). Can decline in adult intellectual functioning be reversed? *Developmental Psychology, 22,* 223–232.

Scogin, F., & Bienias, J. L. (1988). A three-year follow-up of older adult participants in a memory-skills training program. *Psychology and Aging, 3,* 334–337.

Skinner, B., & Vaughan, M. (1983). *Enjoy old age.* New York: Warner.

Stigsdotter Neely, A., & Bäckman, L. (1993a). Long-term maintenance of gains from memory training in older adults: Two 3 1/2 years follow-up studies. *Journals of Gerontology: Psychological Sciences, 48,* P233–237.

Stigsdotter Neely, A., & Bäckman, L. (1993b). Maintenance of gains following multifactorial and unifactorial memory training in late adulthood. *Educational Gerontology, 19,* 105–117.

Stigsdotter Neely, A., & Bäckman, L. (1995). Effects of multifactorial memory training in old age: Generalizability across tasks and individuals. *Journals of Gerontology: Psychological Sciences, 50,* P134–P140.

Verhaeghen, P., & Kliegl, R. (1998). *The effects of learning a new algorithm on asymptotic accuracy and execution speed in old age: A reanalysis of Baltes and Kliegl (1992).* Manuscript submitted for publication.

Verhaeghen, P., & Marcoen, A. (1996). On the mechanisms of plasticity in young and older adults after instruction in the method of loci: Evidence for an amplification model. *Psychology and Aging, 11,* 164–178.

Verhaeghen, P., Marcoen, A., & Goossens, L. (1992).Improving memory performance in the aged through mnemonic training: A meta-analytic study. *Psychology and Aging, 7,* 242–251.

Verhaeghen, P., & Salthouse, T. A. (1997). Meta-analyses of age-cognition relations in adulthood: Estimates of linear and non-linear age effects and structural models. *Psychological Bulletin, 122,* 231–249.

Willis, S. L. (1989). Improvement with cognitive training: Which old dogs learn what tricks? In L. W. Poon, D. C. Rubin, & B. A. Wilson (Eds.), *Everyday cognition in adulthood and late life* (pp. 545–569). Cambridge: Cambridge University Press.

Willis, S. (1990). Introduction to the special section on cognitive training in later adulthood. *Developmental Psychology, 26,* 875–878.

Willis, S. L., Blieszner, R., & Baltes, P. B. (1981). Training research in aging: Modification of performance on the fluid ability of figural relations. *Journal of Educational Psychology, 73,* 41–50.

Willis, S. L., Cornelius, S. W., Blow, F. C., & Baltes, P. B. (1983). Training research in aging: Attentional processes. *Journal of Educational Psychology, 75,* 257–270.

Willis, S. L., & Schaie, K. W. (1986). Training the elderly on the ability factors of spatial orientation and inductive reasoning. *Psychology and Aging, 1,* 239–247.

Wilson, B. A., & Watson, P. C. (1996). A practical framework for understanding compensatory behaviour in people with organic memory impairment. *Memory, 4,* 465–486.

Wong, B. Y. L. (1989). Musing about cognitive strategy training. *Intelligence, 13,* 1–4.

Yesavage, J. (1982). Degree of dementia and improvement with memory training. *Clinical Gerontologist, 1,* 77–81.

Yesavage, J. A., Sheikh, J. I., Friedman, L., & Tanke, E. (1990). Learning mnemonics: Roles of aging and subtle cognitive impairment. *Psychology and Aging, 5,* 133–137.

Zarit, S. H., Zarit, J. M., & Reever, K. E. (1982). Memory training for severe memory loss: Effects on senile dementia patients and their families. *Gerontologist, 4,* 373–377.

2

Theoretical and Methodological Issues in Memory Training

ROBERT HILL

LARS BÄCKMAN

A difficult issue that adults typically face as they as they grow older, and especially as they move into very late life, is declining memory function. However, the magnitude of age-related memory deficits varies across different forms of memory. Specifically, whereas performance in tasks assessing semantic memory, primary memory, procedural memory, and various forms of priming tends to be relatively little affected by the normal aging process, age-related impairments are legion in tasks assessing episodic memory (see Bäckman, Small, & Larsson, in press; Craik & Jennings, 1992, for reviews). Specific examples of this kind of memory loss include forgetting names and faces, misplacing important objects (e.g., house keys), forgetting telephone numbers, missing appointments, and even losing the train of a conversation in a social setting (e.g., Bolla, Lindgren, Bonaccorsy, & Bleecker, 1991).

Episodic memory deals with conscious retrieval of information that is encoded in a particular place at a particular time (Tulving, 1983). This form of memory is typically assessed by having subjects recall or recognize information acquired in the laboratory (e.g., a list of words or a series of faces). To the extent that age-related deficits are particularly likely to be observed in episodic memory, it is not surprising to find that attempts to enhance memory in old age have focused primarily on this form of memory. An example of this kind of memory deficit is age-related cognitive decline (see Larabee, 1996; Rediess & Caine, 1996), which has been labeled in the fourth edition of the *Diagnostic and Statistical Manual for Mental Disorders* as a psychological factor affecting a medical condition (American Psychiatric Association, 1996, p. 684).

This chapter will focus primarily on issues related to the efficacy of memory training as a psychological intervention for remediating memory loss in old age. Research has documented that modest gains in verbal and name-face recall are achievable in community-dwelling, high-functioning older adults through memory-training interventions (for an overview, see the chapter by Paul Verhaegen, in this volume). Focused short-term interventions in which older adults are taught specific mnemonic strategies (e.g., the method of loci) to facilitate encoding of to-be-remembered items (e.g., high-imagery nouns) represent the major training paradigm.

A central goal of this chapter is to examine the memory-training literature to ascertain whether such an approach to cognitive rehabilitation can be extended to a wider range of older adults, as well as to a broader spectrum of cognitive problems in everyday living. In this regard, we will explore several methodological and theoretical issues underlying memory training: (a) the unique strengths of a mnemonic device for addressing the kinds of deficits that are inherent in cognitive changes associated with old age, (b) the role that individual characteristics play in mediating training outcomes, (c) The extent to which mnemonic techniques can be effectively applied to everyday problems, and (d) The degree to which training can be extended beyond traditional contexts (e.g., computer-based instruction).

Mnemonic Training for the Acquisition and Retention of Information

It is our belief that to take full advantage of training in utilizing a mnemonic technique, its nature and purpose should be clearly delineated. In this section, we explore how mnemonic techniques are used to improve acquisition of information and to facilitate retention (or minimize forgetting). *Acquisition* refers to the initial encoding, of information at a specific point in time. This might consist of an item (e.g., a name) that is to be remembered when one is confronted with a stimulus cue (e.g., a face). *Retention,* on the other hand, refers to the ability to encode information in such a way that it can be recalled at a later point in time (e.g., remembering a newly learned phone number several weeks after it was initially learned). The extent to which a mnemonic device is designed for these purposes and its influence on acquisition and retention in an older adult population are described below.

Issues in the Acquisition of Information

One of the more highly publicized features of a mnemonic device is that it represents a kind of encoding that facilitates retrieval of large amounts of information. Highly practiced users of mnemonics (called *mnemonists*) have demonstrated that it is possible to encode large amounts of information (e.g., a complete list of phone numbers in a local phone book, line and verse from the Bible, and very long strings of random numbers) using mnemonic procedures (Cermak, 1975; Higbee, 1988). It is also noteworthy that such feats of "memory power" can be achieved by persons of average intellectual ability who learn to use a mnemonic proficiently. For example, Belleza, Six, and Phillips (1992) trained two individuals to produce nearly perfect recall of 80-digit number strings after only a few minutes of study.

In a meta-analysis of research studies with older adults where mnemonic strategies were employed to enhance acquisition, Verhaeghen, Marcoen, and Goossens (1992) concluded that, on average, active memory training produces a very modest gain of

10% over placebo training. This magnitude of gain was associated with brief interventions that varied in terms of the number of training sessions and the amount of material covered in each session. Training typically involved limited exposure and practice in using a specific technique (e.g., the method of loci), as well as additional skills to facilitate its use (e.g., imagery pretraining).

As a way to enhance acquisition, more intensive interventions employing the same subject selection procedures, but increasing the number of training sessions, have also been tried (Stigsdotter & Bäckman, 1989; Stigsdotter Neely & Bäckman 1993a, 1995), and reviews of this research appear in several chapters of this volume (see chapter 4 by Anna Stigsdotter Neely). Interestingly, these studies have reported only slight performance advantages over briefer interventions, suggesting that training intensity itself may not be the most important component for achieving skill competency, but characteristics of the mnemonic strategy, as well as the subjects, should also be considered. As a demonstration of this point, Kliegl, Smith, and Baltes (1989, 1990) utilized an intensive training approach to determine the limits of age differences in cognitive reserve capacity for learning verbal material via the method of loci. In these studies, not only were training procedures intensive, but participants were also specifically selected who were intellectually high-functioning, motivated, and in optimal physical health. In addition, training was designed to ensure that participants achieved competence in utilizing the mnemonic procedure; that is, they could not progress through the training until they had achieved predetermined levels of performance proficiency. These studies demonstrated that with properly designed training, high-functioning older adults can substantially alter their baseline memory performance by applying mnemonic procedures to the material to be remembered. In fact, some of their subjects showed more than 10-fold increases in acquisition. From this research, it appears that simply providing additional training is not, in and of itself, sufficient to appreciably change an individual's ability to acquire information. What needs additional consideration is more systematic examination of how the specific characteristics of those being trained can influence the degree to which training leads to the actual mastery of the mnemonic itself, and the extent to which the mnemonic can be applied to acquiring material in question.

Issues in Retention and Forgetting

Perhaps the most powerful feature of a mnemonic device is its ability to facilitate the retention of information even after a long time. For example, Bellezza (1981) argued that one of the most useful characteristics of a mnemonic device is that it produces a kind of encoding that prohibits forgetting of information even without continual rehearsal. Specifically, a mnemonic produces a more distinctive encoding (Craik & Jennings, 1992; Craik & Simon, 1980; Hill, Storandt, & Simeone, 1989) by connecting to-be-remembered information with information stored in permanent memory. The stronger this connection, the greater the likelihood that acquired information will be retained for longer periods.

From a practical standpoint, a mnemonic device should help the individual retain important information (e.g., names and faces, phone numbers) over longer intervals even though the material may not be frequently used (Higbee, 1988). Thus, what is important in this regard is not the sheer quantity of information that can be retrieved, but the relative permanence (or durability) of a specific memory trace.

Although little information is available that has investigated the role of mnemonics in facilitating retention of information in older adults, there is a large body of research on younger-aged groups that has examined the nature of the forgetting process (see Bogartz, 1990; Loftus, 1985; Slameka, 1985; Slameka & McElree, 1983; Wixted & Ebbesen, 1991) and the role that mnemonics play in minimizing forgetting (Belleza, 1981; Higbee, 1988). In this regard, the operational definition of *forgetting* is the performance difference between two or more retention intervals, *retention* being a memory measure that is obtained at a single point in time. Analysis of the forgetting rate, then, has involved examining the slope of the line that connects these different points of measurement.

In some samples, data suggest that older individuals may forget information at a faster rate than young adults (Brainerd, Reyna, Howe, & Kingma, 1990). Giambra and Arenberg (1993) also reported that in their sample of adults over 60 years there may be small and, depending on statistical power, reliable age-related differences in forgetting rate for longer retention intervals. Some research in both old and young adults indicates that both the quantity of learned material and the rate of forgetting, particularly when the retention interval is long, may be influenced by mnemonic skill (Boltwood & Blick, 1970; Bower & Clark, 1969).

In a study examining the impact of naturally occurring memory strategies on the rate of forgetting in older adults, Hill, Allen, and Gregory (1990) documented that those who spontaneously employed a mnemonic to encode a list of high-imagery nouns experienced less forgetting than did those who reported using no memory strategy (or only rote rehearsal). This study suggests that some older adults can spontaneously generate and utilize mnemonic strategies to facilitate retention. For example, nearly half the subjects in this study reported spontaneously using first-letter pegword techniques, categorizing the words, or creating stories that incorporated the words, and it is noteworthy that these strategy users outperformed those who reported using no strategy at each follow-up. Note also that this was a highly educated and relatively young group of older adults. Thus, the extent to which mnemonics are effectively employed in old age for the purpose of retention of information may depend, in part, on individual characteristics such as education and previous exposure to mnemonic strategies.

Most of the research investigating the retention effects of memory training in older adults has examined only retention of the mnemonic strategy itself (see Anschutz, Camp, Markley, & Kramer, 1985; Scogin & Bienias, 1988; Stigsdotter & Bäckman, 1989; Stigsdotter Neely & Bäckman, 1993a, 1993b, 1995) rather than maintenance of the materials encoded at study via the mnemonic. Thus, the forgetting rate of learned material has not been systematically explored in this literature. From a cognitive rehabilitation standpoint this is a serious omission, because what matters most in many everyday situations is remembering encoded information (e.g., a name or a telephone number) over an extended time rather than retrieving only information about the mnemonic procedure itself (e.g., the steps necessary to encode a telephone number).

Individual Differences as a Mediating Factor in Memory Training

This section examines the extent to which individual difference variables mediate response to memory training. As alluded to previously, individual differences with regard to motivation and intellectual abilities can be an important factor in influencing gains associated with more intensive training (see Kliegl et al., 1989, 1990). Thus, by way of background, we will first highlight research that has documented the relationship between individual difference variables and episodic memory performance. We will then examine the role that individual differences play in mediating the utilization of cognitive support (e.g., the provision of retrieval cues; see Bäckman & Larsson, 1992) in experimental memory tasks. Finally, we will highlight those studies that have investigated individual difference variables in memory-training interventions with adults.

Individual Differences in Episodic Memory

A well-known phenomenon regarding aging and episodic memory is the influence of subject-related characteristics on performance. Studies have consistently found that subject-related variables within demographic, cognitive, lifestyle-related, and health-related domains can mediate episodic memory performance in old age (see Bäckman, Mäntylä, & Herlitz, 1990; Hultsch & Dixon, 1990; Salthouse, 1991b, for reviews). Exploring how specific characteristics of the individual covary with memory performance may yield important theoretical information regarding the optimization and modifiability of memory in late life (e.g., Hill, Wahlin, Winblad, & Bäckman, 1995; Zelinski, Gilewski, & Schaie, 1993). Although there are a wide range of potential individual-difference variables, those that most frequently appear in the published literature can be roughly classified within four general content domains: (a) demographics, (b) cognitive factors, (c) lifestyle, and (d) disease.

Demographics

In this section, age and education are highlighted as subject demographics; however, it should be noted that other demographics have been found to mediate episodic memory performance, including gender (Herlitz, Nilsson, & Bäckman, 1997). Only age and education are highlighted in this section because they are the two most commonly cited demographic variables predicting episodic memory performance.

It is well known that there are reliable declines in episodic memory performance from early to late adulthood (see Kausler, 1991; Salthouse, 1991b, for reviews). In addition, comparisons of older adults of different ages suggest that age-related deterioration of episodic memory continues into very late life (e.g., Bäckman, 1991; Bäckman & Larsson, 1992; Wahlin et al., 1993; West, Crook, & Barron, 1992), with marked declines after 70 years of age (Christensen, Mackinnon, Jorm, Henderson, & Korten, 1994; Colsher & Wallace, 1991; Giambra, Arenberg, Zonderman, Kawas, & Costa, 1995; Johansson, Zarit, & Berg, 1993). However, it has been suggested that chronological age per se may be only a marker of other, more critical variables related to memory performance (e.g., education, intellectual ability, health). Some studies have found that age may play a relatively minor role in change in episodic memory when factors such as health and intellectual ability are controlled (see Hill et al., 1995). Thus, disentangling the true effects of age on episodic memory has been a difficult research issue, particularly in advanced age.

The relationship between education and episodic memory has also been extensively evaluated (Kausler, 1991; Perlmutter, 1978; Salthouse, 1991b). Education has generally been defined as the number of years of formal schooling, and in this context, it has been a potent ordinal predictor of memory performance (Hultsch & Dixon, 1990; Salthouse, 1993; West et al., 1992; Zelinski et al., 1993). Likewise, studies that have grouped individuals according to educational attainment have reported education-related advantages across various memory tasks (Craik, Byrd, & Swanson, 1987; Inouye, Albert, Mohs, Sun, & Berkman, 1993; Wiederholt et al., 1993). Educational status may also be linked to a variety of factors, including genetic selection, neuronal growth during critical periods in life, cognitive stimulation during active work periods, physical health, and use of memory strategies (Hill et al., 1995; Mortimer & Graves, 1993).

Cognitive Factors

This section highlights three cognitive variables and their relationship to episodic memory: verbal ability, working memory, and processing speed, all of which have been found to influence memory performance. Verbal ability has received attention in this context as a component of crystallized intellectual function that is positively associated with episodic memory. Zelinski and Gilewski (1988) found that across 3 years, older adults with high vocabulary scores declined less on a measure of episodic memory than those with lower scores. West et al. (1992) reported that vocabulary mediated the degree to which age influenced performance across all of their measures of episodic memory. Similarly, Craik et al. (1987) found that in a sample of older adults who were trichotomized according to vocabulary scores, those in the highest vocabulary grouping outperformed the two lower groupings.

Both working memory (Foos, 1989; Hartley, 1986; Morris, Gick, & Craik, 1988) and speed of processing (Salthouse, 1985a, 1985b, 1991a, 1992, 1993) also exert a strong influence on episodic memory performance. With regard to working memory, distinctions between capacity and efficiency have been made with the notion that working memory capacity may show the greatest age-related declines, and that working memory efficiency may be less influenced by age and more likely to be amenable to modification (see Foos, 1989). Processing speed, as described by Salthouse (1996), has received considerable attention as a theoretical construct that involves the speed with which an individual can perform the requisite operations to negotiate a given cognitive task. Since episodic memory is defined as a higher order cognitive process, processing speed has been examined as an elementary factor in memory performance (Salthouse, 1985a, 1991b; Salthouse & Coon, 1993; Salthouse & Kersten, 1993) and in gauging the benefits of memory training (Kliegl et al., 1990).

Lifestyle

Lifestyle variables examined in this section include behavioral indices, such as level of physical and social activity and use of substances such as alcohol and tobacco. It is well documented that these variables are highly interrelated; however, they have also been evaluated individually for their relative contribution to the prediction of memory performance

Research indicates that level of social participation is positively associated with memory performance (Cockburn & Smith, 1991; Craik et al., 1987). Furthermore, self-reported physical exertion has been found to predict performance on memory tasks, although its predictive value may be restricted to relatively strategy-free tasks (Christensen & Mackinnon, 1993; Stones & Kozma, 1989). Although the use of substances such as tobacco and alcohol have not shown a consistent relationship to episodic memory, self-report measures of these indices may not be adequate to detect subtle differences in memory performance (Hill, 1989; Hill, Storandt, & Malley, 1993). What seems to be the case, however, is that those older adults who are actively engaged in demanding, cognitively stimulating pursuits and who avoid lifelong patterns of substance abuse tend to be advantaged with respect to episodic memory (Hultsch, Hammer, & Small, 1993). It should be noted, however, that the causal direction of the relationship between activity and cognitive performance is unclear. As much as social activities may be beneficial to intellectual functioning, it may also be that persons who are cognitively adept tend to engage more in social activities than those who have lower cognitive functioning.

Disease

Although the individual difference variables discussed hitherto influence episodic memory in old age, it is clear that the most powerful characteristic is the presence or absence of disease. Dementia is the most prominent in this regard, and studies document that in dementia, episodic memory performance deteriorates markedly across the disease process (e.g., Almkvist & Bäckman, 1993; Herlitz, Adolfsson, Bäckman, & Nilsson, 1991; Herlitz & Viitanen, 1991; Welsh, Butters, Hughes, Mohs, & Heyman, 1992). M. M. Baltes, Kuhl, Gutzmann, and Sowarka (1995) have proposed that changes in cognitive processes due to Alzheimer's disease (AD) may most prominently display themselves in terms of a reduced cognitive reserve capacity. More specifically, older adults who are at high risk for developing AD may show deficiencies in developmental reserve capacity, or in the ability take advantage of opportunities for optimizing episodic memory function in supportive task conditions.

Research has also identified clinical depression as a strong predictor of memory performance in elderly adults (Hart, Kwentus, Hamer, & Taylor, 1987; La Rue, 1989; Lichtenberg, Ross, Millis, & Manning, 1995), especially in task situations requiring expenditure of cognitive effort and self-initiated operations at encoding and retrieval (Bäckman & Forsell, 1994; Weingartner, Cohen, Murphy, Martello, & Gerdt, 1981). These findings have been extended to mood and motivational characteristics of aspects of depression in nondepressed older adults, particularly with regard to motivational factors (Bäckman, Hill, & Forsell, 1996).

Individual Differences in Utilization of Cognitive Support

In this section, a theoretical framework involving the influence of the provision of cognitive support on cognitive reserve capacity (see Baltes, 1987; Baltes, Dittmann-Kohli, & Kliegl, 1986) is examined. Special attention is given to examining the impact of the previously highlighted individual difference variables on the size of gains following the provision of cognitive support.

Although the aging process exerts a negative influence on episodic memory functioning, most older adults also possess substantial cognitive reserve capacity—a potential for memory improvement. Specifically, when different forms of cognitive support are provided (e.g., directed encoding instructions, item organizability, motor activity at learning, a rich material, retrieval cues), older adults typically exhibit sizable performance gains relative to control conditions in which these forms of support are lacking (for reviews, see Bäckman et al., 1990; Craik & Jennings, 1992).

An interesting question concerns whether there are individual differences among older adults with regard to the ability to benefit from cognitive support in episodic memory tasks. Most research addressing this issue has compared groups of elderly individuals who suffer from dementia or depression with normal elderly adults in tasks varying in the level of cognitive support provided. Results indicate pronounced dementia-related deficits in the ability to utilize cognitive support for remembering (see Bäckman & Herlitz 1996; Herlitz, Lipinska, & Bäckman, 1992, & Bäckman 1995, for reviews); demented patients require a substantial amount of cognitive support in both encoding and retrieval in order to demonstrate memory facilitation. In clinical depression, the empirical picture is less clear (see the chapter by Pachana, Marcopulos, and Takagi in this book), although there is research indicating that depressed older adults may show deficits in utilizing item organizability (Bäckman & Forsell, 1994; Watts, Dagleish, Bourke, & Healy, 1990), visual imagery (Hart et al., 1987), and an increased presentation rate (Bäckman & Forsell, 1994) to improve memory performance.

Other research has examined the influence of demographic and lifestyle variables on the ability to utilize cognitive support within samples of healthy older adults. There is evidence to suggest that the level of support required to demonstrate memory improvement may increase from early to later portions of the late adult life span (Bäckman, 1991; Bäckman & Larsson, 1992; Hill et al., 1995). In addition, older individuals who are highly educated and socially active have been found to benefit more from cognitive support than less educated and less active individuals (Craik et al., 1987; Hill et al., 1995). In contrast, self-reported exercise habits, as well as gender, have not been found to be related to the size of performance gains from the provision of support in episodic memory tasks (Hill et al., 1995). Thus, it appears that individual difference variables may affect not only general level of episodic memory functioning in old age, but also the degree to which memory performance can be modified by means of supportive task conditions. The relationship between overall memory function and potential for memory improvement is further discussed in the next section, which reviews current approaches to memory-training research with older adults that have specifically examined the effects of various individual difference variables on the size of training-related gains.

Mnemonic Training for Modifying Episodic Memory Performance

Investigations have examined the extent to which subject characteristics are predictive of performance gains from memory training. In brief, these have included age (Rose & Yesavage, 1983), verbal ability (Yesavage, Sheikh, Decker-Tanke, & Hill, 1988), mental status (as measured by the MMSE; Hill, Yesavage, Sheikh, & Friedman, 1989; Yesavage, Sheikh, Friedman, & Tanke, 1990), cognitive factors such as processing speed (Kliegl et al., 1990), and personality characteristics (Gratzinger, Sheikh, Friedman, & Yesavage, 1990). These studies have suffered from various problems, including limited range of variation in the predictors, inadequate sample size, and a lack of theoretical rationale for guiding variable selection. In spite of these deficiencies, what follows is a review of how these studies have examined individual characteristics in memory-training interventions.

Age has received the most attention as an individual characteristic that could influence memory-training outcomes. As noted previously (e.g., Bäckman, 1991; Bäckman & Larsson, 1992; Craik et al., 1987; Hill et al., 1995), age has been found to be a critical characteristic determining the utilization of cognitive support to improve episodic memory. With regard to memory-training research, age has been specifically manipulated by contrasting old and young adults (Kliegl et al., 1989; Rose & Yesavage, 1983; Yesavage & Rose, 1984). Results indicate that young adults may gain more than older adults from mnemonic training even when both groups achieve a similar level of skill competency (Kliegl et al., 1989). Thus, this research supports the contention that cognitive reserve capacity may decrease with advancing age.

Level of education, primarily defined as years of formal schooling, has also been found to predict utilization of cognitive support to improve memory even after controlling for the effects of age (Hill et al., 1995). Interestingly, education as a control variable has been included in virtually every memory-training study to equate treatment and control groups. Although it has never been formally evaluated as a mediator of memory-training gains, most researchers believe that it could exert sufficient impact on training gains to be experimentally manipulated as a between-groups factor.

Verbal ability, as measured primarily by vocabulary proficiency, has been found to be a strong predictor of memory performance. In one study, Yesavage et al. (1988) found that verbal ability predicted response to memory training inasmuch as those who were high in verbal ability benefited more from training in the method of loci than low-verbal-ability subjects.

Individual characteristics that may have the most promise for influencing memory-training outcomes are processing speed and working memory. Some theorists have postulated that processing speed may supersede other subject characteristics, including age, education, and verbal ability, in accounting for age-related performance deficits in episodic memory (Salthouse, 1993, 1996). Processing speed may also be a critical component for accessing a mnemonic strategy, as well as decoding stored information in order to retrieve stimulus material, particularly under paced performance conditions. In one study, processing speed, as measured by the digit symbol substitution test, was found to predict response to memory training (Kliegl et al., 1990), although the percentage of the variance explained by this variable was minimal. The same may be true of working memory, which may play a critical role in mnemonic training, since it can be anticipated that learning and accessing a mnemonic require the individual to mentally transfer and recode information (e.g., change numbers to letters), as well as to refer back to transformed information as a way to decode the stimulus material (Baddeley, 1981). To date, working memory has not been used to predict response to memory training.

As described earlier, clinical depression has been found to negatively influence episodic memory performance, as well as the ability to benefit from cognitive support in old age (e.g., Bäckman & Forsell, 1994; Hart et al., 1987; La Rue, 1989). Like education, depression has not been specifically examined as a predictor of response to memory training; however, it is clear that clinical depression in late life affects motivational processes. Therefore, it is conceivable that older individuals with depressive symptoms may also be deficient in accessing sufficient processing resources to utilize a mnemonic (as a form of cognitive support) even when they have learned and practiced the procedure via a specific intervention. Bäckman et al. (1996) observed that nondepressed individuals who experience depressive symptoms showed deficits in the ability to utilize cognitive support (e.g., more study time) to improve memory.

In summary, subject-related characteristics range along a continuum where the anchor points are represented by young versus old, highly versus poorly educated, high versus low verbal ability, active versus inactive, fast versus slow processing speed, efficient versus inefficient working-memory capability, and positive versus negative mood states. Intermediate positions on this continuum would be occupied by individuals who vary on these and other characteristics. As one progresses in the negative direction along this continuum, there is a gradual decrease in episodic memory functioning, a decrease in the ability to benefit from memory-training interventions for improving memory, and a concomitant increase in the degree of support required to show memory improvement. Thus, the observed relationship between memory proficiency and memory plasticity points to specific individual difference variables that may exert a direct influence on memory-training outcomes.

Expanded Application of Mnemonic Techniques

Mnemonics as a Number Memory Aid

As described earlier, the vast majority of memory-training interventions have focused on remediating two kinds of memory loss: verbal material (e.g., word lists composed of high-imagery nouns) and name-face associations (e.g., recalling the names of faces). One area that has received relatively little attention in older adult samples is the potential benefit of mnemonic training for numeric material. In their meta-analytic review of memory interventions, Verhaegen et al. (1992) highlighted over 30 published research papers. Of these, 20 were exclusively designed to facilitate recall of word lists, and 9 targeted name-face recall; the remaining 2 involved both word and name-face mnemonic training.

From a practical standpoint, it is evident that in contemporary society, gaining access to essential goods and services requires remembering personalized number sequences (e.g., four-digit personal identification numbers [PINs], lock combinations, telephone access codes, door codes to senior housing complexes, home-based security systems). As an example, the pervasiveness of automated banking services is dramatic. There are over 105,000 automated teller machines (ATMs) in the United States, and 480,000 worldwide, and it has been estimated that a typical homeowner will hold PINs for three different credit and/or debit cards (Harrow, 1995). While it is possible to preselect these security numbers, most are randomly generated in order to prevent the possibility of theft. With the proliferation of ATMs (Engley, 1995), it is becoming increasingly difficult to access banking services without ready access to a PIN, and the degree to which older adults use such services may depend, in part, on their ability to retrieve specific number sequences from memory at the point of service (e.g., standing in front of a bank teller machine; Bulkeley, 1995).

Although studies exist examining the effectiveness of mnemonic procedures for nonverbal material including random number strings, addresses, and phone numbers (Bellezza et. al., 1992; Higbee, & Kunihira, 1985; Kilpatrick, 1985; Kliegl, Smith, Heckhausen, & Baltes, 1987; Slak, 1970, 1971), such research has been confined to younger groups. For example, Kliegl et al. (1987) trained two young adults in an intensive procedure that involved number and letter transformation, as well as a method of linking numbers to familiar dates. They found large increases in number recall in these two individuals. As has been reported in related research with verbal material, special selection of subjects, a high frequency of sessions, and assurance that participants would achieve skill competency may have been critical factors in producing these large performance gains. Thus, in addition to providing novel stimuli to test theoretical assumptions about the role of individual differences in memory training, improving recall of numbers may be useful in enhancing day-to-day functioning in older adults.

Several recent studies have examined the efficacy of specialized mnemonic techniques as a way to improve both the acquisition and the retention of numerical material in older adults. In one study, Hill, Campbell, Foxley, and Lindsay (1997) utilized a visual imagery mnemonic that involved the linking of numbers to letters in the alphabet and the forming of meaningful words that could be decoded to the numbers. Participants were randomized into a placebo and a training group. Participants in both groups committed four six-digit number strings to memory at posttesting. Those in the training group were instructed to use the mnemonic procedure. There were no differences in recall between the groups at the immediate posttest; however, differences appeared at a 3-day follow-up favoring the mnemonic group and were highly significant at 7 days. This study provides preliminary evidence not only that older adults can benefit from number mnemonic training, but such training is effective in facilitating retention of numerical material. It is important to note that subjects trained in this study were "high-functioning" older adults, and although individual difference variables were not assessed for predicting training gains, such characteristics may be very important in determining whether an older adult can learn such a strategy and utilize it in novel contexts.

Mastering Components of the Mnemonic

A general problem in the published memory-training literature is the lack of research examining the extent to which individuals can learn the mnemonic procedure itself, and as alluded to earlier, learning a mnemonic procedure has often been confounded with proficient use of the mnemonic once it is learned. As the focus of many memory-training studies has been to compare memory interventions with placebo training, the degree to which specific components of the mnemonic are mastered has been of secondary importance.

In this regard, consider the well-known name-face mnemonic described by McCarty (1980) and later by Yesavage and Rose (1983; see also Yesavage, Lapp, & Sheikh, 1989), and described in detail in the the chapter by Stigsdotter in this book, in reference to older adults. To utilize this mnemonic the learner must successfully accomplish several steps: The first step requires identifying a prominent facial feature (e.g., a large nose). Although this may seem simple at the outset, such identification involves a number of abilities, including visual acuity and good visual search capability. The second step involves the mental transformation of this facial characteristic into a familiar image ("His nose reminds me of a Hill"). It is important to note that this step not only requires abstract reasoning and feature integration but must be performed in a time-limited context (e.g., meeting other people at a party). In the third step, this new image must be linked to the person's last name. Here, the older adult must have sufficient verbal knowledge to form such a link. Finally, the person must decode the integrated image in reverse order to retrieve the name. McCarty (1980) provided the following example that describes how this mnemonic should work:

> To pair a face with the name *Conrad,* a person might choose the nose as the prominent facial feature, select the words *con rat* as the name transformation, and create a visual image in which a man wearing a prisoner's uniform (a con) rides on a rat that slides down the nose. (p. 145)

What is clear from this brief description is that failure to execute any one of these component steps will result in a breakdown of the total mnemonic procedure itself. Interestingly, most mnemonic procedures involve multiple concrete steps that may require very different kinds of cognitive skills. In fact, training curricula for mnemonic procedures are often organized around such steps. For example, Hill et al. (1997) used a multistep training procedure for utilizing the number-consonant mnemonic to encode number sequences.

It may be critical in future research to assess the degree to which the older learner is able to master each step, and the training that is needed to ensure competency in performing each step quickly as well as in the correct sequence. It is this kind of research that may ultimately determine whether a given mnemonic is useful as a practical cognitive rehabilitation tool. Only a few studies have examined the level of training necessary to master specific steps of the mnemonic and the extent to which individual differences can predict overall performance competency within and across steps. Not surprisingly, findings from these few studies suggest that those who are more proficient in learning component skills underlying the mnemonic gain more from training (Hill, Sheikh, & Yesavage, 1989; Kliegl et al., 1990).

Novel Training Methods and Individual Differences

This final section describes the potential benefits of incorporating advanced technology to enhance memory-training interventions and issues that may be associated with the application of such technology to older adults. We noted earlier in this chapter that tailored instruction that ensures skill mastery yields the greatest benefits from training. We also noted that the effectiveness of mnemonic training depends, in part, on the characteristics of those being trained and on the match of those characteristics with the training format. The question arises, then: What additional benefit might be accrued from an instructional format that can capitalize on the unique strengths of the individual learner?

Since the late 1980s, there has been an explosion in computer-based systems designed to facilitate individualized training objectives. Finkel and Yesavage (1990) were, perhaps, the first to test the idea that computer-based programming could be applied to memory training in older adults as well. Specifically, they evaluated the effectiveness of a computerized tutorial for training older adults in the method of loci. Their results provide evidence that computer-based training was at least as effective as in vivo training and had the added benefit that a computer tutorial was more efficient in presenting the material, could be modified to fit the individual's learning pace, and required less face-to-face instruction than in vivo training. More recent research has demonstrated that it is possible to extend this method of training by using CD-ROM technology in contexts that may be even more familiar to the older adult than the computer terminal (e.g., a television set; see Baldi, Plude, & Schwartz, 1996).

There are multiple advantages to incorporating computer-based technology into memory-training programs for older adults: First, the interactive and user-paced nature of contemporary computer programs allows the older adult to tailor the training experience to his or her specific learning needs (e.g., speed of presentation, level of complexity). Such flexibility has been shown to maximize concept learning and mastery (Baldi et al., 1996). Second, it is possible, using programming features such as graphics animation and interactive presentation mediums, to augment the learning environment with more supportive conditions, such as extra practice opportunities and varied support in the form of additional retrieval cues. Further, practice can be modified to conform more closely to real-world contexts. For example, a name could be presented on-screen by an actor who states, "Hi, my name is Robert McDougal. I am from Salt Lake City, Utah. What is your name?"

From the point of view of the experimenter, computerized testing also has several inherent advantages. For example, multiple learning parameters (e.g., the number of items correct, the amount of time required to complete a task) can be measured simultaneously. Further, the learner can provide continuous input as to what does and does not work in training (computer training has the distinct advantage of preventing the learner from progressing through steps in the mnemonic before previous steps are mastered). This input is very important, given that research has shown that skill mastery is a critical aspect of effective training (see Kliegl et al., 1990).

As such technology becomes more common in memory-training research, a number of additional issues will arise. Prominent in this regard are the added individual difference variables associated with computer familiarity. For example, a 60-year-old adult who was born in the 1930s will not have had the benefit of exposure to the computer at an early age. Thus, initial exposure to computers will vary widely across older adults, with some having virtually no experience in using computers. Finally, attitudes (and/or fears) associated with computer usage may be influential in predicting both comfort in using and willingness to experiment with computer-aided technology. Thus, although computer-aided instruction represents a new and promising horizon for memory-training interventions for older adults, the ability to utilize such technology to improve memory may vary greatly across individuals. As in our previously articulated conceptual scheme, those who possess greater facility and confidence in computer use are likely to gain the most from memory training that incorporates this kind of technology as part of the training format. To date, training studies employing computer-based formats as the instructional medium (see Baldi et al., 1996; Finkel & Yesavage,

1990) have not examined these individual difference variables; therefore, these variables represent a new avenue for testing the role of individual differences in memory-training efficacy.

Summary and Implications

This chapter highlighted a number of theoretical and methodological issues to consider when developing memory-training interventions for older adults. Foremost among these concerns is the kinds of outcomes from training that are important to measure, that is, the acquisition as well as the retention of information. Most of the research to date has focused on issues of acquisition, leaving retention (or forgetting) of learned material relatively unexplored. We also reviewed the role that individual characteristics play in influencing training gains, including demographic, lifestyle, cognitive competencies, and disease-related variables. In particular, these characteristics were examined for their ability to influence gains from training interventions. Finally, we highlighted several future directions for memory intervention research, including the application of techniques to a broader range of stimuli (e.g., numbers) and the incorporation of advanced technology in training regimens (e.g., computer-assisted training tutorials). The future of memory training is likely to involve extending what is learned theoretically and methodologically in the controlled classroom environment to issues and problems facing older adults in the everyday world.

References

Almkvist, O., & Bäckman, L. (1993). Progression in Alzheimer's disease: Sequencing of neuropsychological decline. *International Journal of Geriatric Psychiatry, 8,* 755–763.

American Psychiatric Association (1996). *Diagnostic and statistical manual of mental disorders* (4th ed.). Washington, DC: American Psychiatric Association.

Bäckman, L. (1991). Recognition memory across the adult life span: The role of prior knowledge. *Memory and Cognition, 19,* 63–71.

Bäckman, L. (1995). Cognitive support and episodic memory in normal aging and Alzheimer's disease: A continuity view of the modifiability of memory performance in old age. In R. Cacabelos, H. Frey, & B. Winblad (Eds.), *Neurogerontology and Neurogeriatrics* (Vol. 1, pp. 85–106). Barcelona: Prous.

Bäckman, L., & Forsell, Y. (1994). Episodic memory functioning in a community-based sample of very old adults with major depression: Utilization of cognitive support. *Journal of Abnormal Psychology, 103,* 361–370.

Bäckman, L., & Herlitz, A. (1996). Knowledge and memory in Alzheimer's disease: A relationship that exists. In R. G. Morris (Ed.), *The cognitive neuropsychology of Alzheimer's disease* (pp. 89–104). Oxford: Oxford University Press.

Bäckman, L., Hill, R. D., & Forsell, Y. (1996). Affective and motivational symptomatology as predictors of episodic recall among very old depressed adults. *Journal of Abnormal Psychology, 105,* 97–105.

Bäckman, L., & Larsson, M. (1992). Recall of organizable words and objects in adulthood: Influences of instructions, retention interval, and retrieval cues. *Journal of Gerontology: Psychological Sciences, 47,* 273–278.

Bäckman, L., Mäntylä, T., & Herlitz, A. (1990). The optimization of episodic remembering in old age. In P. B. Baltes & M. M. Baltes (Eds.), *Successful aging: Perspectives from the behavioral sciences* (pp. 118–163). Cambridge: Cambridge University Press.

Bäckman, L., Small, B. J., & Larsson, M. (in press). Memory. In J. G. Evans, T. F. Williams, B. L. Beattie, J.-P. Michel, & G. K. Wilcock (Eds.), *Oxford textbook of geriatric medicine* (2nd ed.). Oxford: Oxford University Press.

Baddeley, A. D. (1981). The concept of working memory: A view of its current state and probable future development. *Cognition, 10,* 17–23.

Baldi, R. A., Plude, D. J., & Schwartz, L. K. (1996). New technologies for memory training with older adults. *Cognitive Technology, 1,* 25–35.

Baltes, M. M., Kuhl, K.-P., Gutzmann, H., & Sowarka, D. (1995). Potential of cognitive plasticity as a diagnostic instrument: A cross-validation and extension. *Psychology and Aging, 10,* 167–172.

Baltes, P. B. (1987). Theoretical propositions of life-span developmental psychology: On the dynamics between growth and decline. *Developmental Psychology, 23,* 611–626.

Baltes, P. B., Dittmann-Kohli, F., & Kliegl, R. (1986). Reserve capacity of the elderly in aging-sensitive tests of fluid intelligence: Replication and extension. *Psychology and Aging, 1,* 172–177.

Bellezza, F. S. (1981). Mnemonic devices: Classification, characteristics, and criteria. *Review of Educational Research, 51,* 247–275.

Bellezza, F. S., Six, L. S., & Phillips, D. S. (1992). A mnemonic for remembering long strings of digits. *Bulletin of the Psychonomics Society, 30,* 271–274.

Bogartz, R. S. (1990). Evaluating forgetting curves psychologically. *Journal of Experimental Psychology: Learning, Memory, and Cognition, 16,* 138–148.

Bolla, K. I., Lindgren, K. N., Bonaccorsy, C., & Bleecker, M. L. (1991). Memory complaints in older adults: Fact or fiction? *Archives of Neurology, 48,* 61–64.

Boltwood, C. E., & Blick, K. A. (1970). The delineation and application of three mnemonic techniques. *Psychonomics Science, 20,* 339–341.

Bower, G. H., & Clark, M. C. (1969). Narrative stories as mediators for serial learning. *Psychonomics Science, 14,* 181–182.

Brainerd, C. J., Reyna, V. F., Howe, M. L., & Kingma, J. (1990). Development of forgetting and reminiscence. *Monographs for the Society for Research in Child Development, 55,* v–93.

Bulkeley, W. M. (1995, April 19). To read this, give us the password . . . Ooops! Try it again. *Wall Street Journal,* pp. A1, A8.

Cermak, L. (1975). *Improving your memory.* New York: McGraw-Hill.

Christensen, H., & Mackinnon, A. (1993). The association between mental, social and physical activity and cognitive performance in young and old subjects. *Age and Ageing, 22,* 175–182.

Christensen, H., Mackinnon, A., Jorm, A. F., Henderson, L. R. S., & Korten, A. E. (1994). Age differences in interindividual variation in cognition in community-dwelling elderly. *Psychology and Aging, 9,* 381–390.

Cockburn, J., & Smith, P. T. (1991). The relative influence of intelligence and age on everyday memory. *Journal of Gerontology: Psychological Sciences, 46,* 31–36.

Colsher, P. L., & Wallace, R. B. (1991). Longitudinal application of cognitive function measures in a defined population of community-dwelling elders. *Annals of Epidemiology, 1,* 215–230.

Craik, F. I. M., Byrd, M., & Swanson, J. M. (1987). Patterns of memory loss in three elderly samples. *Psychology and Aging, 2,* 79–86.

Craik, F. I. M., & Jennings, J. M. (1992). Human memory. In F. I . M. Craik & T. A. Salthouse (Eds.), *The handbook of aging and cognition* (pp. 51–110). Hillsdale, NJ: Erlbaum.

Craik, F. I. M., & Simon, E. (1980). Age differences in memory: The roles of attention and depth of processing. In L. W. Poon, J. L. Fozard, L. S. Cermak, D. Arenberg, & L. W. Thompson (Eds.), *New directions in memory and aging: Proceedings of the George A. Talland Memorial Conference* (pp. 95–112). Hillsdale, NJ: Erlbaum.

Engley, H. L. (1995, October 2). ATM turns 30: What did we do without it. *Salt Lake Tribune*, p. C2.

Finkel, S. I., & Yesavage, J. A. (1990). Learning mnemonics: A preliminary evaluation of a computer-aided instruction package for the elderly. *Experimental Aging Research, 15,* 199–201.

Foos, P. W. (1989). Adult age differences in working memory. *Psychology and Aging, 4,* 269–275.

Giambra, L. M., & Arenberg, D. (1993). Adult age differences in forgetting sentences. *Psychology and Aging, 8,* 451–462.

Giambra, L. M., Arenberg, D., Zonderman, A. B., Kawas, C., & Costa, P. T. (1995). Adult life-span changes in immediate visual memory and verbal intelligence. *Psychology and Aging, 10,* 123–139.

Gratzinger, P., Sheikh, J. I., Friedman, L., & Yesavage, J. A. (1990). Cognitive interventions to improve face-name recall: The role of personality trait differences. *Developmental Psychology, 26,* 889–893.

Harrow, R. O. (1995, November 17). You must remember this: Passwords are easy to forget. *Salt Lake Tribune*, p. A1.

Hart, R. P., Kwentus, J. A., Hamer, R. M., & Taylor, J. R. (1987). Selective reminding procedure in depression and dementia. *Psychology and Aging, 2,* 111–115.

Hartley, J. T. (1986). Reader and text variables as determinants of discourse memory in adulthood. *Psychology and Aging, 1,* 150–158.

Herlitz, A., Adolfsson, R., Bäckman, L., & Nilsson, L.-G. (1991). Cue utilization following different forms of encoding in mildly, moderately, and severely demented patients with Alzheimer{{acute}}s disease. *Brain and Cognition, 15,* 119–130.

Herlitz, A., Lipinska, B., & Bäckman, L. (1992). Utilization of cognitive support for episodic remembering in Alzheimer's Disease. In L. Bäckman (Ed.), *Memory functioning in dementia* (pp. 73–96). Amsterdam: Elsevier.

Herlitz, A., Nilsson, L-G, & Bäckman, L. (1997). Gender differences in episodic memory. *Memory and Cognition, 25,* 801–811.

Herlitz, A., & Viitanen, M. (1991). Semantic organization and verbal episodic memory in patients with mild and moderate Alzheimer's disease. *Journal of Clinical and Experimental Neuropsychology, 13,* 559–574.

Higbee, K. L. (1988). *Your memory: How it works and how to improve it* (2nd ed.). Englewood Cliffs, NJ: Prentice Hall.

Higbee, K. L., & Kunihira, S. (1985). Cross-cultural applications of yodai mnemonics in education. *Educational Psychologist, 20,* 57–64.

Hill, R. D. (1989). The residual effects of cigarette smoking on cognitive performance in normal aging. *Psychology and Aging, 4,* 251–254.

Hill, R. D., Allen, C., & Gregory, K. (1990). Self-generated mnemonics for enhancing free recall performance in older learners. *Experimental Aging Research, 16,* 141–145.

Hill, R. D., Campbell, B. W., Foxley, D., & Lindsay, S. (1997). Effectiveness of the number-consonant mnemonic for retention of numeric material in community-dwelling older adults. *Experimental Aging Research, 23,* 275–286.

Hill, R. D., Sheikh, J., & Yesavage, J. (1989). Pretraining enhances mnemonic training in elderly adults. *Experimental Aging Research, 14,* 207–211.

Hill, R. D., Storandt, M., & Malley, M. (1993). The effect of long-term aerobic training on psychological function in older adults. *Journal of Gerontology, 48,* 12–17.

Hill, R. D., Storandt, M., & Simeone, C. (1989). The effects of memory skills training and incentives on free recall in older learners. *Journal of Gerontology: Psychological Sciences, 45,* 227–242.

Hill, R. D., Wahlin, Å., Winblad, B., & Bäckman, L. (1995). The role of demographic and lifestyle variables in utilizing cognitive support for episodic remembering in very old adults. *Journal of Gerontology: Psychological Sciences 50B,* 219–227.

Hill, R. D., Yesavage, J. A., Sheikh, J., & Friedman, L. (1989). Mental status as a predictor of response to memory training in older adults. *Educational Gerontology, 15,* 633–639.

Hultsch, D. F., & Dixon, R. A. (1990). Learning and memory in aging. In J. E. Birren & K. W. Schaie (Eds.), *Handbook of the psychology of aging* (3rd ed., pp. 258–274). San Diego: Academic Press.

Hultsch, D. F., Hammer, M., & Small, B. J. (1993). Age differences in cognitive performance in later life: Relationships to self-reported health and active life style. *Journal of Gerontology: Psychological Sciences, 48,* 1–11.

Inouye, S. K., Albert, M. S., Mohs, R., Sun, K., & Berkman, L. F. (1993). Cognitive performance in a high-functioning community-dwelling elderly population. *Journal of Gerontology: Medical Sciences, 48,* 146–151.

Johansson, B., Zarit, S. H., & Berg, S. (1993). Changes in cognitive function of the oldest old. *Journal of Gerontology: Psychological Sciences, 47,* 75–80.

Kausler, D. H. (1991). *Experimental psychology, cognition, and human aging* (2nd ed.). New York: Springer-Verlag.

Kilpatrick, J. (1985). Doing mathematics without understanding it: A commentary on Higbee and Kunihira. *Educational Psychologist, 20,* 65–68.

Kliegl, R. K., Smith, J., & Baltes, P. B. (1989). Testing-the-limits and the study of adult age differences in cognitive plasticity of a mnemonic skill. *Developmental Psychology, 25,* 247–256.

Kliegl, R., Smith, J., & Baltes, P. B. (1990). On the locus and process of magnification of age differences during mnemonic training. *Developmental Psychology, 6,* 894–904.

Kliegl, R., Smith, J., Heckhausen, J., & Baltes, P. B. (1987). Mnemonic training for the acquisition of skilled digit memory. *Cognition and Instruction, 4,* 203–223.

Larabee, G. L. (1996). Age associated memory impairment: Definition and psychometric characteristics. *Aging, Neuropsychology, and Cognition, 3,* 118–131.

La Rue, A. (1989). Patterns of performance on the fuld object memory evaluation in elderly inpatients with depression or dementia. *Journal of Clinical and Experimental Neuropsychology, 11,* 409–422.

Lichtenberg, P. A., Ross, T., Millis, S. R., & Manning, C. A. (1995). The relationship between depression and cognition in older adults: A cross-validation study. *Journal of Gerontology: Psychological Sciences, 50B,* 25–32.

Loftus, G. R. (1985). Evaluating forgetting curves. *Journal of Experimental Psychology: Leaning, Memory, and Cognition, 11,* 397–406.

McCarty, D. L. (1980). Investigation of a visual imagery mnemonic device for acquiring face-name association. *Journal of Experimental Psychology: Human Learning and Memory, 6,* 145–155.

Morris, R. G., Gick, M. L., & Craik, R. I. M. (1988). Processing resources and age differences in working memory. *Memory and Cognition, 16,* 362–366.

Mortimer, J. A., & Graves, A. B. (1993). Education and other socioeconomic determinants of dementia and Alzheimer's disease. *Neurology, 43,* 39–44.

Perlmutter, M. (1978). What is memory aging the aging of? *Developmental Psychology, 14,* 330–345.

Rediess, S., & Caine, E. D. (1996). Aging, cognition, and DSM IV. *Aging, Neuropsychology, and Cognition, 3,* 105–117.

Rose, T. L., & Yesavage, J. A. (1983). Differential effects of a list-learning mnemonic in three age groups. *Gerontology, 29,* 293–298.

Salthouse, T. A. (1985a). Speed of behavior and its implications for cognition. In J. E. Birren & K. W. Schaie (Eds.), *Handbook of the psychology of aging* (2nd ed., pp. 400–426). New York: Van Nostrand.

Salthouse, T. A. (1985b). *A theory of cognitive aging.* Amsterdam: Elsevier Science Publishers.

Salthouse, T. A. (1991a). Mediation of adult age differences in cognition by reductions in working memory and speed of processing. *Psychological Science, 2,* 179–183.

Salthouse, T. A. (1991b). *Theoretical perspectives on cognitive aging.* Hillsdale, NJ: Erlbaum.

Salthouse, T. A. (1992). *Mechanisms of age-cognition relations in adulthood.* Hillsdale, NJ: Erlbaum.

Salthouse, T. A. (1993). Speed mediation of adult age differences in cognition. *Developmental Psychology, 29,* 722–738.

Salthouse, T. A. (1996). The processing-speed theory of adult age differences in cognition. *Psychological Review, 103,* 403–428.

Salthouse, T. A., & Coon, V. E. (1993). Influence of task-specific processing speed on age differences in memory. *Journals of Gerontology: Psychological Sciences, 48,* 245–255.

Salthouse, T. A., & Kersten, A. W. (1993). Decomposing adult age differences in symbol arithmetic. *Memory and Cognition, 21,* 699–710.

Scogin, F., & Bienias, J. L. (1988). A three-year follow-up of older adult participants in a memory-skills training program. *Psychology and Aging, 3,* 334–337.

Slak, S. (1970). Phonemic recoding of digital information. *Journal of Experimental Psychology, 86,* 398–406.

Slak, S. (1971). Long-term retention of random sequential digital information with the aid of phonemic recoding: A case report. *Perceptual and Motor Skills, 22,* 455–460.

Slamecka, N. J. (1985). On comparing rates of forgetting: Comment on Loftus. *Journal of Experimental Psychology: Learning, Memory, and Cognition, 11,* 812–816.

Slamecka, N. J., & McElree, B. (1983). Normal forgetting of verbal lists as a function of their degree of learning. *Journal of Experimental Psychology: Learning, Memory, and Cognition, 9,* 384–397.

Stigsdotter, A., & Bäckman, L. (1989). Multifactorial memory training with older adults: How to foster maintenance of improved performance. *Gerontology, 35,* 260–267.

Stigsdotter Neely, A., & Bäckman, L. (1993a). Long-term maintenance of gains from memory training in older adults: Two 3-year follow-up studies. *Journal of Gerontology: Psychological Sciences, 48,* 233–237.

Stigsdotter Neely, A., & Bäckman, L. (1993b). Maintenance of gains following multifactorial and unifactorial memory training in late adulthood. *Educational Gerontology, 19,* 105–117.

Stigsdotter Neely, A., & Bäckman, L. (1995). Effects of multifactorial memory training in old age: Generalizability across tasks and individuals. *Journal of Gerontology: Psychological Sciences, 50B,* 209–215.

Stones, M. J., & Kozma, A. (1989). Age, exercise, and coding performance. *Psychology and Aging, 4,* 190–194.

Tulving, E. (1983). *Elements of episodic memory.* New York: Oxford University Press.

Verhaeghen, P., Marcoen, A., & Goossens, L. (1992). Improving memory performance in the aged through mnemonic training: A meta-analytic study. *Psychology and Aging, 7,* 242–251.

Wahlin, Å., Bäckman, L., Mäntylä, T., Herlitz, A., Viitanen, M., & Winblad, B. (1993). Prior knowledge and face recognition in a community-based sample of healthy, very old adults. *Journal of Gerontology: Psychological Sciences, 48,* 54–61.

Watts, S. N., Dagleish, T., Bourke, P., & Healy, D. (1990). Memory deficit in clinical depression: Processing resources and the structure of materials. *Psychological Medicine, 20,* 345–349.

Weingartner, H., Cohen, R. M., Murphy, D. L., Martello, J., & Gert, C. (1981). Cognitive processes in depression. *Archives of General Psychiatry, 38,* 42–47.

Welsh, K. A., Butters, N., Hughes, J. P., Mohs, R. C., & Heyman, A. (1992). Detection and staging of dementia in Alzheimer's disease: Use of the neuropsychological measures developed for the consortium to establish a registry for Alzheimer's disease. *Archives of Neurology, 49,* 448–452.

West, R. L., Crook, T. H., & Barron, K. L. (1992). Everyday memory performance across the life span: Effects of age and noncognitive individual differences. *Psychology and Aging, 7,* 72–82.

Wiederholt, W. C., Cahn, D., Butters, N. M., Salmon, D. P., Kritz-Silverstein, D., & Barrett-Connor, E. (1993). Effects of age, gender and education on selected neuropsychological tests in an elderly community cohort. *Journal of the American Geriatrics Society, 41,* 639–647.

Wixted, J. T., & Ebbesen, E. B. (1991). On the form of forgetting. *Psychological Science, 2,* 409–415.

Yesavage, J. A., Lapp, D., & Sheikh, J. I. (1989). Mnemonics as modified for use by the elderly. In L. W. Poon, D. C. Rubin, & B. A. Wilson (Eds.), *Everyday cognition in adulthood and late life* (pp. 598–611). New York: Cambridge University Press.

Yesavage, J. A., & Rose, T. L. (1983). Concentration and mnemonic training in the elderly with memory complaints: A study of combined therapy and order effects. *Psychiatry Research, 9,* 157–167.

Yesavage, J. A., & Rose, T. L. (1984). Semantic elaboration and the method of loci: A new trip for older learners. *Experimental Aging Research, 3,* 155–159.

Yesavage, J. A., Sheikh, J., Decker-Tanke, E., & Hill, R. (1988). Response to memory training and individual differences in verbal intelligence and state anxiety. *American Journal of Psychiatry, 145,* 636–639.

Yesavage, J. A., Sheikh, J. L., Friedman, L., & Tanke, E. D. (1990). Learning mnemonics: Roles of aging and subtle cognitive impairment. *Psychology and Aging, 5,* 133–137.

Zelinski, E. M., & Gilewski, M. J. (1988). Memory for prose and aging: A meta-analysis. In M. L. Howe & C. J. Brainerd (Eds.), *Cognitive development in adulthood* (pp. 133–158). New York: Springer-Verlag.

Zelinski, E. M., Gilewski, M. J., & Schaie, K. W. (1993). Individual differences in cross-sectional and 3-year longitudinal memory performance across the adult life span. *Psychology and Aging, 8,* 176–186.

3

Cognitive Skill Acquisition, Maintenance, and Transfer in the Elderly

MICHAEL K. GARDNER

DAVID L. STRAYER

DAN J. WOLTZ

ROBERT D. HILL

Skills refer to knowledge of "how to" perform some action rather than "knowledge of" some facts or events (Schmidt & Bjork, 1992). These two forms of knowledge are in some cases independent of one another. A person can know how to drive an automobile without factual knowledge of how the automobile works. Conversely, a person could study technical manuals and learn about how the various components of an automobile function, but this knowledge would not be of much help in driving if that person had not practiced the skill of driving. People often do not think of everyday skills as knowledge, and older individuals may be much more conscious of their memory for factual information than of their memory for skills (see Kausler, 1991). Yet, it is likely that their proficiency in relatively simple cognitive skills is a greater determinant of their life satisfaction than is the extent of their factual knowledge base.

As the population ages, the problem of skill usage becomes abundantly clear. In order to maintain a normal, active life, older individuals need to do three things: (a) maintain skills acquired during earlier life, (b) transfer these skills to new settings and situations, and (c) acquire new skills to deal with problems that existing skills cannot handle. Some examples will make these categories clear.

Most individuals learn to find their way around their neighborhood during their younger years. During later years, the navigation skills that they developed earlier are equally important. Indeed, with retirement, one could assume that older individuals may spend more time out and about in their local neighborhoods. Thus, they must maintain their implicit knowledge of local geography and transportation systems (see Atchley, 1980).

Likewise, during young adulthood, individuals acquire a knowledge of how to create a schedule and monitor adherence to it. During later adulthood, this skill may need to be maintained even though the demand for scheduling formal appointments and meetings may not be as high. For example, an older adult may require one or more medications to control various medical conditions. In this regard, scheduling and timing of the taking of medications may require the application of the learned skills described above.

Banking and financial management is another area where skills are acquired during youth and middle age and must continue to be applied during old age. The ability to budget spending is often most important in later life, when income is more limited and fixed (see Atchley, 1980). These are just a few everyday examples that demonstrate the importance of skill maintenance. Skills acquired early in life must be kept active and well honed so that they can continue to be used in later life.

Sometimes changes in the environment and situation require more than simple skill maintenance: They require that a skill be slightly modified and/or transferred to conditions that differ to some degree from the conditions that existed when the original skills were acquired (Salomon & Perkins, 1989). Finding one's way around the neighborhood requires developing a cognitive map of the neighborhood, including salient landmarks. One who later moves to a retirement community will need to develop a new cognitive map to find his or her way about. Failure to develop one may result in a significant decrease in the enjoyment of a new environment. As noted, the schedule-monitoring skill may also require some updating. Declines in health may increase the number and frequency of medication administrations. Not only will the actual medications change, but the skills that relied on internal cues ("remembering" to take a pill) may need to be supplemented by external cues (a digital watch that "beeps" as a reminder to take a pill; see Park et al., 1994). Likewise, banking and financial management skills may need to be transferred to new institutions and situations. An example of a common financial task frequently encountered by most people is withdrawing money from an automatic teller machine (ATM). Because ATMs have replaced many of the person-to-person banking processes (e.g., providing a paper withdrawal request to a bank teller), older adults must transfer their traditional banking skills to this new context (inserting an ATM card into a machine and entering a personal access code number) if they desire maximum access to their money.

Skill transfer may also occur in subtle situations. Older adults may need to change the way they interact with those around them as caregivers change and friends move or die. Interpersonal skills that were effective in dealing with one individual may be ineffective with another. In short, an older person may be required to adapt to his or her environment, and adaptation often means transferring skills to new and different situations.

Sometimes skills learned long ago must be called upon or relearned. After the loss of a spouse, an older widower may find that he has responsibilities in everyday life that were taken care of by the departed spouse (e.g., cooking, banking). These may be skills that he learned and used decades earlier but has used infrequently in recent years.

Even if individuals can maintain and transfer their existing skills, changes in the environment will require that new skills be learned. The ever-quickening pace of change in our society, especially in the area of technology, requires that we learn to do things that were unheard of only 20 years ago (Michio, 1997; Pickover, 1992).

Computers now permeate almost all areas of commerce and information dispersal. Finding books in many libraries requires a computer search. Many individuals communicate via electronic mail, use the Internet to arrange travel plans and lodging, and conduct electronic banking. These operations require an understanding of how to operate a computer: how to "log on," how to use a modem, and how to save and print files. For many older adults, these are new skills that must be acquired.

Technology and the new skill it requires, has also spilled over into how citizens (including older adults) interact with the government. Many businesses and government agencies are experimenting with new technologically based means of dispersing payments and services (e.g., "smart cards"; see Fancer, 1996; Gauthier, 1996). These changes will require that older adults learn how utilize the new technologies or possibly miss out on their fair share of opportunities for obtaining goods and services.

As the population not only ages but also expands, transportation systems change. Those who once drove on highways may find themselves taking light rail systems instead of more familiar buses. These new transportation systems may require understanding how to get and use fare cards, such as those used in Washington's Metro railway, and reading maps of systemwide connections and transfers.

New skills will also be required as the elderly engage in new hobbies and work endeavors. As their interests and employment opportunities shift, they will be faced with new challenges that their current skill repertoire may only partially address. Thus, the ability to acquire new skills will in part determine the degree of satisfaction (e.g., the ability to engage in hobbies) and the standard of living (e.g., the ability to make changes that allow one to remain in the workforce) of older individuals.

The Distinction Between Declarative and Procedural Knowledge

To understand cognitive skills, it's important to understand the distinction between declarative knowledge and procedural knowledge. We introduced this distinction earlier as "knowledge of" and "how to." This distinction (using slight variants in terminology) is made in several prominent theories of learning and memory (e.g., Anderson, 1983; Fitts & Posner, 1967; Schneider & Shiffrin, 1977; Shiffrin & Schneider, 1977; Squire, 1987). Declarative knowledge consists of sets of facts or lists of words or sentences. Declarative knowledge is what we are testing when we ask someone to remember a list of words or the list of things we need at the supermarket. Declarative knowledge is *knowledge of*, for instance, (a) What did you do yesterday? (b) What is your nephew's name? (c) What is the capital of North Dakota?

Procedural knowledge is memory for the procedures used to do things. We usually demonstrate procedural knowledge by performing a skill, rather than retrieving a set of facts. Procedural knowledge asks *how to* rather than requiring *knowledge of*. Procedural skills include (a) how to ride a bicycle, (b) how to balance a checkbook, and (c) how to find one's way home from the doctor's office.

Another important distinction is between explicit and implicit memory (Squire, 1987). Explicit memory is open to conscious introspection and is usually volitional (that is, it involves a conscious attempt to recall or recognize something). Declarative knowledge is usually associated with explicit memory. Implicit memory is not open to conscious introspection and is nonvolitional (that is, it does not require a conscious attempt to recall or recognize something). Procedural knowledge is usually associated with implicit memory.

In this chapter, we describe methods of improving cognitive skills that are procedural, and the parameters that affect such methods. Thus, we deal with procedural knowledge and implicit memory. In the real world, however, the distinction is not as clear-cut as it might seem at first. Even though cognitive skills are primarily procedural knowledge in the form of implicit memory, these skills must make use of and interact with declarative knowledge in the form of explicit memory. Thus, deficits in both kinds of knowledge (and types of memory) are relevant to the acquisition, maintenance, transfer, and performance of the skill. In this chapter, we focus our discussion on cognitive skill issues relating to the normal course of aging. We do not address problems related to neuropsychological conditions such as Alzheimer's disease, stroke, and dementia. While such conditions undoubtedly affect cognitive skills, an analysis of their impact on skill acquisition, maintenance, and transfer is beyond the scope of this chapter.

Cognitive Problems Associated With Normal Aging

A number of cognitive problems are associated with normal aging. We briefly review them in this section because these deficits impact what strategies are effective in training cognitive skills in the elderly.

Fluid Versus Crystallized Abilities

Cattell and Horn (Cattell, 1963, 1971; Horn, 1970, 1982; Horn & Cattell, 1966) proposed a theory of intelligence that divides general intelligence into two related types: fluid intelligence and crystallized intelligence. Fluid intelligence represents the basic biological capacity to learn (including the ability to acquire new skills), and crystallized intelligence represents the products of acculturation or acquired knowledge (Gardner & Clark, 1992; Kausler, 1991). Horn and Cattell (1966) initially reported different developmental courses for fluid and crystallized intelligence. Fluid intelligence peaks somewhere during the 20s, and declines thereafter, while crystallized intelligence appears to increase in the 20s and 30s then remain stable throughout the life span (Gilinksy & Judd, 1994; Sternberg & Powell, 1983), although some research has suggested that in very late life (70+ years), even crystallized intelligence declines (Bäckman & Nilsson, 1996; Giambra, Arenberg, Zonderman, Kawas, & Costa, 1995; Lindenberger & Baltes, 1997). The evidence in support of the fluid-crystallized intelligence distinction comes primarily from cross-sectional studies using traditional intelligence tests (LaRue, 1992; Lindenberger & Baltes, 1997), such as the various Wechsler scales (Wechsler, 1944, 1955, 1981). More specifically, the performance subtests (e.g., Picture Completion, Picture Arrangement, Block Design, Object Assembly, and Digit Symbol) have been taken as measures of fluid ability, while the Information, Vocabulary, Similarities, and Comprehension subtests have been taken as measures of crystallized intelligence (see Kausler, 1991; LaRue, 1992; Salthouse, 1991b). Note that "fluid" tests generally place a premium on speed of correct responding, while "crystallized" tests tend to place greater emphasis on correctness of the response.

The decline in fluid ability is important to the extent that it indicates a reduced capacity to acquire new cognitive skills. The Horn and Cattell theory attributes this reduced capacity to a deterioration of the underlying neural systems that support new learning. However, the true state of affairs is considerably more complicated. First, does the picture that Horn and Cattell initially presented reveal itself in longitudinal studies as well as in the cross-sectional studies that gave rise to the theory? The answer is not exactly. Longitudinal studies (e.g., Schaie, 1979, 1983a, 1983b; Schaie & Hertzog, 1986; Schaie & Strother, 1968) have found that many fluid abilities are relatively stable in young adulthood—in some instances until age 50—and then decline in very old age (Schaie & Willis, 1991). As noted earlier, research suggests that in very old age, even crystallized abilities appear to decline (see Bäckman & Nilsson, 1996; Hultsch, Hertzog, Small, McDonald-Miszczak, & Dixon, 1992; Giambra et al., 1995).

Cohort effects may influence changes in fluid ability performance (see Kausler, 1991). Cohort effects refer to the fact that in a cross-sectional study, the age of the participant is confounded with the date of birth. For instance, individuals in their 60s were all born approximately 60 years ago and had different environmental influences from those born 40 years ago. This is not the case in a longitudinal study because we follow individuals born at different times until they become a given age. The cohort effect can be important if, during certain periods of time, certain skills were emphasized by society or, conversely, were neglected by society. In that case, effects that we would wish to attribute to aging might really be due to differences in the sociocultural context over time. Schaie (1990; see also Schaie & Willis, 1991; Nilsson et al., 1997) has shown that cohort effects do indeed exist, with some abilities increasing over cohorts as we move toward the present, some decreasing, and others remaining relatively stable. The existence of these cohort effects argues for caution in drawing too strong a conclusion from the cross-sectional data that indicate a decline in fluid ability after early adulthood.

Given that there is a precipitous decline in fluid ability in very old age particularly, at least after age 60, any attempt to teach new cognitive skills must take this decline into account. This decline cannot be attributed solely to older individuals' having a slower rate of processing. Two studies (Doppelt & Wallace, 1955; Storandt, 1977) compared older and younger samples on timed and untimed versions of the performance subtests of the WAIS. Although older samples benefited more than younger subjects from the removal of the time constraints, their performance level did not reach that of the younger sample (LaRue, 1992); likewise, performance in timed and untimed conditions was highly correlated (greater than 0.85). Some hope is offered by training studies that have intervened in an attempt to improve the fluid ability performance of the elderly (e.g., Plemons, Willis, & Baltes, 1978; Willis, Blieszner, & Baltes, 1981). These studies have generally shown an improvement in the fluid ability measure after training. While these studies are promising, it is often difficult to assess what led to the performance improvement: new strategies for performing the skill, increased motivation, or a genuine improvement in a more basic underlying ability.

Working Memory and Attention

Memory and attention are important cognitive resources utilized in learning new skills. These resources also decline with increasing age. With regard to attention, Stankov (1988) performed a factor-analytic study investigating changes in attention over the ages of 20–70. He administered numerous traditional and experimental tests to his subjects, including the WAIS-R, 9 tests believed to tap fluid or crystallized intelligence, and 11 tests of attention. His factor analysis identified three dimensions of attention—search, concentration, and attentional flexibility—that were different from the dimensions of fluid and crystallized intelligence. All three attentional factors declined with advancing age. Indeed, Stankov (1988) concluded that the decline in attentional flexibility was primarily responsible for the decrease in fluid intelligence over age. When attentional flexibility was held constant, fluid ability was no longer negatively correlated with age.

Working memory, or one's immediate capacity to store and manipulate information, is another aspect of attention that shows a decline with advancing age. Working memory is strongly related to general intelligence (Kyllonen & Christal, 1990) and fluid ability in particular (see Kausler, 1991). The model of working memory accepted by most researchers in cognition is the one put forth by Alan Baddeley (1986, 1990; Baddeley & Hitch, 1974). According to Baddeley, working memory consists of three components: (a) a visuospatial sketchpad for dealing with visual images; (b) an auditory phonological loop for maintaining auditory/verbal information; and (c) a central executive that directs attention for the processing of information and oversees and coordinates the visuospatial and auditory subsystems. According to Baddeley (1986), it is the central executive that is negatively impacted by aging. He noted that forward digit span (primarily indexing the phonological loop) shows relatively little decline (e.g., Craik, 1977), while backward digit span (which involves both the phonological loop and manipulation by the central executive) shows a much greater decline (e.g., Bromley, 1958). Other experiments are consistent in showing that tasks that require either reorganization of the material before output or coordinating attention over different channels (i.e., time-sharing attentional resources) display declining performance with advancing age. As an example of the former, Talland (1965) studied performance on a task that required subjects to listen to sequences of words. Every word in the first half of the presentation was repeated in the second half, except one. Subjects were to output the single word first and then repeat the sequence of words. Older subjects performed this task more poorly than younger subjects did. As an example of the latter, Broadbent and Heron (1962) had subjects cross out certain target digits in a display while simultaneously listening to sequences of 10 letters and responding when a sequence repeated itself. Older subjects were capable of performing the two tasks separately, but their performance declined much more than younger subjects' when the two tasks were performed in tandem (Baddeley, 1986). These results are in agreement with Stankov's (1988) finding of a decline in attentional flexibility in old age.

This possible age-related decline in attentional ability may also be linked to declines in performance flexibility. The elderly seem less able to make use of feedback to modify their performance, which is critical in learning a new skill. Rabbit (1981) has shown that individuals use error feedback in reaction time tasks to modify and optimize their performance. Individuals typically speed up until they make an error and then slow down. This process continues until some optimal trade-off between speed and accuracy is achieved. Rabbit (1981) found that while the elderly can respond as quickly as younger subjects, their responses to error are much less finely tuned (Baddeley, 1986). As a group, older adults are more likely to make more errors and have longer reaction times. As Baddeley (1986) pointed out, this finding is consistent with the view that the working-memory central executive is impaired with advancing age. Although it seems able to monitor performance, its ability to intervene to successfully modify performance is reduced. Such an inability to modify performance on the basis of error feedback would have to be accommodated in any cognitive skill-training program.

Explicit Memory

Memory difficulties associated with aging are not limited to working memory. The elderly also exhibit difficulty remembering things over more extended periods of time, and this is particularly problematic when older adults are attempting to learn the content contained within new skill sequences (e.g., remembering the street address to a doctor's office). Indeed, the memory complaints of older adults that are most likely to affect skill acquisition usually center on these kinds of memory problems. In this section, we discuss memory problems within the context of explicit memory (or declarative knowledge; see Anderson, 1983).

Older subjects appear to have problems encoding information for storage in explicit memory (Schaie & Willis, 1991). For instance, the elderly do not spontaneously organize information that is to be recalled later (Craik & Rabinowitz, 1984; Gillund & Perlmutter, 1988), even though such organization is strongly correlated with amount recalled. However, if older subjects are trained in organizational techniques (Hill, Storandt, & Simeone, 1989; Hultsch, 1971; Schmitt, Murphy, & Sanders, 1981) or other kinds of mnemonic strategies (e.g., Hill, Allen, & McWhorter, 1991; Kliegl, Smith, & Baltes, 1989; Robertson-Tchabo, Hausman, & Arenberg, 1976; Stigsdotter Neely & Bäckman, 1989, 1993a, 1993b, 1995; Yesavage, Lapp, & Sheikh, 1989, see also the chapters by Hill & Bäckman, as well as Stigsdotter Neely and Verhaegen in this text), they seem to improve their recall ability.

Older individuals also have difficulty with retrieval of information from explicit memory. These retrieval difficulties are revealed in comparisons between performances on free recall and recognition memory tests (e.g., Craik, 1986; Craik & McDowd, 1987; Kaszniak, Poon, & Riege, 1986; Poon, 1985) and between performances on free recall and cued memory tests (Craik, 1986; Hultsch, 1985; Poon, 1985). In both cases, the relative advantage of either recognition (in which the items themselves are cues) or cued recall (in which a relevant cue is used to stimulate retrieval) over free (or unsupported) recall is greater for older subjects than for younger subjects (Bäckman, Mäntylä, & Herlitz, 1990). This finding indicates that older individuals are less likely than younger individuals to generate effective retrieval cues on their own—either because they have not adequately encoded the material, or because they are unable or unwilling to generate cues.

One hypothesis advanced to explain the retrieval difficulties experienced by older adults, and particularly the very old, involves the role that the aging process plays in limiting the amount of processing resources required to successfully complete the task relative to the amount required by younger subjects (see Bäckman et al., 1990; Craik, 1977, 1986). According to this hypothesis, the elderly will be disadvantaged at any task that requires a high outlay of cognitive resources or effort (e.g., Craik, 1983; Craik & Byrd, 1982; Hasher & Zacks, 1979, 1984). As an example, free recall requires a higher effort level, during both encoding and retrieval, than recognition and cued recall, which are more heavily supported tasks (Wahlin et al., 1993; Wahlin, Bäckman, & Winblad, 1995). Some evidence has been found for this hypothesis in dual-task studies where subjects engaged in both recognition and recall while performing a secondary task such as choice reaction time (e.g., Craik & McDowd, 1987; Macht & Buschke, 1983). Reaction times are slower for both older and younger subjects during recall than during recognition, but the relative effect is much greater for older subjects, a finding indicating a greater mental cost for free recall of declarative information for older subjects (see Kausler, 1991; Salthouse, 1991a).

Speed of Information Processing

Salthouse (1985, 1991a, 1991b, 1993, 1996) has proposed that many of the decrements in cognitive ability associated with aging are the result of a reduction in the speed of performing basic information processes such as comparing two items or incrementing position in a serial list. Through detailed structural equation analyses of ability test data, Salthouse (1993, 1996) has demonstrated that the negative relationship between age and fluid ability, and between age and explicit memory, is attenuated when speed of performing elementary information processes is held constant. Furthermore, he has demonstrated that the controlling variable is not simply motor speed, but speed of performing elementary cognitive operations.

The reduction in the speed of performing elementary cognitive operations with increasing age is also related to working memory ability. Salthouse (1991a) found that age was strongly predictive of processing speed, and that processing speed was predictive of working memory, but that age was only mildly to moderately predictive of working memory. In our opinion, it is difficult to conclusively disentangle the effects of processing speed, working memory, and attentional flexibility. It may be that a reduction in processing speed increases demands upon working memory to keep information available for ongoing processes, thus stressing working memory. Or it may be that declines in the working memory executive make it difficult to execute sets of basic information processes quickly and efficiently. A third possibility is that a reduction in attentional flexibility both impairs the working memory executive and reduces the ability to move among basic information processes, the result being an effective reduction in their average speed of execution. In any case, a reduction in the speed of basic information processes, for whatever reason, needs to be taken into account in designing skills-training programs for the elderly, especially when one is setting the "pace" at which skills are initially learned by older adults.

Summary

The normal course of aging includes declines in many cognitive abilities. Such declines must be taken into account by any cognitive skill acquisition program aimed at this population. The following general points should be kept in mind:

1. There appears to be a decline in fluid ability, which is necessary for new learning. There is, however, some debate about the size of this decline after controlling for confounding factors such as cohort effects. The locus of the decline may be a reduction in attentional flexibility.
2. There is a decline in at least three aspects of attention: search, concentration, and attentional flexibility. The decline in attentional flexibility may be particularly problematic, as the acquisition of new skills often involves attending to many aspects of the new task until performance automaticity is achieved.
3. There is a decline in working-memory ability that appears to be localized in the central executive. This may in fact be describing the attentional flexibility problem in different terms. Since the central executive is associated with active manipulation of information in working memory, as well as with time-sharing of attentional resources, impairment of this function will limit the capacity of older adults to learn a skill at any single point in time.
4. With regard to explicit memory, there is a decline in the extent to which "to-be-remembered" material is encoded during study time, and there is a corresponding decline in the extent to which effective retrieval cues are self-generated. However, when the older learner is induced to encode effectively and/or is provided support in the form of cues at study or test (see Bäckman et al., 1990), recall should improve.
5. There is a reduction in the speed of performing basic information processes. This is tied to the decline in working memory and attentional flexibility (the direction of causality is not completely certain) and impacts fluid ability, which can be critical in the initial acquisition of declarative information contained in a given skill.

Strategies for Skill Training in Older Populations Derived From Traditional Approaches

In this section, we will explore several recommendations for the development of skill-training programs for older populations. These recommendations are drawn broadly from the traditional literature in skill acquisition and task analysis. We begin by considering the interaction between diversity and complexity of training environment, on the one hand, and the learner's amount of available cognitive resources (described in the previous section), on the other.

The Paradox of Skill Training

When training a new skill, the number and variety of procedures and situations used during training plays an important role in the subsequent level and quality of the skill performance. If small numbers of procedures and situations are used during training, skill acquisition will be fast and relatively error-free. Furthermore, training will engender relatively low levels of frustration in the learner. While these would seem to be desirable attributes of any training program, the ultimate level of skill acquisition will be relatively circumscribed, leading to good performance in situations that were similar to training, but with relatively little generalization to different situations. In addition, focused training is likely to lead to relatively high levels of transfer errors, that is, mistakes made in situations where we would hope to find generalization (see Salomon & Perkins, 1989). Oddly enough, many skill-training programs that are designed in just this way often produce disappointing results inasmuch as the learner is unable to use his or her new skills to deal with a variety of issues in everyday living (e.g., skill training for using a computer does not generalize to accessing one's account through an ATM machine).

The alternative to a limited training program would be training involving a large number of procedures and situations. Such a program leads to slower acquisition of the trained skill and higher error rates during training, but it results in far greater generalization and fewer transfer errors (e.g., learning the fundamentals of organizing one's day by prioritizing the most important tasks). What are the problems in such programs? They take longer for the learner to complete, and they tend to lead to higher levels of frustration on the part of the learner. They also sometimes require prerequisite levels of cognitive skill on the part of the learner. If the program is too difficult (i.e., requires more cognitive skills than the learner has), the learner may never complete the program.

The last point suggests that the complexity of the skill-training program is not a variable that can be considered in isolation. It interacts with the level of cognitive resources of the learner. An ideal skill-learning program matches the complexity of the training to the cognitive level of the learner; that is, it is adaptive. With a high level of cognitive resources available, it is possible to increase the complexity of the training environment, and therefore to increase generalizability and reduce transfer errors. With a low level of cognitive resources available, we may need to reduce the level of complexity of the training environment, at least during early acquisition. Later, after early skills have been mastered, greater complexity may be introduced without overloading the learner's cognitive resources. Such an individualized training strategy would require a thorough task analysis of the skill to be learned. We provide an example of this kind of training below.

In sum, the paradox of skill training is this: Those training environments that tend to maximize acquisition tend to minimize generalization. In general, we want to begin at the highest level of complexity possible, while not overloading the learner's cognitive system, and while not producing unacceptably high levels of frustration. Two things help achieve this goal: (a) a detailed evaluation of the cognitive resources of the learner (e.g., neuropsychological tests, traditional psychometric instruments, and possibly laboratory-based measures of relevant cognitive capabilities) and (b) a flexible training system that can be adjusted to the cognitive resource level of the learner.

Task Analysis

The traditional approach to providing flexibility in the training environment is known as *task analysis*. Task-analytic approaches have been proposed from both behavioral (e.g., Briggs, 1968, 1970; Gagne, 1962, 1967, 1970a, 1970b; Gagne & Briggs, 1979) and cognitive (e.g., Gardner, 1985; M. D. Merrill, 1973; P. F. Merrill, 1978, 1980) theoretical perspectives. The essence of task analysis is to analyze the to-be-trained skill into its underlying prerequisite skills, knowledge components, and/or behaviors. These underlying components may either be trained directly or be further analyzed into a hierarchy of prerequisites. Eventually the trainer understands what pieces are required to perform the skill and can determine which pieces the learner already has and which pieces need to be taught. Training is then aimed at two goals: (a) imparting missing component skills, knowledge, and/or behaviors and (b) blending the components into a fluid performance of the high-level skill.

The latter point needs to be stressed. It is quite possible to possess all the component skills and still be unable to combine them into the higher level skill (see Anderson, 1983). For instance, in tennis one may know how to toss a ball and swing a racket for serve but may be unable to produce an acceptable serve due to the inability to perform the toss and swing in synchrony and with the correct timing. Often a good deal of training is devoted to putting the parts together into an acceptable whole.

There has been a debate in psychology over what has been termed *part/whole learning* (Carlson, Khoo, & Elliot, 1990; Schneider & Detweiler, 1988). Under what circumstances is it better to teach a skill as a whole rather than to teach the skill via the teaching of its component parts? In general, it is better to teach a skill as a whole because the problem of how to blend components is avoided (the blending is implicit in the instruction of the whole skill; see Lintern, & Gopher, 1980). However, there are circumstances that would favor the part skill approach (see Ash, & Holding, 1990; Carlson, Sullivan, & Schneider, 1989). If the learner has an insufficient repertoire of underlying component skills to allow direct training of the whole skill, part skill training would be preferable. Also, if the skill being taught is infrequent in the context of some larger training program, direct instruction in the infrequent skill would be likely to produce competence in the skill, given the small number of chances for practice within the larger training program. Finally, if the cognitive resources of the learner are too few for her or him to learn the skill as a whole, part skill training might be the only feasible route to skill acquisition. The first and last of these situations are applicable to older learners.

Concrete Suggestions

In this section, we will make some concrete suggestions based on the traditional (primarily decomposition) approaches to skill learning. These suggestions should foster more effective skill-learning programs for the elderly. To illustrate the suggestions, we will apply them to a hypothetical problem: teaching older individuals how to utilize a city bus system. We should point out that we have not actually developed such a training program; we merely wish to show how the suggestions could be applied.

To facilitate skill acquisition, early instructions in the skill-training program should be kept to a minimum. For instance, when older people are beginning to be taught to use a bus system, they might be taken on a bus ride rather than be given verbal instructions on the necessary steps. During the early phases of skill training, individuals are attempting to take declarative knowledge (i.e., rules about how to perform the skill) and apply it to problems at hand. It is this process of repeated application of the declarative rules that builds procedural knowledge of the skills themselves. But the declarative knowledge takes up working memory and attentional resources that may already be in short supply in the elderly. Minimizing instructions will help to free up these cognitive resources for use in building the skill. Later in training, instructions may have to be lengthened, especially as the training program encounters more complex situations needed to establish generalization, but by this time, the procedural skill should be well established, and more working memory and attention should be available for dealing with the heavier verbal instruction load. For example, after older individuals have mastered the basics of bus riding, the process of obtaining and utilizing bus transfers might have to be explained.

Feedback is an important component of our skill acquisition example. To acquire a skill correctly, the learner must know when he or she has succeed and/or failed. Early sessions of training should include high levels of performance feedback. This is beneficial to all learners, but especially to the elderly, who may not modify their behavior as readily to comply with performance feedback (see the findings of Rabbit, 1981, discussed above). As training continues, feedback must eventually be reduced, and finally eliminated, because most skills require performance in an environment that does not provide direct feedback. High levels of feedback early ensure efficient skill acquisition; low levels of feedback later ensure skill transfer to the environment. With regard to our bus-riding example, early bus rides might be with a trainer who follows a checklist (e.g., "Does the person know the intended destination? Does the person know when the next bus is scheduled to arrive? Does the person have the exact fare?"), while later rides might require only spot checks prior to departure.

Variability needs to be programmed into skill learning. Without this variability, the skill acquired may be overly specific and may not generalize to new environments and tasks. Early in training, variability should be relatively limited. For instance, training conditions might be blocked within sessions, with each session representing a unique skill or subskill. Keeping variability limited early in the training minimizes the strain on cognitive resources and thus allows these resources to be available for acquiring the skill. When people are learning to ride the bus system, early rides might all be on one particular route. Later in training, variability should be systematically increased. For instance, training conditions might be mixed so that each new trial or problem requires a different skill or subskill. This variability will increase the likelihood of transfer and generalization from the conditions of training to the real world. Later in the process of learning to ride the bus system, bus rides would probably encompass several connecting bus routes.

Variability in the scheduling of training sessions is also important for facilitating maintenance of the to-be-learned skill. In general, it's been found that distributed practice produces superior recall over massed practice (Bahrick & Phelps, 1987; Ebbinghaus, 1885; Glenberg, 1977, 1979; Leicht & Overton, 1987). It is for this reason that students who "cram" for an exam typically have poor memory for the material after the course is over. The superiority of distributed practice seems to be linked to multiple opportunities to encode new material in slightly different contexts. Each of these contexts provides an additional retrieval cue that may be useful in retrieving the material. To maximize retention, one wants to have relatively short practice sessions spaced with intervening rest periods. This may be especially important for the older learner because, as we noted earlier in the chapter, aging is associated with reduced information-processing resources. While these findings are based primarily on memory for verbal declarative material, we believe they apply equally to the early stages of skill learning that involve translating declarative knowledge into procedural skills. For example, when older people are trained to ride the bus, training sessions should be limited to 30 minutes but could be scheduled during different days of the week and different times of day. These differences in day and time should provide additional retrieval cues to stimulate appropriate processes to maximize retrieval of necessary information.

Several other things can be done to improve skill maintenance. First, any skill taught must be used regularly if it is to be maintained. The old adage "Practice makes perfect" is close to the mark. Practice makes for better fluid skill performance and facilitates skill maintenance. In our bus-riding example, elderly trainees should be encouraged (health permitting) to take one bus ride a week. Skills that do not have high baseline usage in the real world may require "booster sessions" of training. These would involve bringing individuals back at prespecified intervals (such as 6 and 12 months) for additional training on the skill. An example of such a skill might be financial planning: It might be used only once or twice a year, but doing it correctly is crucial; therefore booster sessions might be necessary. Thus, encouraging our older learners to make bus travel a regular part of their daily routine would be important to preserving their newly acquired skills.

To maintain a skill after training, prompts for the skill should be gradually faded into the environment. At first, the skill might have to be prompted explicitly by instruction to use it. Eventually, the prompt for the skill should be the situation in real life that calls for the skill. The process of fading must be gradual, however, with instruction about when to use the skill. Hopefully, the skill will be instrumentally conditioned through the reinforcement inherent in being able to accomplish tasks successfully. With regard to bus riding, the environment of the bus stop should eventually lead the elderly individual to mentally go through the checklist of bus-riding steps that were previously explicitly covered by the trainer. If riding the bus leads to the accomplishment of important personal goals, we would expect that the bus-riding environment would come to cue bus-riding skills in memory.

Finally, using external memory aids to prompt usage of the skill can enhance maintenance. The individual can be given something as simple as a sheet of paper with the steps of the skill written on it. Given the encoding and retrieval difficulties of the elderly, external memory aids form a viable adjunct to direct skill training. Without skill training, the steps could not be performed fluidly and competently, but, the "cheat sheet" can serve to initiate skill usage. We would point out that even the most seasoned bus rider, young or old, keeps a bus schedule in case he or she needs to catch a bus at an unusual time.

Several things can also be done to improve skill generalization and transfer. First, it is important to teach individuals where and when the skill will (and won't) be useful. This is essentially teaching the parameters of acceptable skill application. Without direct instruction in generalization, the trainer leaves the issue up to induction on the part of the learner. This is a poor practice for all but the most able of learners. In teaching an older person how to ride the bus, we would probably point out which steps would transfer to riding a subway train, and which wouldn't (e.g., how fares are paid might be through exact change on the bus, but by fare card on a train).

Of course, generalization should be built into the skill training itself. The training should encompass many different types of problems and contexts of skill usage. The greater the universe of problem types and contexts encountered in training, the greater the degree of generalizability built into the skill. In bus riding, for example, we would

Table 3.1 A Skill-Training Framework for Learning How to Travel by Bus

Skill domain	Training element	Bus example
Acquisition	Minimize explicit instructions early	Start by simply riding the bus
	Provide regular feedback	Provide information about errors and successes negotiating the route
Maintenance	Programmed variability	Change routes and times periodically
	Distributed practice	Ride the bus regularly
	Faded prompting	Slowly take away maps
	Booster sessions	Provide periodic review of training
Generalizability	Train in different contexts	Make changes between the bus and the subway
	Review skills	Provide regular progress reports
	Give external aids	Develop easy-to-read bus schedule prompts

want individuals to practice catching the bus at many locations, including bus stations, in addition to bus stops.

Just as booster sessions encourage maintenance, periodic review of the individual's current skill needs can encourage transfer. A yearly meeting with each of the elderly residents of a retirement home might point out different problems for different people. The meeting would be an opportunity for reminding individuals which of their current skills might be applicable to their current problems, as well as pointing out new areas that require new training. In the case of riding the bus, just where does the individual want or need to go? Is there a bus route to the desired destination? Or is there some alternative means of transportation for reaching that destination (e.g., taxi)? The use of external memory aids is also relevant to generalization. A list of a "bag of tricks" that one can make periodic reference to makes it easier to decide which trick to apply to which problem situation.

Summary

Table 3.1 outlines the strategies we have previously described, above and we have linked them to specific bus-usage training examples. What is highlighted in this table is the overarching concept that when providing skill-based training it is useful to think of three fundamental domains: acquisition, maintenance, and generalizability. As we noted in the beginning of this chapter, it is important to keep in mind that older adults may have some unique attributes by virtue of the aging process that should be considered when applying a skills-training approach to their everyday problems. However, we believe that utilizing principles from the skill-training literature may represent the kind of approach to training that will lead to the most usable, durable, and transferable kinds of learning for the older adult in our contemporary society.

References

Anderson, J. R. (1983). *The architecture of cognition*. Cambridge, MA: Harvard University Press.

Ash, D. W., & Holding, D. H. (1990). Backward versus forward chaining in the acquisition of a keyboard skill. *Human Factors, 32,* 139–146.

Atchley, R. (1980). *The social forces in later life: An introduction to social gerontology* (3rd Ed.) Belmont, CA: Wadsworth.

Bäckman, L., & Nilsson, L.-G. (1996). Semantic memory functioning across the adult life span. *European Psychologist, 1,* 27–33.

Bäckman, L., Mäntylä, T., & Herlitz, A. (1990). The optimization of episodic remembering in old age. In P. B. Baltes & M. M. Baltes (Eds.). *Successful aging: Perspectives from the behavioral sciences* (pp. 118–163). New York: Cambridge University Press.

Baddeley, A. D. (1986). *Working memory*. Oxford: Oxford University Press.

Baddeley, A. D. (1990). *Human memory: Theory and practice*. Boston: Allyn & Bacon.

Baddeley, A. D., & Hitch, G. (1974). Working memory. In G. A. Bower (Ed.), *Recent advances in learning and motivation* (Vol. VIII, pp. 47–90). New York: Academic Press.

Bahrick, H. P., & Phelps, E. (1987). Retention of Spanish vocabulary over eight years. *Journal of Experimental Psychology: Learning, Memory, and Cognition, 13,* 344–349.

Briggs, L. J. (1968). Sequencing of instruction in relation to hierarchies of competence. *AIR Monograph, No. 3.*

Briggs, L. J. (1970). Handbook of procedures for the design of instruction. *AIR Monograph, No. 4.*

Broadbent, D. E., & Heron, A. (1962). Effects of a subsidiary task on performance involving intermediate memory in younger and older men. *British Journal of Psychology, 53,* 189–198.

Bromley, D. B. (1958). Some effects of age on short-term learning and memory. *Journal of Gerontology, 13,* 398–406.

Carlson, R. A., Khoo, H., & Elliot, R. G. (1990). Component practice and exposure to a problem-solving context. *Human Factors, 32,* 267–286.

Carlson, R. A., Sullivan, M. A., & Schneider, W. (1989). Component fluency in a problem-solving context. *Human Factors, 31,* 489–502.

Cattell, R. B. (1963). Theory of fluid and crystallized intelligence: An initial experiment. *Journal of Educational Psychology, 54,* 105–111.

Cattell, R. B. (1971). *Abilities: Their structure, growth, and action*. Boston: Houghton Mifflin.

Craik, F. I. M. (1977). Age differences in human memory. In J. E. Birren & K. W. Schaie (Eds.), *Handbook of the psychology of aging*. New York: Van Nostrand Reinhold.

Craik, F. I. M. (1983). On the transfer of information from temporary to permanent memory. *Philosophical Transactions of the Royal Society, London, Series B, 302,* 341–359.

Craik, F. I. M. (1986). A functional account of age differences in memory. In F. Klix & H. Hagendorf (Eds.), *Human memory and cognitive capabilities*. Amsterdam: Van Nostrand Reinhold.

Craik, F. I. M., & Byrd, M. (1982). Aging and cognitive deficits: The role of attentional processes. In F. I. M. Craik & S. Trehub (Eds.), *Aging and cognitive processes* (pp. 191–211). New York: Plenum Press.

Craik, F. I. M., & McDowd, J. M. (1987). Age differences in recall and recognition. *Journal of Experimental Psychology: Learning, Memory, and Cognition, 13,* 474–479.

Craik, F. I. M., & Rabinowitz, J. C. (1984). Age differences in the acquisition and use of verbal information. In J. Long and A. Baddeley (Eds.), *Attention and performance X*. Hillsdale, NJ: Erlbaum.

Doppelt, J. E., & Wallace, W. L. (1955). Standardization of the Wechsler Adult Intelligence Scale for older persons. *Journal of Abnormal and Social Psychology, 51,* 312–330.

Ebbinghaus, H. (1885). *Uber das Gedächtnis.* Leipzig, Germany: Duncker & Humblot.

Fancher, C. (1996, August). Smart Cards. *Scientific American,* pp. 30–35.

Fitts, P. M., & Posner, M. I. (1967). *Human performance.* Belmont, CA: Brooks/Cole.

Gagne, R. M. (1962). The acquisition of knowledge. *Psychological Review, 69,* 355–365.

Gagne, R. M. (Ed.). (1967). *Learning and individual differences.* A symposium of the Learning Research and Development Center, University of Pittsburgh, Columbus, OH: Charles E. Merrill.

Gagne, R. M. (1970a). *The conditions of learning.* New York: Holt, Rinehart, & Winston.

Gagne, R. M. (1970b). Some new views of learning and instruction. *Phi Delta Kappan, 51,* 468–472.

Gagne, R. M., & Briggs, L. J. (1979). *Principles of instructional design* (2nd ed.). New York: Holt, Rinehart, & Winston.

Gardner, M. K. (1985). Cognitive psychological approaches to instructional task analysis. In E. W. Gordon (Ed.), *Review of research in education* (Vol. 12, pp. 157–195). Washington, DC: American Educational Research Association.

Gardner, M. K., & Clark, E. (1992). The psychometric perspective on intellectual development in childhood and adolescence. In R. J. Sternberg & C. A. Berg (Eds.), *Intellectual development* (pp. 16–43). Cambridge: Cambridge University Press.

Gauthier, P. (1996, May). Get Set! Smartcards are coming to America. *Portable Design, 1,* 31–34, May.

Giambra, L. M., Arenberg, D., Zonderman, A. B., Kawas, C., & Costa, P. T. (1995). Adult life span changes in immediate visual memory and verbal intelligence. *Psychology and Aging, 10,* 123–139.

Gilinsky, A. S., & Judd, B. B. (1994). Working memory and bias in reasoning across the adult lie span. *Psychology and Aging, 9,* 356–371.

Gillund, G., & Perlmutter, M. (1988). Episodic memory and knowledge interactions across adulthood. In L. L. Light & D. M. Burke (Eds.), *Language, memory and aging.* Cambridge: Cambridge University Press.

Glenberg, A. M. (1977). Influences of retrieval processes on the spacing effect in free recall. *Journal of Experimental Psychology: Human Learning & Memory, 3,* 282–294.

Glenberg, A. M. (1979). Component-levels theory of the effects of spacing of repetitions on recall and recognition. *Memory & Cognition, 7,* 95–112.

Hasher, L., & Zacks, R. T. (1979). Automatic and effortful processes in memory. *Journal of Experimental Psychology: General, 120,* 301–309.

Hasher, L., & Zacks, R. T. (1984). Automaticity processing of fundamental information: The case of frequency of occurrence. *American Psychologist, 39,* 1372–1388.

Hill, R. D., Allen, C., & McWhorter, P. (1991). Stories as a mnemonic aid for older learners. *Psychology and Aging, 6,* 484–486.

Hill, R. D., Storandt, M., & Simeone, C. (1989). The effects of memory skills training and incentives on free recall in older learners. *Journal of Gerontology: Psychological Sciences, 45,* 227–242.

Horn, J. L. (1970). Organization of data on life-span development of human abilities. In L. R. Goulet & P. B. Baltes (Eds.), *Life-span developmental psychology: Research and theory* (pp. 423–466). New York: Academic Press.

Horn, J. L. (1982). The aging of human abilities. In B. B. Wolman (Ed.), *Handbook of developmental psychology* (pp. 267–300). New York: Wiley.

Horn, J. L., & Cattell, R. B. (1966). Refinement and test of the theory of fluid and crystallized general intelligences. *Journal of Educational Psychology, 51,* 253–270.

Hultsch, D. (1971). Adult age differences in free classification and free recall. *Developmental Psychology, 4,* 338–342.

Hultsch, D. (1985). Adult memory: What are the limits? In E. M. Gee & G. M. Gutman (Eds.), *Canadian gerontological collection V* (pp. 20–52). Winnipeg: Canadian Association on Gerontology.

Hultsch, D. F., Hertzog, C., Small, B. J., McDonald-Miszczak, L., & Dixon, R. A. (1992). Short-term longitudinal change in cognitive performance in later life. *Psychology and Aging, 7,* 571–584.

Kaszniak, A. W., Poon, L. W., & Riege, W. (1986). Assessing memory deficits: An information-processing approach. In L. W. Poon (Ed.), *Handbook for clinical memory assessment of older adults* (pp. 168–188). Washington, DC: American Psychological Association.

Kausler, D. H. (1991). *Experimental psychology, cognition, and human aging* (2nd ed.). New York: Springer-Verlag.

Kliegl, R., Smith, J., & Baltes, P. B. (1989). Testing the limits and the study of adult age differences in cognitive plasticity of a mnemonic skill. *Developmental Psychology, 25,* 247–256.

Kyllonen, P. C., & Christal, R. E. (1990). Reasoning ability is (little more than) working-memory capacity?! *Intelligence, 14,* 389–433.

LaRue, A. (1992). *Aging and neuropsychological assessment.* New York: Plenum Press.

Leicht, K. L., & Overton, R. (1987). Encoding variability and spacing repetitions. *American Journal of Psychology, 100,* 61–68.

Lindenberger, U., & Baltes, P. B. (1997). Intellectual functioning in old and very old age: Cross-sectional results from the Berlin Aging Study. *Psychology and Aging, 12,* 410–432.

Lintern, G., & Gopher, D. (1980). Adaptive training of perceptual-motor skills: Issues, results, and future directions. *International Journal of Man-Machine studies, 10,* 521–551.

Macht, M. L., & Buschke, H. (1983). Age differences in cognitive effort in recall. *Journal of Gerontology, 38,* 695–700.

Merrill, M. D. (1973). Content and instructional analysis for cognitive transfer tasks. *A. V. Communications Review, 21,* 109–125.

Merrill, P. F. (1978). Hierarchical and information processing task analysis: A comparison. *Journal of Instructional Design, 1,* 35–40.

Merrill, P. F. (1980). Analysis of a procedural task. *NSPI Journal, 19,* 11–15.

Michio, K. (1997). Visions: How science will revolutionize the 21st century. New York: Anchor Books.

Nilsson, L.-G., Bäckman, L., Erngrund, K., Nyberg, L., Adolfsson, R., Bucht, G., Karlsson, S., Widing, M., & Winblad, B. (1997). The Betula prospective cohort study: Memory, health, and aging. *Aging, Neuropsychology, and Cognition, 4,* 1–32.

Park, D. C., Willis, S. L., Morrow, D., Diehl, M. et al. (1994). Cognitive function and medication usage in older adults. *Journal of Applied Gerontology, 13,* 39–57.

Pickover, C. A. (1992). *Visions of the future: Art, technology, and computing in the twenty-first century.* New York: St. Martin's Press.

Plemons, J. K., Willis, S. L., & Baltes, P. B. (1978). Modifiability of fluid intelligence in aging: A short-term longitudinal training approach. *Journal of Gerontology, 33,* 224–231.

Poon, L. W. (1985). Differences in human memory with aging: Nature, causes, and clinical implications. In J. E. Birren & K. W. Schaie (Eds.), *Handbook of the psychology of aging* (2nd ed.). New York: Van Nostrand Reinhold.

Rabbit, P. (1981). Cognitive psychology needs models for changes in performance with old age. In J. B. Long & A. D. Baddeley (Eds.), *Attention and performance X.* Hillsdale, NJ: Erlbaum.

Robertson-Tchabo, E. A., Hausman, C. P., & Arenberg, D. A. (1976). A classic mnemonic for old learners: A trick that works. *Educational Gerontology, 1,* 215–226.

Salomon, G., & Perkins, D. N. (1989). Rocky roads to transfer: Rethinking mechanisms of a neglected phenomenon. *Educational Psychologist, 24,* 113–142.

Salthouse, T. A. (1985). *A theory of cognitive aging.* Amsterdam: North-Holland.

Salthouse, T. A. (1991a). Mediation of adult age differences in cognition by reductions in working memory and speed of processing. *Psychological Science, 2,* 179–183.

Salthouse, T. A. (1991b). *A theory of cognitive aging.* Amsterdam: Elsevier.

Salthouse, T. A. (1993). Speed mediation of adult age differences in cognition. *Developmental Psychology, 29,* 722–738.

Salthouse, T. A. (1996). The processing-speed theory of adult age differences in cognition. *Psychological Review, 103,* 403–428.

Schaie, K. W. (1979). The primary mental abilities in adulthood: An exploration in the development of psychometric intelligence. In P. B. Baltes & O. G. Brim, Jr. (Eds.), *Life-span development and behavior* (Vol. 2). New York: Academic Press.

Schaie, K. W. (Ed.). (1983a). *Longitudinal studies of adult psychological development.* New York: Guilford Press.

Schaie, K. W. (1983b). The Seattle Longitudinal Study: A twenty-one year exploration of psychometric intelligence in adulthood. In K. W. Schaie (Ed.), *Longitudinal studies of adult psychological development.* New York: Guilford Press.

Schaie, K. W. (1990). Intellectual development in adulthood. In J. E. Birren & K. W. Schaie (Eds.), *Handbook of the psychology of aging* (3rd ed., pp. 291–309). New York: Academic Press.

Schaie, K. W., & Hertzog, C. (1986). Toward a comprehensive model of adult intellectual development: Contributions of the Seattle Longitudinal Study. In R. J. Sternberg (Ed.), *Advances in human intelligence* (Vol. 3, pp. 79–118). Hillsdale, NJ: Erlbaum.

Schaie, K. W., & Strother, C. R. (1968). A cross-sectional study of age changes in cognitive behavior. *Psychological Bulletin, 70,* 671–680.

Schaie, K. W., & Willis, S. L. (1991). *Adult development and aging* (3rd ed.). New York: HarperCollins.

Schmitt, F. A., Murphy, M. D., & Sanders, R. E. (1981). Training older adult free recall rehearsal strategies. *Journal of Gerontology, 36,* 329–337.

Schneider, W., & Detweiler, M. (1988). The role of practice in dual-task performance: Toward workload modeling in a connectionist/control architecture. *Human Factors, 30,* 539–566.

Schneider, W., & Shiffrin, R. M. (1977). Controlled and automatic human information processing: 1. Detection, search, and attention. *Psychological Review, 84,* 1–66.

Shiffrin, R. M., & Schneider, W. (1977). Controlled and automatic human information processing: 2. Perceptual learning, automatic attending, and a general theory. *Psychological Review, 84,* 127–190.

Squire, L. R. (1987). *Memory and brain.* Oxford: Oxford University Press.

Stankov, L. (1988). Aging, attention, and intelligence. *Psychology and Aging, 3,* 59–74.

Sternberg, R. J., & Powell, J. S. (1983). The development of intelligence. In J. H. Flavell & E. M. Markman (Vol. Eds.), *Handbook of child psychology: Vol. III. Cognitive development* (4th ed., pp. 341–419). New York: Wiley.

Stigsdotter Neely, A., & Bäckman, L. (1989). Multifactorial memory training with older adults: How to foster maintenance of improved performance. *Gerontology, 35,* 260–267.

Stigsdotter Neely, A., & Bäckman, L. (1993a). Long-term maintenance of gains from memory training in older adults: Two 3 ½ years follow-up studies. *Journals of Gerontology: Psychological Sciences, 48,* 233–237

Stigsdotter Neely, A., & Bäckman, L. (1993b). Maintenance of gains following multifactorial and unifactorial memory training in late adulthood. *Educational Gerontology, 19,* 105–117.

Stigsdotter Neely, A., & Bäckman, L. (1995). Effects of multifactorial memory training in old age: Generalizability across tasks and individuals. *Journals of Gerontology: Psychological Sciences, 50B,* 209–215.

Storandt, M. (1977). Age, ability level, and method of administering and scoring the WAIS. *Journal of Gerontology, 37,* 602–603.

Talland, G. (1965). Three estimates of the word span and their stability over the adult years. *Quarterly Journal of Experimental Psychology, 17,* 301–307.

Wahlin, Å., Bäckman, L., & Winblad, B. (1995). Free recall and recognition of slowly and rapidly presented words in very old age. A community-based study. *Experimental Aging Research, 21,* 251–271.

Wahlin, Å., Bäckman, L., Mäntylä, T., Herlitz, A., Viitanen, M., & Winblad, B. (1993). Prior knowledge and face recognition in a community-based sample of healthy, very old adults. *Journal of Gerontology: Psychological Sciences, 48,* P54–P61.

Wechsler, D. (1944). *The measurement of adult intelligence.* Baltimore: Williams & Wilkins.

Wechsler, D. (1955). *Wechsler Adult Intelligence Scale.* New York: Psychological Corporation.

Wechsler, D. (1981). *Wechsler Adult Intelligence Scale—Revised.* New York: Psychological Corporation.

Willis, S. L., Blieszner, R., & Baltes, P. B. (1981). Intellectual training research in aging: Modification of performance on the fluid ability of figural relations. *Journal of Educational Psychology, 73,* 41–50.

Yesavage, J. A., Lapp, D., & Sheikh, J. A. (1989). Mnemonics as modified for use by the elderly. In L. W. Poon, D. Rubin, & B. Wilson (Eds.), *Everyday cognition in adulthood and late life.* Cambridge: Cambridge University Press.

PART II

COGNITIVE REHABILITATION STRATEGIES IN NORMAL AGING

4

Multifactorial Memory Training in Normal Aging:

In Search of Memory Improvement Beyond the Ordinary

ANNA STIGSDOTTER NEELY

From everyday functioning ("Where did I put those car keys?") to the fundamentals of existence ("Who am I?), our ability to remember a previous episode is perhaps one of the most important cognitive assets we have. Throughout human history, possession of a proficient memory has been treasured. The ancient Greeks were devoted to memory improvement, an interest that led to the development of the first memory techniques (Yates, 1966). In addition to the practical advantages of having good memory skills, the fact is that rapid and accurate retrieval of information almost always impresses, whether it is the slick car salesperson who remembers you from an earlier visit or your grandmother who can rattle off the name of nearly every plant and tree in the forest. Good memory can be an important social tool. Thus, it is no wonder that concerns about memory decrements are raised as we get older and begin to experience changes in memory functioning. This concern, in turn, often triggers an interest in what can be done to improve remembering.

In recent years, a fair amount of focus has been on examining how memory can be improved in late life (Verhaeghen, Marcoen, & Goossens, 1992). Some researchers have taken a developmental perspective by addressing questions about age-related differences in terms of memory gain or plasticity (Kliegl, Smith, & Baltes, 1989, 1990; see Verhaeghen in this volume for a detailed review of plasticity research). In the memory-training literature, however, the majority of research conducted on people over 60 has been pragmatic, examining the effects of different memory-training programs (Stigsdotter Neely, 1994; Verhaeghen, 1993). Of particular interest since the late 1970s have been programs that have included training in several memory-relevant skills. The purpose of this chapter is to describe and evaluate these multifactorial approaches to memory improvement in old age, including a final section that briefly describes the most common memory techniques and skills that have been used in these programs.

A Multifactorial Approach to Memory Training in Old Age

A common theme in memory-training studies is the acknowledgment that memory improvement, as well as remembering in general, may be determined not only by a limited number of encoding and retrieval processes, but also by other cognitive (attention; Stigsdotter Neely & Bäckman, 1993b; Yesavage & Rose, 1983) and non-cognitive factors (self-efficacy beliefs, stress and anxiety levels; Stigsdotter & Bäckman, 1989; Lachman, 1991; McEvoy & Moon, 1988; Yesavage, 1985). One of the most influential examples of this contextualistic approach to remembering is the tetrahedral model devised by Jenkins (1979). In short, this model emphasizes that a full understanding of memory performance requires consideration of four basic factors: encoding activities (e.g., organization, repetition, mnemonics), subject characteristics (skills, verbal ability, attention abilities, beliefs, emotional state), retrieval factors (e.g., type of memory test), and the nature of the materials (e.g., verbal, visual). Of particular importance in this model is the notion that these sources of variation interact with each other; delineating the nature of these interactions is thought to optimize the understanding of human memory. In memory-training research, similar models have been advanced emphasizing the multiple origins of memory improvement (see Herrmann & Searleman, 1992, for more details). In this literature, a memory-training program that includes training in several critical areas in addition to training in encoding and retrieval skills is commonly referred to as a *multifactorial training program* (Herrmann & Searleman, 1992; Stigsdotter & Bäckman, 1989).

Many researchers have been enthusiastic about the possibilities of a multifactorial approach to remediating memory loss in old age (Stigsdotter & Bäckman, 1989; see West and Lachman, chapters 5 and 6 in this volume). To design a memory-training program addressing several memory-relevant and critical factors is considered more beneficial to memory performance gains in old age than the more dominant approach taken to memory improvement, where only encoding and retrieval skills are trained. In essence, it is hoped that the multifactorial approach can demonstrate performance gains that are stronger, more durable, and generalizable to other tasks and situations than those produced by traditional memory training (Herrmann, Rea, & Andrzejewski, 1988; Herrmann & Searleman, 1992; Stigsdotter & Bäckman, 1989). In addition to memory skills, three particular factors that are relevant to memory improvement have caught the attention of researchers interested in the multifactorial view: emotional states (stress and anxiety levels), belief structures (self-efficacy beliefs), and attention skills. A brief presentation follows that outlines these lines of research and explores the effectiveness of memory-training programs in which the multiple origins of memory improvement have been acknowledged. This review will focus on the assumed superiority of multifactorial over traditional training in improving memory performance in old age.

Investigating the Effectiveness of Pretraining

During the early and mid 1980s, a research team under the direction of Yesavage and Sheikh at the Palo Alto Veterans Administration Medical Center set out to investigate ways to facilitate the learning of mnemonic techniques for older adults. This learning was accomplished by providing pretraining—that is, training in a number of different memory-relevant processes—before introducing the mnemonic technique. The mnemonic device used most frequently in this work was the face-name mnemonic, which is an imagery-based technique (this and other techniques will be discussed in a later section). The rationale for including pretraining, according to the authors, is exemplified in the following quote from Yesavage, Lapp, and Sheikh (1989): "The mnemonic systems commonly used often are confusing, complicated and anxiety-producing for the elderly. It is assumed that preliminary training may prepare them for the task of learning these mnemonics" (p. 601). In other words, with mnemonic-relevant pretraining, mnemonic acquisition will be facilitated, and subsequent memory performance should be enhanced. The four pretraining activities investigated were imagery, semantic judgment, relaxation training, and a combination of the two first skills (Hill, Sheikh, & Yesavage, 1988). Both imagery and semantic judgment are critical encoding skills that promote a deep and elaborate processing of the to-be-remembered information (Craik & Lockhart, 1972). Furthermore, these skills are also relevant for augmenting the efficacy of the face-name mnemonic. The ability to form vivid mental images is a crucial aspect of the face-name mnemonic. Making a semantic judgment, which in these studies consisted of producing statements concerning the pleasantness of the face, was believed to increase the elaboration of the to-be-remembered name and face. Relaxation, on the other hand, is thought to enhance attention and reduce high stress or anxiety levels and thereby improve memory (Yesavage, 1984, 1985; Yesavage & Jacob, 1984).

The results of this research demonstrated that pretraining in imagery and semantic judgment improved memory performance more than control group conditions that consisted either of being retested or of hearing lectures on memory and aging designed to promote a positive attitude toward aging—an outcome that would be predicted from the extensive literature stemming from the levels of processing tradition (Yesavage, 1983; Yesavage, Rose, & Bower, 1983). What is noteworthy about this research is not the result that pretraining in encoding skills gave rise to improved memory performance following training, but the finding that relaxation training was as effective as imagery and semantic judgment pretraining in facilitating mnemonic acquisition (Hill et al., 1988; Sheikh, Hill, & Yesavage, 1986). Reduced anxiety levels were shown to be especially effective for people who were initially highly anxious (Yesavage, Sheikh, Decker Tanke, & Hill, 1988). These results are in agreement with the notion of a multifactorial view of gain in memory performance in old age, showing that training in cognitive as well as noncognitive skills can have a positive effect on memory gain.

The Relevance of Pretraining to Efficient Mnemonic Learning

From a practical standpoint, it is important to ask whether these results indicate that pretraining is a necessary prerequisite for efficient mnemonic learning. From the above results, it is not possible to answer this question with any certainty. They do, however, suggest that the benefits of pretraining are minimal. When interpreting results, one has to consider the context of how the issue at stake was investigated. The positive effects of pretraining are probably restricted to very defined situations. As will be elaborated on further in the next section, pretraining may be especially useful when the mnemonic is complex and the training program is rather brief, as was the case in the above studies, where only 8 hours of training were provided. With more training and cognitively less taxing mnemonics, pretraining may not be as beneficial. Another issue is whether pretraining plus mnemonic training, as conducted in the above studies, actually results in better performance gains than simply receiving the same amount of only mnemonic training, a comparison not made in the above research (the mnemonic group employed in these studies received only 4 hours of training). From a practical point of view, it would be interesting to know how 8 hours of training should be organized to obtain the best improvements on our ability to remember names and faces. For example, is it better to focus exclusively on the complex face-name mnemonic for 8 hours, or is it better to first provide 4 hours of pretraining in imagery, semantic judgment, or relaxation and then to introduce the face-name mnemonic. It is unfortunate that this comparison has not been made because it is a rather critical test of the pretraining notion as a facilitative aid for learning a complex mnemonic. As it stands now, there is no evidence to suggest that 8 hours of task-specific training is less (or for that matter more) effective than a program employing 4 hours of pretraining and 4 hours of mnemonic training; thus, it is hard to make a recommendation one way or the other.

Finally, concerns could be raised about the motivation behind introducing the pretraining notion. As cited above, the motivation for providing pretraining was to facilitate the learning of complex and frustrating mnemonic techniques. An interesting solution to the problem of complexity is to develop strategies to cope with the stress that it produces, as was done in the pretraining approach described above. Another and, considering the target group, perhaps more logical solution would be to try to avoid complex and frustrating techniques all together.

In conclusion, for the purposes of this review, the most interesting and noteworthy aspect of the pretraining studies reviewed here is the introduction of training in non-cognitive factors by addressing emotional states with relaxation training in conjunction with memory training. This work has inspired many other research endeavors, especially the next series of studies to be presented.

Multifactorial Versus Unifactorial Memory Training

Influenced by the work of Yesavage and colleagues, Stigsdotter Neely and Bäckman at the Stockholm Gerontology Research Center also conducted a series of studies based on the notion of the multifactorial nature of memory improvement. Like the previously described work, this research examined the effectiveness of a multifactorial memory-training program involving training in encoding skills, attention, and relaxation. The major difference between the two approaches is the role of pretraining as a means of improving mnemonic learning. In this regard, the work by Stigsdotter Neely and Bäckman emphasizes to a much greater extent the multifactorial nature of improvement by combining several critical abilities into one training program with less or no emphasis on pretraining per se.

The rationale for developing a multifactorial program was based on two lines of reasoning. First, efficient application of the above-mentioned skills is beneficial for learning and memory in general. Having efficient encoding skills and good control over attentional functions in conjunction with optimal levels of stress and anxiety have been shown in several studies to exert a positive effect on memory performance (Eysenck, 1985, 1988; Kausler, 1991). Second, these key processes for efficient remembering have also been shown to be age-sensitive (Salthouse, 1991). Older subjects have been shown to use less optimal encoding skill (see Bäckman, Mäntylä, & Herlitz, 1990, for a review), to have decrements in attention (see McDowd & Birren, 1990, for a review), and to be more susceptible to stress than younger adults (Bäckman & Molander, 1986; Molander & Bäckman, 1989). From this perspective, we argued that efforts to alleviate decline in episodic memory performance should be multifactorial; that is, these efforts should include training in several critical cognitive and noncognitive factors if they are to obtain reliable, durable, and generalized gains (see Stigsdotter Neely, 1994, for a review).

To examine the effectiveness of our multifactorial training program, we compared it to a more traditional unifactorial training program, where only encoding skills were practiced and no attention and relaxation training were provided. We also compared our program to a cognitive activation training program comprising training in problem-solving skills (Stigsdotter & Bäckman, 1989; Stigsdotter Neely & Bäckman, 1993a, 1993b, 1995). Thus, the questions of primary interest addressed in these studies were whether multifactorial training gives rise to immediate and more pronounced gains than unifactorial and cognitive activation training and whether these positive gains generalize over time and tasks.

The results of these studies indicated that both multifactorial and unifactorial training produced improved memory performance immediately after training, whereas those in the cognitive activation training and a control group did not show any improvement between assessments. This pattern of results was maintained 6 months as well as 3.5 years after completion of training. Further, the transfer of gains was limited to tasks very similar to the criterion task. The similar patterns of performance following multifactorial and unifactorial training indicate that attentional and relaxation training may not contribute to an improvement in memory performance above training in specific encoding skills (Stigsdotter Neely, 1994).

Our data indicate rather strongly that training-related gains after this rather brief intervention are task-specific. The following findings provide converging evidence for this view. First, training in only encoding skills results in improved memory performance; the skills trained were especially beneficial in mastering a list recall task. Second, the fact that cognitive activation, attention, and relaxation training did not improve memory performance as measured by list recall of concrete words strongly suggests the specificity of brief memory intervention. And finally, transfer was found only for those tasks most closely related to the criterion task.

As discussed in the previous section, it is important to view results in their appropriate context because conclusions depend on how the issue of interest was examined. First, the above conclusions hold true within the boundaries of how these studies evaluated the effectiveness of the multifactorial program. In other words, the findings are contingent on how the training was conducted, the type of memory tests used to measure gains, and so forth. Thus, although attention and relaxation training as conducted in our multifactorial memory training program may not be beneficial in improving memory performance, other forms of attention and relaxation training may still show improved memory performance following multifactorial training.

Second, one might ask why we did not obtain any additional effects from relaxation training like those that Hill et al. (1988) documented. In line with the above contextualization of our findings, the discrepancies in results might be due to methodological differences between the studies. As alluded to earlier, it may be that relaxation training has its primary effects early in training when subjects are unfamiliar with the training context and the task. Hence, the subjects benefit more from reduced levels of stress in shorter programs. In the present case, the multifactorial training program was longer and provided more training in less complex encoding skills than the program used in the Hill et al. (1988) study. This state of affairs might have reduced the stress levels, thus eliminating the potential benefits of relaxation training.

Changing Self-Efficacy Beliefs

The third line of research with a multifactorial approach to memory improvement in old age is studies examining the effectiveness of a program involving training that enhances self-efficacy beliefs and promotes positive and adoptive self-conceptions of memory. This research has been conducted primarily by Lachman and collaborators at Brandeis University (in this volume) and by West and colleagues at the University of Florida (in this volume), but it has lately engaged many researchers (see Floyd & Scogin, 1997, for a review). Since this work is presented in great detail elsewhere in this volume, this chapter will only briefly highlight some of the results that are relevant to the multifactorial approach to training.

In short, the rationale behind this approach is that older adults are not as confident about their memory functioning as the young (Lachman, 1990, 1991). Older adults who believe that there is nothing they can do to prevent memory decline may not have the motivation or desire to apply the new strategies to other problems in other settings (Elliott & Lachman, 1989). Further, there is also ample evidence that memory self-assessments and performance in general are positively related, a finding indicating that people holding negative, self-defeating attitudes also perform more poorly (Bandura, 1984, 1989). Hence, it is suggested that a memory-training program designed to identify and improve negative self-efficacy beliefs and dysfunctional attributional patterns, as well as to improve encoding skills, may improve memory functioning to a greater extent than programs addressing only encoding skills.

Memory-training studies targeting these belief structures have looked at (a) how memory training affects self-efficacy beliefs, (b) how self-efficacy training affects beliefs as well as memory performance, and (c) how a multifactorial approach including training in both encoding skills and self-efficacy beliefs affects memory performance as well as memory beliefs. Results concerning the first two issues have been mixed; some studies have found that memory or self-efficacy training has a positive effect on beliefs and memory performance, while others have not (see West and Lachman in this volume for a more thorough review of these studies).

Of particular interest from a multifactorial perspective is the last approach, investigating whether an integrated approach that simultaneously targets beliefs and encoding skills results in stronger, more durable, and generalized memory gains than only memory training. In the few studies addressing this issue, multifactorial training programs have yielded memory performance improvements similar to those in programs that trained encoding skills (Lachman, Weaver, Bandura, Elliott, & Lewkowicz, 1992; Weaver, Lachman, & Dick, 1990). Additionally, the multifactorial training program has shown greater beneficial effects on sense of control and perceived ability to improve memory, recall confidence, and attributions than traditional memory training (Lachman et al.,1992; Weaver et al.1990). In only one study did the multifactorial training show greater immediate, as well as maintained, gains than traditional memory training (Caprio-Prevette & Fry, 1996). Again, the majority of the results show no advantage for a multifactorial view in attaining stronger memory gains that are generalized over time, tasks, and situations. Noteworthy is that the multifactorial training led to greater increases in beliefs than did training targeting only beliefs and only memory training, a finding supporting the use of multifactorial training to improve self-efficacy beliefs (see Floyd & Scogin, 1997 for a review; Lachman et al, 1992).

The Multifactorial Approach: Expectations of Gains Beyond the Ordinary?

In this brief summary of research endeavors focusing on the multiple origins of memory improvement in late life, the targeting of self-efficacy beliefs, attention, stress, or anxiety levels in conjunction with memory techniques has predominated. The outcome of this research has revealed that memory improvements following multifactorial training are not distinct from those obtained after traditional memory training with respect to the magnitude of immediate, long-term, and generalized memory improvements. What has become rather evident is that the majority of studies have shown task-specific effects from training (e.g., improvement is seen only in the tasks or abilities trained). Given these less encouraging results of the multifactorial approach, what should be concluded about the viability of this notion as a guiding principle for memory-training programs for older adults? Evidently, to design a training program with the "multi" notion in order to improve memory beyond the ordinary (e.g., to produce stronger, more durable, and generalized gains) is not justified according to the reviewed literature. Rather, the task-specificity notion might be a more viable option to model training after; the implication is that a multifactorial approach should be used when improvements in several cognitive and noncognitive functions are desired. Hence, if the main goal is to improve older adults' beliefs and attitudes about the aging process and their memory performance on names, then teaching self-efficacy skills in addition to a memory technique for remembering names is justified.

Of course, the limited impact of the multifactorial approach on memory performance may be a function of multiple factors, including (a) the choice of dependent measures for criterion tasks and/or (b) the limited scope of the intervention relative to the difficulty in changing abilities such as emotion (stress and anxiety levels), beliefs, and thought patterns that have become firmly rooted in the individual's self-concept. Before we discard the multifactorial notion, we need more carefully designed studies that include a broader variety of dependent measures of the specific components trained and measures of generalizability over time, tasks, and situations. It is actually remarkable that given the optimism concerning memory improvements of a more durable and general nature following multifactorial intervention that more studies have not incorporated tests of long-term maintenance and transfer.

In conclusion, multifactorial training has not given rise to memory improvements over and beyond those resulting from more traditional approaches targeting only memory techniques. It should be pointed out that all of the programs reviewed here, multi- or unifactorial, involved training in encoding and retrieval skills; thus, these skills may be the dominant contributor to improvements in memory performance. The next part of this chapter will primarily review the most common memory techniques used in memory intervention research with older adults.

Memory Strategies: The Common Denominator for Memory Improvements

That memory skills are the common denominator in training programs is, of course, not surprising. Numerous studies have shown that efficient encoding and retrieval processes are of great importance in explicit memory functioning. Efficient or elaborate processing is accomplished when the to-be-remembered information is thought about by semantically or visually integrating the new information with what one already knows. There are many ways in which material can be elaborately processed. For example, this morning I suddenly remembered that I had to call the bank during my lunch hour. This realization came to me during my usual, hectic morning routine of getting myself and my children fed, cleaned, dressed, and ready to meet the new day. I knew that without some sort of elaboration, I was doomed to forget to make the phone call. Unfortunately, a search for a pen and some paper to write myself a reminder would have been as futile at this point in the morning as trying to convince my 2-year-old to keep her cereal either in her bowl or in her mouth. Instead, I chose a mental strategy: I imagined a financial crisis had hit and people were frantically trying to get into the bank to sell their stocks and take out their savings, while I sat idly by and ate my lunch. I hoped that this drastic scene would trigger my memory later at lunch, and it did.

In his excellent book, *Searching for Memory: The Brain, the Mind, and the Past* (1997), Daniel Schacter wrote:

> If we want to improve our chances of remembering an incident or learning a fact, we need to make sure that we carry out elaborative encoding by reflecting on the information and relating it to other things we already know. Laboratory studies have shown that simply intending to remember something is unlikely to be helpful, unless we translate that intention into an effective elaborative encoding. (p. 45)

In my example, the probability of remembering to call the bank increased substantially after my rather sketchy elaboration of this episode. If, instead, I had just told myself without any further elaboration that I had to remember to call the bank at lunch, I would have been left with a more impoverished memory of this episode and most likely a decreased likelihood of later recollection than my elaborated encoding of that same episode. So, in order to foster a rich and long-lived memory of the past, the importance of elaborative encoding cannot be underestimated.

The vast majority of memory-training studies with older adults have focused on investigating the effectiveness of internal memory strategies as opposed to external strategies such as note-taking skills and the use of diaries and beepers (Intons-Peterson & Newsome, 1992). The most frequently used memory strategies in this literature are the face-name mnemonic and the method of loci (Stigsdotter Neely, 1994; Verhaeghen, 1993). Recently, a fair amount of research has been devoted to the number mnemonic, and several studies have used a variety of more basic memory-encoding skills such as visual imagery and organization. Elaborative encoding is a critical ingredient of nearly all memory improvement techniques. Memory techniques generate rich and detailed encodings that are tightly linked to preexisting knowledge and yet are distinctly different from other items in memory. The remarkable memory feats observed after employing a mnemonic such as the method of loci are certainly due to the technique's capacity to produce elaborate encodings.

In the section that follows, I will give a brief presentation of the most frequently used mnemonics and the more basic memory skills used in this research for remembering single-item information, names, and numbers.

Methods That Improve Memory for Single-Item Information

The method of loci is among the most widely used techniques in the aging literature on memory improvement. It is also one of the oldest techniques known: It was developed by the ancient Greek orators exclusively for memorizing speeches (Yates, 1966). In present time and context, the method of loci has been used to remember specific single-item information in sequence, such as items on a shopping list or things that one has to do during the day (Lorayne & Lucas, 1974). The first step in learning this technique consists of generating a list of distinct places (loci), such as places in one's own apartment or specific locations in town. This sequence of locations is fundamental to this mnemonic and must be overlearned in order for the technique to be useful. To encode information, the first to-be-remembered item is associated with the first locus on the list, the second item to the second locus, and so forth. At retrieval, one "returns" to the first place in one's mental list of loci, which then serves as a cue for recalling the to-be-remembered item that was placed there. One then goes on to retrieve the second locus, and so forth.

To take a concrete example, let's say that I have to do three things today: call the bank, buy milk, and return a book to the library. My three first loci are on the stove, on the living-room sofa, and in the freezer. I then place the first item I have to remember—calling the bank—on the stove. Here I picture the turmoil of the stock market taking place on a burning stove, hundreds of people running around screaming, "Sell" and "Buy." The second item to remember is the milk, so I picture a sofa cover with the pattern of cows and pillows designed to look like milk cartons. Finally, in the freezer, I put the books. Later, during the day I consult my loci list. I revisit the stove, the sofa, and the freezer, and hopefully these cues will be efficient enough to take me back to my mental pictures of the things that I needed to get done, namely, banking, buying milk, and returning books.

As mentioned earlier, the first step in learning the method of loci is devoted to generating and memorizing the loci list. The list of loci can either consist of self-generated loci or be provided by the teacher; both types of lists have been used in the literature with positive results (Baltes & Kliegl, 1992; Stigsdotter & Bäckman, 1989). On one hand, a self-generated list may be preferred over an externally provided list. The reasons are twofold. First, the fact that the list was self-generated is, from a memory perspective, a beneficial and desirable feature since self-generated items are for the most part easier to recall (Bäckman & Mäntylä, 1988; Mäntylä, 1986). Second, the familiarity of self-generated items is an aspect that would increase the likelihood of long-term maintenance of the loci.

On the other hand, there are two aspects worth emphasizing concerning the advantages of a teacher-provided list. First, with a fixed set of loci, it is easier to monitor progress in acquiring the loci list, which is an important feature in a training context. Second, it is a great advantage that the predetermined nature of the loci list lends itself more easily to experimental manipulations, where the association between the loci and the to-be-remembered item can be varied (e.g., Thompson & Kliegl, 1991). The choice of using either a self-generated or a teacher-provided list should be guided by the intention of the training.

There are other less cognitively demanding means of remembering item-specific information, such as executing elaborative encoding on the items or events that one would like to remember, much as is described in the initial example of elaborative processing (calling the bank at lunch). By using visual imagery, a more basic encoding skill, I created a very vivid mental scenario involving a hypothetical, although in these days likely, situation in the bank. Another common method used to remember several items is the link method. In this technique, one associates each to-be-remembered item with its predecessor by having them interact. Imagine that three errands have to be run: mailing a letter, getting a new key made, and dropping some film off for developing. Picture a mailbox with a huge key protruding from the box opening. Then form an association between the key and film developing, such as seeing your pictures being developed portraying only keys, keys, and keys. This technique does not provide the same amount of retrieval support as the method of loci. Here, remembering one item will trigger the memory of the others. These two latter methods can be varied to suit the user and the task by mentally picturing several interacting items in one picture instead of imagining them one by one or two by two (Stigsdotter Neely & Bäckman, 1993b). Another common instruction to facilitate recall of item-specific information is to form category organization, like organizing a grocery shopping list in terms of food categories, dishes, and/or menus. This method is used frequently in everyday life.

Finally, the most obvious means of remembering item-specific information is to write the information down on a piece of paper. Efficient note taking should by no means be underestimated as a proficient memory device, as it is perhaps the most prevalent method for remembering single-item information in everyday life used by both young and old. When teaching older adults the techniques described here it is important to emphasize that internal techniques such as the method of loci should not replace external techniques. Rather, they are complementary. Sometimes note taking is to be preferred over internal techniques, but in other situations, the knowledge of elaborative encoding can come in handy, particularly in those situations when one does not have the time to write the to-be-remembered information down (Intons-Peterson & Fournier, 1986).

In this literature on memory intervention in normal aging, mnemonics such as the method of loci have been seriously questioned as rehabilitative memory aids for older people. This criticism has been based on the premise that mnemonics are difficult to apply and are inappropriate in most everyday situations. Research has also shown that memory experts, like cognitive psychologists themselves, do not use mnemonics to any great extent in everyday life (Park, Smith, & Cavanaugh, 1990). Despite this criticism, there are some important reasons for including training in mnemonics such as the method of loci for elderly people.

One of the advantages of using the method of loci, for example, is the possibility of demonstrating rather impressive performance improvements in a fairly short time, such as recalling words in serial order both forward and backward—certainly a skill of little practical value, but the point here is to be able to demonstrate that great gains can be achieved by engaging in elaborate encoding. This demonstration is an encouraging experience for the learner and important for training success. If training can build confidence by showing that improvements can come about when information is processed elaboratively, that is in and of itself as good as any reason for addressing mnemonics in a training context. Further, the method of loci provides a convenient way to talk about the importance of efficient encoding and retrieval processes in explicit remembering. The source of the memory gains is easily explained to the subject by referring to the rich and elaborate type of processing engaged in at encoding and also by focusing on the list of loci serving as a preexisting knowledge structure that provides retrieval support.

Methods That Improve Memory for Names

To be able to remember names is a valued skill for people of all ages. Names are rather difficult to remember partly due to their abstract nature. Many different techniques are used to improve the ability to remember names (Higbee, 1988). These range from rather complex mnemonics to fairly simple recommendations of use-it-or-lose-it. The more complex techniques usually rely on imagery transformations, such as the name-face mnemonic used in the studies by Yesavage and colleagues described earlier (McCarty, 1980; Yesavage, 1983). This name-face mnemonic consists of three steps: First, select a prominent feature of the face; second, make a concrete imagery transformation of the person's name; and third, form an interactive visual image linking the name transformation to the prominent facial feature. This could be done in the following way: I have a colleague with distinctively blue eyes and her name is Pernilla Hegg. To make a mental picture of her name, I take the initial letter from her first name, *P* and the three last letters of her surname, *(H)egg,* and combine them into a new word that could be pictured as a gigantic Peg(g). Then I merge Steps 1 and 2 by hanging her distinctively blue eyes on the giant peg. The next time I encounter Pernilla, I will most likely pay attention to her blue eyes, which will then serve as a retrieval cue for my mental representation of her name, blue eyes hanging from a giant peg. Then, I must decode the image to retrieve the name, *P* for "Pernilla" and *eg* for "Hegg." This is memory acrobatics at its best! While this method is initially very time-consuming and sometimes difficult, it is usually fun, especially when one creates these images together with other people.

There are many ways in which this complex technique can be simplified without jeopardizing improvements. One version consists of only performing the second step in the above sequence. Usually, the problem is to remember the name and not who the name belongs to. Hence, the first as well as the third step may be redundant and could be omitted. The purpose of associating a prominent facial feature with the name is just to guarantee that the name will be given to the right person. So it may be enough for later successful recollection to execute only Step 2, elaborating the name by transforming the name into a visual representation, a concrete picture.

Other less cognitively demanding strategies often used are different strategies for elaborating the to-be-remembered name by associating it with previous knowledge, such as thinking of somebody you know who has that same name. Further elaboration upon this association is also recommended by either reflecting upon the nature of the association or to extend the elaboration to include information that would facilitate later recollection of the information. For example, today when I called my son's dentist, she introduced herself as Gun Persson. Not having a pen around, I thought of my high school friend called Gunnel and another friend who also has Persson as her family name. I imagined the two of them together, dressed as dentists with drills in their hands and scary smiles.

Perhaps the best advice is given by the slogan "Use it or lose it." Compliance with the beautiful simplicity of this rather rough statement actually has shown to result in remarkable memory improvements in people with rather severe brain pathologies (Bird & Kinsella, 1995; Camp & McKitrick, 1992). To retrieve the name as soon as you have learned it and to repeat the name at increasingly longer intervals is a technique known as spaced retrieval. This technique is described in great detail by both Camp, Bird, and Cherry and Bird in this volume and is a valuable method that can be easily combined with any of the described memory techniques in this chapter.

The described methods of improving name recall are all effective. However, they do differ in their ease of applicability in everyday life. The first name-face technique described in this section is obviously the most cognitively demanding technique and is not recommended in situations requiring attention to some other source of information than remembering the name. The reason is that for most of us, it comes at the cost of either losing track of the attended information while executing the three steps in the face-name mnemonic or hindering our ability to efficiently perform all three steps. Although this is an excellent method when enough time is available, the less cognitively demanding techniques presented are a better choice in more cognitively challenging situations such as social gatherings.

Methods That Improve Memory for Numbers

Dependency on number codes has increased dramatically in our society since the late 1980s. To gain access to essential services requires remembering personalized number sequences (e.g., four-digit personal identification numbers, door codes). In the memory-training literature, relatively few studies have examined the effectiveness of different number techniques compared to techniques for verbal material. However, recently, a fair amount of work has been conducted in our laboratory investigating, among other things the effectiveness of different methods of remembering numbers (Derwinger, Persson, Hill, Bäckman, Stigsdotter Neely, 1999; Hill, Campbell, Foxley, & Lindsay, 1997).

The number mnemonic used in our research was described by Higbee (1988) and is called the *number-consonant* or *number-phonetic system*. Like the method of loci, this is an old technique, which requires a sequence of information to be overlearned for successful recall. The number-consonant technique consists of four steps. The first step requires the memorization of a series of digit-letter pairs, $0 = S$ or Z; $1 = T$ or D; $2 = N$; $3 = M$; $4 = R$; $5 = L$; $6 = J$; $7 = K$ or G; $8 = F$ or V; $9 = P$ or B. It is essential that these digit-letter pairs be overlearned, and several methods of memorization are possible, such as linking a physical characteristic or sound that is common to both the letter and the number. For example, in the case of the number 1, both T and D involve one downward stroke. The second step is the word generation step, which involves transforming the to-be-remembered number string into letters and then joining the letters with placeholder vowels to form a word or series of words. For example, from the number sequence 2194 the letters $N\ T\ P\ R$ are used. A word or word series is then created from this letter combination (e.g., NoT PooR). The third step is to memorize the generated word or word series. Several techniques may be used to facilitate this process, including selecting words that are connected to the number sequence in some meaningful way (e.g., for a bank code with the PIN 0832, the word SaVe MoNey could be created). The fourth step consists of obtaining the original number sequence from the generated word by retracing from Step 3 to Step 1.

In our research, we compared the number-consonant mnemonic with a self-taught program where a group of subjects developed their own techniques for remembering four-digit numbers by using more basic encoding skills, such as visualization and association with previous knowledge. For example, in order to remember the code 4512, the subjects might associate 45 with the end of World War II and 12 with a dozen red roses, creating the mental image of celebrating the end of the war by giving 12 beautiful flowers to a dear friend. Preliminary results of this study showed that both groups improved memory performance after training, but that the number-consonant mnemonic group gained significantly more. This study included a number of transfer tests and a long-term maintenance test. Among the transfer tests that have not yet been analyzed are data pertaining to transfer to everyday life. These data will, of course, be important in evaluating the pros and cons concerning both these methods of remembering numbers.

From a practical perspective, in what situations should this rather complex number-consonant mnemonic be used? From my experience of being a dedicated user and also from reports of a majority of the 120 persons who underwent training with this technique, its greatest use is in remembering critical four-digit codes that are not used every day. Number codes that are used daily quickly become overlearned and proceduralized, which are potent means of long-term remembering, reducing the need for complex elaborative processing.

Aspects to Consider When Designing a Memory-Training Program

When designing and conducting a memory-training program for healthy older adults, there are many things to consider. What behaviors, skills, and processes should be addressed? How much training should be given? What types of tests should be used to measure treatment gains?

Regarding which components should be targeted in memory training, it was concluded in the first part of this chapter that multifactorial memory training has not yet proven to be a more potent means of obtaining durable and general gains than more traditional approaches focusing exclusively on memory processes. In essence, the majority of research results are task-specific, indicating that the memory improvement is most evident in the task you received training in. This finding suggests that the notion of task specificity might be a viable principle to guide training, meaning that training should specifically focus on improving memory performance on particular tasks and/ or behaviors in particular situations and with particular methods. Thus, if the goal is to improve memory of four-digit numbers, then adequate techniques should be chosen for that purpose, such as the number-consonant mnemonic and/or a less cognitively demanding method such as visual imagery elaboration. However, this does not mean that training need target only one particular task with one particular method. A wider range of tasks, skills, and methods could be used in training, such as memory for names, numbers, and noncognitive factors such as self-efficacy beliefs, but this wider focus has to be accompanied by task-specific training in those particular tasks and skills.

Applying the notion of task specificity when designing a memory-training program also determines the intention behind the intervention, which is to improve memory performance on particular tasks, in particular situations with particular methods, a definition that does not emphasize the generality of results. To have a clearly defined goal as well as the means to obtain that goal is important when introducing the program to the participants. Though our experiences in life tend to support the fact that few skills or improvements come easy, many participants in a memory-training program still have the hope that memory improvement will come easily and lead to general improvements. These positive and unrealistic expectations have to be addressed early in the training program by clearly stating what is going to be accomplished through the training. To adjust beliefs about memory training to the actual intention of training, by stressing that memory training comes at the cost of time and effort and does not lead to general gains, is important for the success of a training program.

Two other issues to consider when designing a memory-training program are the amount of training given and the type of tasks used to measure treatment gains. Concerning how much training is needed, the training phase differs quite extensively in memory-training studies in this area. Usually a training session lasts between 1 and 1.5 hours and the program itself runs anywhere from 1 to 32 sessions, with a mean of around 6 sessions (see Stigsdotter Neely, 1994, for a review). From a practical perspective, six to eight sessions of 60 to 90 minutes each are recommended to adequately master most of the described mnemonics and memory skills. As I pointed out previously, most studies in this area have included only tests of immediate gains in the criterion task and less frequently have used tests measuring transfer over time, tasks, and situations. In order to capture the effectiveness of a memory-training program, all of these measures are important to include.

Finally, the research portrayed in this chapter concerns only healthy aged persons and indicates that most of these people are, cognitively speaking, well functioning compared to subjects with early signs of dementia. To introduce training in cognitively demanding memory techniques for people who experience early signs of dementia or forgetfulness beyond the normal is not advisable (see Bird in this volume; Bäckman, Josephsson, Herlitz, Stigsdotter, & Viitanen, 1991). A good rule of thumb when designing a memory-training program for practical purposes is to build the training around the interests and cognitive skills of the participants and to calibrate the amount of training accordingly.

Final Conclusions

One of the major goals of applied memory-training research is to understand the complexity of factors behind memory improvement in order to develop efficient memory interventions. As this book attests, memory improvement is a function of several critical factors, such as individual differences, methodological issues, and the skills and processes trained. The aim of this chapter was to focus on the latter of those determinants of memory gain: what skills and processes should be trained to give rise to reliable memory improvements in healthy older adults. I presented research investigating the benefits of a multifactorial approach comprising training in several cognitive and noncognitive factors, compared to memory-training programs where only encoding and retrieval processes have been of primary concern. At this time, the multifactorial approach has not yet given rise to gains beyond the ordinary. As a matter of fact, the critical factor accounting for gains in terms of the skills or processes trained is most likely training of encoding and retrieval operations. This result, in addition to the specificity of gains in other tasks trained, points to the intimate relation between gains and the task trained. To ensure positive benefits from memory interventions, a good piece of advice is to guide training after the notion of task specificity—focusing the training specifically on those particular tasks, skills, and behaviors that are of primary interest to the learner.

Reference

Bäckman, L., Josephsson, S., Herlitz, A., Stigsdotter, A., & Viitanen, M. (1991). The generalizability of training gains in dementia: Effects of an imagery-based mnemonic on face-name retention duration. *Psychology and Aging, 6,* 489–492.
Bäckman, L., & Mäntylä, T. (1988). Effectiveness of self-generated cues in younger and older adults: The role of retention interval. *International Journal of Aging and Human Development, 26,* 163–167.
Bäckman, L., Mäntylä, T., & Herlitz, A. (1990). The optimization of episodic remembering in old age. In P. B. Baltes & M. M. Baltes (Eds.), *Successful aging: Perspectives from the behavioral sciences* (pp. 118–163). New York: Cambridge University Press.
Bäckman, L., & Molander, B. (1986). Adult age differences in the ability to cope with situations of high arousal in a precision sport. *Psychology and Aging, 2,* 133–139.
Baltes, P. B., & Kliegl, R. (1992). Further testing of limits of cognitive plasticity: Negative age differences in a mnemonic skill are robust. *Developmental Psychology, 1,* 121–125.
Bandura, A. (1984). Recycling misconceptions of perceived self-efficacy. *Cognitive Therapy and Research, 8,* 231–255.
Bandura, A. (1989). Regulation of cognitive processes through perceived self-efficacy. *Developmental Psychology, 25,* 729–735.

Bird, M., & Kinsella, G. (1995). Long-term cued recall of tasks in senile dementia. *Psychology and Aging, 11,* 45–56.

Camp, C. J., & McKitrick, L. A. (1992). Memory interventions in DAT populations: Methodological and theoretical issues. In R. L. West & J. D. Sinnott (Eds.), *Everyday memory and aging: Current research and methodology* (pp.155–172). New York: Springer-Verlag.

Caprio-Prevette, M. D., & Fry, P. S. (1996). *Experimental Aging Research, 22,* 281–303

Craik, F. I. M., & Lockhart, R. S. (1972). Levels of processing: A framework for memory research. *Journal of Verbal Learning and Verbal Behavior, 11,* 671–684.

Derwinger, A., Persson, M., Hill, R. D., Bäckman, L., & Stigsdotter Neely, A. (1999). *Remembering numbers in old age: An investigation of the benefits of mnemonics vs. self-generated memory techniques.* Manuscript in preparation. Umeå University.

Elliot, E., & Lachman, M. E. (1989). Enhancing memory by modifying control beliefs, attributions, and performance goals in the elderly. In P. S. Fry (Ed.), *Psychological perspectives of helplessness and control in the elderly* (pp. 339–367). North Holland: Elsevier Science Publishers.

Eysenck, M. W. (1985). Anxiety and cognitive-task performance. *Personality and Individual Differences, 6,* 579–585.

Eysenck, M. W. (1988). Anxiety and attention. *Anxiety Research, 1,* 9–15.

Floyd, M., & Scogin, F. (1997). Effects of memory training on the subjective memory functioning and mental health of older adults: A meta-analysis. *Psychology and Aging, 12,* 150–161.

Herrmann, D. J., Rea, A., & Andrzejewski, S. (1988). The need for a new approach to memory training. In M. M. Gruneberg, P. E. Morris, & R. N. Sykes (Eds.), *Practical aspects of memory: Current research and issues* (Vol. 2, pp. 415–420). Chichester, UK: Wiley.

Herrmann, D. J., & Searleman, A. (1992). Memory improvement and memory theory in historical perspective. In D. J. Herrmann, H. Weingartner, A. Searleman, & C. McEvoy (Eds.), *Memory improvement: Implications for memory theory* (pp. 8–20). New York: Springer-Verlag.

Higbee, K. L. (1988). *Your memory: How it works and how to improve it.* New York: Paragon House.

Hill, R. D., Campbell, B. W., Foxley, D., & Lindsay, S. (1997). Effectiveness of the number-consonant mnemonic for retention of numeric material in community-dwelling older adults. *Experimental Aging Reasearch, 23,* 275–286.

Hill, R. D., Sheikh, J. I., & Yesavage, J. A. (1988). Pretraining enhances mnemonic training in elderly adults. *Experimental Aging Research, 14,* 207–211.

Intons-Peterson, M. J., & Fournier, J. (1986). External and internal memory aids: When and how often do we use them? *Journal of Experimental Psychology: General, 115,* 267–280.

Intons-Peterson, M. J., & Newsome, III, G. L. (1992). External memory aids: Effects and effectiveness. In D. J. Herrmann, H. Weingartner, A. Searleman, & C. McEvoy (Eds.), *Memory improvement: Implications for memory theory* (pp. 101–122). New York: Springer-Verlag.

Jenkins, J. J. (1979). Four points to remember: A tetrahedral model of memory experiments. In J. C. Cermak & F. I. M. Craik (Eds.), *Levels of processing in human memory* (pp. 429–446). Hillsdale, NJ: Erlbaum.

Kausler, D. H. (1991). *Experimental psychology, cognition, and human aging* (2nd ed.). New York: Springer-Verlag.

Kliegl, R., Smith, J., & Baltes, P. B. (1989). Testing-the-limits and the study of adult age differences in cognitive plasticity of a mnemonic skill. *Developmental Psychology, 25,* 247–256.

Kliegl, R., Smith, J., & Baltes, P. B. (1990). On the locus and process of magnification of age differences during mnemonic training. *Developmental Psychology, 6,* 894–904.

Lachman, M. E. (1990). When bad things happen to older people: Age differences in attributional style. *Psychology and Aging, 5,* 607–609.

Lachman, M. E. (1991). Perceived control over memory aging: Developmental and intervention perspectives. *Journal of Social Issues, 47,* 159–175.

Lachman, M. E., Weaver, S. L., Bandura, M., Elliott, E., & Lewkowicz, C. J. (1992). Improving memory and control beliefs through cognitive restructuring and self generated strategies. *Journals of Gerontology, 47,* P293–P299.

Lorayne, E. E., & Lucas, J. (1974). *The memory book.* New York: Stein & Day.

Mäntylä, T. (1986). Optimizing cue effectiveness: Recall of 500 hundred and 600 hundred incidentally learned words. *Journal of Experimental Psychology: Learning, Memory and Cognition, 12,* 66–71.

McCarty, D. L. (1980). Investigation of a visual imagery mnemonic device for acquiring face-name associations. *Journal of Experimental Psychology: Human Learning and Memory, 6,* 145–155.

McDowd, J. M., & Birren, J. E. (1990). Aging and attentional processes. In J. E. Birren & K. W. Schaie (Eds.), *Handbook of the psychology of aging* (3rd ed., pp. 222–233). San Diego: Academic Press.

McEvoy, C. L. (1992). Memory improvement in context: Implications for the development of memory improvement theory. In D. J. Herrmann, H. Weingartner, A. Searleman, & C. McEvoy (Eds.), *Memory improvement: Implications for memory theory* (pp. 210–231). New York: Springer-Verlag.

McEvoy, C. L., & Moon, J. R. (1988). Assessment and treatment of everyday memory problems. In M. M. Gruneberg, P. E. Morris, & R. N. Sykes (Eds.), *Practical aspects of memory: Current research and issues* (Vol. 2, pp. 155–160). Chichester, UK: Wiley.

Molander, B., & Bäckman, L. (1989). Age differences in heart rate patterns during concentration in a precision sport: Implications for attentional functioning. *Journal of Gerontology, 44,* P80–P87.

Park, D. C., Smith, A. D., & Cavanaugh, J. C. (1990). Metamemories of memory researchers. *Memory and Cognition, 18,* 321–327.

Salthouse, T. A. (1991). *Theoretical perspectives on cognitive aging.* Hillsdale, NJ: Erlbaum.

Schacter, D. L. (1997). *Searching for memory: The brain, the mind, and the past.* New York: BasicBooks.

Sheikh, J. I., Hill, R. D., & Yesavage, J. A. (1986). Long-term efficacy of cognitive training for age-associated memory impairment: A six-month follow-up study. *Developmental Neuropsychology, 2,* 413–421.

Stigsdotter, A., & Bäckman, L. (1989). Multifactorial memory training with older adults: How to foster maintenance of improved performance. *Gerontology, 35,* 260–267.

Stigsdotter Neely, A. (1994) *Memory training in late adulthood: Issues of maintenance, transfer, and individual differences.* Unpublished doctoral dissertation, Karolinska Institute, Stockholm.

Stigsdotter Neely, A., & Bäckman, L. (1993a). Long-term maintenance of gains from memory training in older adults: Two 3 1/2 years follow-up studies. *Journal of Gerontology, 48,* P233–P237.

Stigsdotter Neely, A., & Bäckman, L. (1993b). Maintenance of gains following multifactorial and unifactorial memory training in late adulthood. *Educational Gerontology, 19,* 105–117.

Stigsdotter Neely, A., & Bäckman, L. (1995). Effects of multifactorial memory training in old age: Generalizability across tasks and individuals. *Journal of Gerontology: Psychological Sciences, 3,* P134–P140.

Thompson, L. A., & Kliegl, R. (1991). Adult age effects of plausibility on memory: The role of time constrains during encoding. *Journal of Experimental Psychology: Learning, Memory, and Cognition, 3,* 542–555.

Verhaeghen, P. (1993). *Teaching old dogs new memory tricks: Plasticity in episodic memory performance in old age.* Unpublished doctoral dissertation, Katholieke University, Leuven, Belgium.

Verhaeghen, P., Marcoen, A., & Goossens, L. (1992). Improving memory performance in the aged through mnemonic training: A meta-analytic study. *Psychology and Aging, 7,* 242–251.

Weaver, S. L., Lachman, M. E., & Dick, L. (1990). *Enhancing memory and self-efficacy: What works and for whom?* Unpublished manuscript.

Yates, F. A. (1966). *The art of memory.* London: Routledge.

Yesavage, J. A. (1983). Imagery pretraining and memory training in the elderly. *Gerontology, 29,* 271–275.

Yesavage, J. A. (1984). Relaxation and memory training in 39 elderly patients. *American Journal of Psychiatry, 141,* 778–781.

Yesavage, J. A. (1985). Nonpharmacologic treatments for memory losses with normal aging. *American Journal of Psychiatry, 142,* 600–605.

Yesavage, J. A., & Jacob, R. (1984). Effects of relaxation and mnemonics on memory, attention and anxiety in the elderly. *Experimental Aging Research, 10,* 211–214.

Yesavage, J. A., Lapp, D., & Sheikh, J. I. (1989). Mnemonics as modified for use by the elderly. In L. W. Poon, D. C. Rubin, & B. A. Wilson (Eds.), *Everyday cognition in adulthood and late life* (pp. 598–611). Cambridge: Cambridge University Press.

Yesavage, J. A., & Rose, T. L. (1983). Concentration and mnemonic training in the elderly with memory complaints: A study of combined therapy and order effects. *Psychiatry Research, 9,* 157–167.

Yesavage, J. A., Rose, T. L., & Bower, G. H. (1983). Interactive imagery and affective judgments improve face-name learning in the elderly. *Journal of Gerontology, 29,* 197–203.

Yesavage, J. A., Sheikh, J. I., Decker Tanke, E. D., & Hill, R. (1988). Response to memory training and individual differences in verbal intelligence and state anxiety. *American Journal of Psychiatry, 145,* 636–639.

5

Innovative Approaches to Memory Training for Older Adults

ROBIN L. WEST

DUANA C. WELCH

MONICA S. YASSUDA

Memory training programs designed to enhance the memory abilities of older adults have been part of the experimental aging literature for decades. The earliest known publication involved the training of mediational strategies for paired-associate learning (Hulicka & Grossman, 1967). Probably long before that, individual clinicians or nurses were offering information about memory to their patients and clients. The purpose of this chapter is not to review the training programs that have been tested over the last three decades, but to focus on recent innovations in the programming of memory interventions for older adults. For the most part, these innovations have been tried but not yet proven, having been applied only in a handful of studies. Our purpose here is to spark the interest of scholars of the aging process, encouraging the pursuit of new directions in cognitive rehabilitation for older adults.

To provide background, we begin with a descriptive overview of previous intervention research, briefly outlining the successes and limitations of that work. We then consider three more recent innovations: (a) videotape training, (b) efficacy-based training, and (c) nondidactic, group study. For each of these, the focus is not on past training data but on future possibilities: What are the characteristic features of this methodology? What empirical evidence suggests that this new approach might have value for older adults? How could this methodology serve to minimize the memory deficits associated with normal aging and/or enhance the impact of training?

What Has Been Learned From Traditional Approaches

Traditional memory intervention programs for older adults have largely consisted of two types: (a) "instant" strategy training—brief training, specific to the recall task (e.g., Hulicka & Grossman, 1967), and (b) extended training involving several sessions and/or several strategies with the full-length intervention lasting from 4 to 15 hours (e.g., Zarit, Cole, & Guider, 1981). The traditional approaches can be characterized by the fact that they were didactic—the experimenter told the trainees what to do and how to do it—and their primary purpose was to teach a strategy (e.g., Treat, Poon, & Fozard, 1981).

These seminal studies provided a solid knowledge base for future cognitive rehabilitation research. We now know that memory strategies, even very complex techniques, can be learned by older adults; that training can lead to improvements that sometimes last for months; and that training tends to be task-specific, with little or no transfer to tasks that were not incorporated in the training regimen. A recent meta-analysis established that training effects are significant when examined across a wide range of studies (Verhaeghen, Marcoen, & Goossens, 1992). Four factors were associated with enhanced training effectiveness: pretraining, group sessions, shorter sessions, and younger participants (Verhaeghen et al., 1992).

At the same time, previous research had limitations, suggesting that new directions might be productive. One limitation of earlier work was that the mechanisms controlling the observed memory improvements were not well understood. Theory took a back seat to empirical issues, and potential mechanisms were not sufficiently explored (Kotler-Cope & Camp, 1990; West & Tomer, 1989; Yesavage, Lapp, & Sheikh, 1989). When improvements occurred after strategy training, it was assumed that the change was due to the learned strategy, even when strategy usage was not assessed (and it rarely has been assessed). But it could be that particular unplanned effects explained or contributed to the impact of training, and these have been studied only rarely (McEvoy, 1992). In a recent training study, Verhaeghen and Marcoen (1996) found that older adults were often noncompliant, not using the imaginal strategy they had learned, especially those older adults who had an effective nonimaginal strategy in their pretest repertoire. Thus, compliance may be an important, unstudied predictor of outcome. Other unplanned or nonstrategic effects could include increased attention or concentration, practice effects (e.g., faster processing, increased familiarity with task requirements), more knowledge about how memory works, reduced depression and improved mood, less anxiety or more confidence during memory testing, enhanced motivation or changed beliefs about one's potential as a memorizer, and superior executive functioning (e.g., better distribution of attention within working memory, improved monitoring and/or self-testing during encoding). Another possible explanation for performance change might be qualitative improvements in the use of association and/or imagery strategies that were already employed before training. Furthermore, trainees could have developed their own idiosyncratic methods of memorizing, unrelated to the trained strategy. Several investigators have begun looking at individual difference factors related to training outcome (e.g., Kliegl, Smith, & Baltes, 1989; Verhaeghen & Marcoen, 1996; Yesavage, Sheikh, Tanke, & Hill, 1988), but relatively few studies have directly addressed the issue of mechanisms: Measurement of pre-post changes in anxiety, mental speed and/or working memory, confidence, memory beliefs, strategy usage, and practice effects (for a nontrained group), in relation to performance outcome, would go a long way toward answering these important questions about mechanisms.

For instance, in order to make the argument that strategies are the mechanism for change, we must be able to demonstrate directly (a) that the trained strategies were used by trainees at posttest, (b) that the training effects did not simply reflect nonspecific practice effects, and (c) that improvements in performance were related to changes in strategy usage. To accomplish goal (b), a practice-only control group must be included in the investigation. To accomplish goal (a), strategy use must be measured, and for goal (c), measured strategy usage must be related to performance at posttest. Most studies in the adult memory-training literature rely exclusively upon improvements in memory to ascertain training effectiveness, without separate measures of strategy use. The exceptions are seven studies that incorporated independent assessment of strategy self-report (e.g., Anschutz, Camp, Markley, & Kramer, 1987; Rankin, Karol, & Tuten, 1984; Rebok & Balcerak, 1989; Verhaeghen & Marcoen, 1996; Wood & Pratt, 1987), overt rehearsal behavior (Murphy, Schmitt, Caruso, & Sanders, 1987; Sanders, Murphy, Schmitt, & Walsh, 1980; Schmitt, Murphy, & Sanders, 1981), or clustering (ARC scores; e.g., Rankin et al., 1984; Sanders et al., 1980; Schmitt et al., 1981). The best of the studies assessing strategy usage was an investigation by Verhaeghen and Marcoen (1996). They provided evidence that preexisting abilities (mental speed, associative memory) were strong predictors of training-related gain, as were posttest strategy behaviors (the number of list rehearsals during test, for both old and young, and correct strategy usage for the young). Correct method-of-loci application was associated to some extent with better performance for older trainees. These data were suggestive about strategy use as a mechanism, but most of the assessments were different at pretest and posttest so it was not possible, in most cases, to see if pre-to-post change in any particular variable predicted gain (Verhaeghen & Marcoen, 1996). Prior investigations can begin to answer questions about strategy utilization as a mechanism for change, but the results were mixed, and none demonstrated directly that pre-post changes in strategy usage predicted pre-post performance changes.

Another limitation of previous work is the lack of evidence concerning strategy maintenance. Tests for strategy maintenance are far less common than tests for maintenance of performance, and often, studies include neither measure. Maintenance of both types must be established if one is to argue for strategic change as the mechanism for improvement. Some studies have demonstrated that memory improvement can be maintained for 1 week to 6 months (see Flynn & Storandt, 1990; Scogin, Storandt, & Lott, 1985; Sheikh, Hill, & Yesavage, 1986; Stigsdotter & Bäckman, 1989, Stigsdotter Neely & Bäckman, 1993a; West & Crook, 1992) or even years (Stigsdotter Neely & Bäckman, 1993b), but the factors explaining successful maintenance are still unclear. Interestingly, the few studies that have directly examined maintenance of strategy use have failed to find it (Anschutz et al., 1987; Schmitt et al., 1981; Wood & Pratt, 1987). Because neither theory nor empirical work has clarified the mechanisms for change, factors that would promote maintenance are poorly understood. The primary motivation for new approaches would be to find an intervention methodology that leads to long-lasting and not just short-term change, so that older adults' deficits can be reduced or eliminated, and so that the mechanisms driving both memory change and maintenance of improved abilities can be understood.

Video-Based Memory Training

The memory limitations of older adults have been studied extensively. Although researchers disagree about the mechanisms that control age differences in memory, the perspectives that have gained widespread acceptance are those that emphasize the working-memory limitations of older adults, their slower processing time, and the fact that older adults require more support for learning (Craik, 1986). Several features of videotaped learning programs may make it possible for older adults to overcome their memory limitations: enhanced support for learning, opportunities for self-paced training and review, and dynamic multimedia representations of strategies. Although videotape has rarely been studied with older adult groups, these benefits are apparent in research with young adults and children.

Rationale for This Innovation

The primary rationale for videotaped instruction is that it is highly effective—often more effective than traditional teaching programs. At one level, videotape can teach people how to use a simple piece of equipment (Le Grice & Blampied, 1994). At a more complex level, a videotape can train therapists, law enforcement personnel, or volunteers to respond appropriately to particular types of crises, through modeling and role playing, without endangering people by placing them in a crisis situation (Holaday & Smith, 1995; Seabury, 1993; Seymour, Stahl, Levine, & Ingram, 1994). Empirical work related to social learning theory has established the advantages of models over traditional didactic learning (Bandura, 1997). Videotape makes it possible for standardized models to be presented at minimum expense. Past uses of videotape for this purpose included teaching students specific therapy techniques (Follette & Callaghan, 1995), teaching disabled or handicapped patients new ways of moving or standing (Dowrick & Raeburn, 1995; Tiong, Blampied, & Le Grice, 1992), and teaching families how to improve social interactions and/or caregiving (Neef, Trachtenberg, Loeb, & Sterner, 1991; Weiner, Kuppermintz, & Guttmann, 1994). In several experimental studies, the video or multimedia approach to training clinicians was much more effective than standard teaching (e.g., Bashman & Treadwell, 1995; Juhnke, 1994).

One of the primary benefits of video is that it takes advantage of the improved learning associated with combined visual and verbal instruction (Banyan & Stein, 1990; Gehring & Toglia, 1988; Slotnick, 1990). Educational psychologists have argued that pictures make text more interesting and motivate learners. More important, visual images may enhance memory. Even at the simplest level (provision of an illustration), reviews of the literature have shown that the combination of visual and verbal information aided retention relative to the case where only text was given (Mayer, 1989). This finding is called the *picture facilitation effect* (Rusted & Hodgson, 1985). The most common theoretical explanation for this effect, Paivio's dual-code theory (1986), emphasizes that the memory system is structured to encode information in combined visual plus verbal modes, whether or not the material is presented in both modalities. When the information provided uses both modalities in the first place, it supports this memory system.

Of course, it is possible to provide visual support for memory rehabilitation classes without using video, but past research has demonstrated that animated pictures are better than static graphics. This topic has been investigated for decades, but only research since the late 1980s will be considered here. Christel (1994) showed that illustrations using motion video were better than static slides for remembering college course material. When study time was controlled, Rieber (1990, 1991) showed that students learned more from animated lessons than from lessons using static pictures. Rieber (1991) also showed that children's intentional learning and incidental learning are both higher when verbal text is combined with animation as opposed to static pictures providing essentially the same information. Rieber suggested that animated sequences should be cued with a voice-over that directs attention to the central features because new learners cannot always identify the critical features on their own (Rieber, 1991). Animation worked better for some students than for others and was particularly beneficial for those with learning difficulties or those who benefited from visual information (Ayersman & von Minden, 1995). Low-ability verbalizers and visualizers unable to translate material from visual to verbal or vice versa benefited especially from both forms being available in a lesson (Riding, Buckle, Thompson, & Hagger, 1989). Although this work was not conducted specifically with older adults, one would expect that older adults would show the same benefits as others with learning deficits, particularly because of some difficulties that older adults may have with generating mental pictures on their own (West, Yassuda, & Welch, 1997).

The strongest case for the "learning value" of video per se was made by the work of Mayer and colleagues (e.g., Mayer & Anderson, 1992). Mayer's work was designed to test the contiguity principle derived from Paivio's dual-coding theory. The contiguity principle argues that learning is best when words and pictures are presented contiguously because simultaneous access to words and pictures enhances the conceptual connections between visual and verbal representations in memory, without taxing working memory (Mayer & Anderson, 1992). In testing this principle, Mayer compared the retention and problem solving of college students after their exposure to simple lessons concerning the internal workings of brakes and air pumps. These lessons were presented under various conditions: successive sections of animation and narration, concurrent animation and narration (the typical videotape format), animation alone, narration alone, and no instruction. Although retention of the basic facts did not differ among formats, application skills did vary. Students given concurrent presentation were better able to identify creative solutions to problems involving brakes and air pumps, suggesting that the highest level of information was gained from the video format. If, in fact, simultaneous presentation of animation and narration enhances learning, without taxing working memory, this would represent an important methodology for older adults who have working-memory limitations (Salthouse, 1990). To our knowledge, there is only one published report demonstrating that older adults learn better with video: Gist, Schwoerer, and Rosen (1989) taught older adults how to use computers by presenting a videotaped middle-aged model and found this approach to surpass text-based instruction.

One potentially important benefit of videotaped training for older adults is that video provides learner control over pacing and total study time. Rieber (1991) emphasized the importance of reviewing videos repeatedly, to reinforce learning. His experimental work (Rieber, 1991) demonstrated the benefits of a feature that has been highly touted in educational circles for older adults (see Sinnott, 1994): student control over presentation. Videotape provides that control. It affords the possibility of stopping, reviewing a concept, pausing to let an idea "sink in," and so forth. Individualized pacing can be especially beneficial for older adults because of the high variability in learning speed (Kausler, 1991).

Newer technologies involving videodisk or interactive computer-based training offer many more options for control over learning, make selective review simpler, and provide individualized feedback on progress. In contrast to video, individuals can sit down at an interactive program and select a particular section to review without having to first view the entire program. The interactive format of the videodisk thus provides more viewer control over content and sequencing. It is important to note, however, that the use of these advanced features may depend on the learning style and computer ability of the learner (e.g., Fitzgerald, 1995; Henry, 1995; Lee, Gillan, & Harrison, 1996), and the results are mixed with respect to the relative value of interactive approaches over noninteractive video (Carrol, Bain, & Houghton, 1994; Lee et al., 1996; Rubenstein, Cherry, & Small, 1993; Yoder, 1993). Videodisk studies with older adults showed that once comfortable with the technology, older adults were able to use the primary interactive features effectively (Baldi, Plude, & Schwartz, 1996; Plude & Schwartz, 1996).

Clearly, then, videotape has demonstrated learning advantages for other populations that could translate into effective learning for older adults as well. But more than that, it has particular advantages for strategy learning, especially imagery-based strategies, effective for recalling names, paired associates, and lists of concrete nouns (McDaniel & Pressley, 1987; Yuille, 1983). Although researchers have discovered many kinds of mnemonics and strategies, the majority of recommended techniques are based on mental imagery. Imaginal strategies—such as the peg system, the keyword method, the link method, the method of loci, and the image-name match method—focus learners on the semantic meaning of items, provide an interactive image link between items (Begg, 1983), and create a potential cueing system whereby one well-learned item, or a distinctive feature, can cue subsequent items in memory, through pictured connections in the mind. Experimental work also suggests that older adults can learn how to use imagery effectively to improve their memory scores (Yesavage et al., 1989).

What do the benefits of imagery have to do with video-based instruction? We would argue that video-based instruction is very valuable for teaching imagery. Mental imagery occurs inside the head. An instructor can stand before a group of trainees and role-play crisis intervention techniques; that is, the instructor can actually show them what to do. For mental imagery, role playing, while helpful, does not demonstrate the method directly. The instructor can describe an image, but an illustration of an effective mental image requires visual media. And although static two-dimensional pictures can be used as illustrations, the addition of animation should enhance the memorability of sample images, as noted earlier (Christel, 1994; Mayer & Anderson, 1992; Rieber, 1991). Furthermore, imagery is more effective when individuals utilize distinctive, elaborated, interactive mental pictures (see discussions of these issues in McDaniel & Pressley, 1987), and an animated presentation can show trainees how to make images more active and interactive. Interestingly, in a recent study in our laboratory, older adults reported substantial increases in utilization of imagery across trials when the testing materials were realistic video representations of people (for a name recall task), even when there were no instructions to utilize imagery of any kind (see West et al., 1997). It is possible that the animated video had a dynamic, realistic quality that may have encouraged the application of imagery.

Finally, videotapes can be seen at home, at relatively low cost. Cost is minimized because no instructor need be present. Videotaping permits homebound and rural older adults to obtain memory training that might not be accessible in other formats. Cost also stays low for older adults who already own VCRs. Approximately three fourths of older adults in the United States have VCRs in their home, whereas many fewer have access to the computer equipment needed for using high-technology interactive programs (Baldi et al., 1996).

Application for Cognitive Rehabilitation

What should one include in a videotaped memory program? First, extant research will be reviewed, followed by a more general list of recommendations. West and Crook (1992) created a 40-minute videotaped training program that described the general benefits of imagery, followed by detailed instruction on the use of imagery to remember names (image-name match method), lists (link method), and object locations (interactive imagery). Vivid animated examples of interactive imagery were provided as the narrator emphasized the importance of images that were active and distinctive, incorporating input from multiple senses. The trained subjects spent one week watching the video at least twice, and they were told to pause the video repeatedly and practice the trained techniques during viewing. The results indicated significant increases on all three target tasks over and above those of a control group, with 1-week maintenance of these gains. More significantly, there was some evidence for generalization to related tasks (such as face recognition), which is rarely shown in the training literature. Generalization may have occurred because the videotaped program enhanced overall learning and made generalization easier, or because the training itself emphasized generalization by illustrating how one basic technique could be applied to several tasks, or because the assessments also used a video format, which may have been a constant reminder to trainees of what they had learned.

Videodisk training, allowing for more interactive learning from a CD-ROM, was employed by Plude and his colleagues (Baldi et al., 1996; Plude & Schwartz, 1996). Their compact-disk interactive (CD-i) program presented the image-name match method for recalling names, as well as the SALT technique, which is based on frequent repetition of a name after hearing it (Plude & Schwartz, 1996). CD-i demonstrated training gains relative to a no-treatment control (Plude & Schwartz, 1996). CD-i has also been compared with a video-based training program similar to the one described above (Baldi et al., 1996). CD-i trainees showed significant gains after a pretest and one training session, but video and control participants did not. After a pretest and a posttest, the control subjects were trained and assessed again and showed gains with both video and CD-i training (Baldi et al., 1996). CD-i trainees maintained their gains on the last assessment, nearly a week after training. Trainees' memory for the strategy was better for CD-i participants than for video participants. These results suggest that the more interactive approach had greater effectiveness for older adults. Plude and his colleagues readily admitted, however, that CD-i technologies are not as accessible to older adults as VCRs, in terms of both equipment availability and personal attitudes (Baldi et al., 1996).

How should researchers proceed? Videotaped instruction could show older adults "how to" create memorable images, and they could learn in a self-paced fashion and review their training regularly. The two studies above showed that older adults improved performance after video-based or CD-i instruction but did not test potential mechanisms for change or long-term maintenance, and neither demonstrated that this particular approach was more effective than traditional instruction. The extant research with children and younger adults, reviewed above, has established the advantages of video-based presentation over traditional lecture presentations, but this research needs to be replicated with older populations. That critical research for older adults remains to be done. Future work with videotaped training needs to extend the maintenance interval to examine strategy usage and performance several weeks or months after training. In addition, as work proceeds, our conceptual understanding of the benefits of video needs to be complemented with more empirical explorations of potential strategic and nonstrategic mechanisms for change.

Researchers interested in videotape for future studies might benefit from guidelines. These recommendations are derived from several reviews of the older-adult-training literature (Dunlosky & Hertzog, 1998; Hertzog, 1992; Kotler-Cope & Camp, 1990; West, 1995; West & Tomer, 1989; Yesavage et al., 1989) as well as more recent research. For older adults, the videotaped information needs to be clear, involving step-by-step instructions for strategies. It is also important to provide evidence for the effectiveness of the techniques for older age groups. To enhance the overall impact of the program, several features of the more effective long-term training programs ought to be included: multiple strategies for the same task (emphasizing that individuals can select the one that will be most effective personally) or multiple tasks for the same strategy (showing the usefulness of the strategy, in general, and encouraging maintenance and generalization). In addition, trainees should be encouraged to work with the materials repeatedly, to master the strategies, and to monitor recall readiness and strategy effectiveness. As we discuss later in this chapter, presentation of memory and aging facts, to promote realistic, nonstereotyped views of one's potential, could be a beneficial component as well. Multifactorial approaches, including beliefs, attentional training, and/or relaxation techniques, are recommended (see Herrmann & Searleman, 1992; Stigsdotter & Bäckman, 1989, Stigsdotter Neely & Bäckman, 1993a).

Changing Memory Beliefs

A second area with high potential for success in memory rehabilitation programs is the area of memory beliefs. Many researchers recognize the importance of memory beliefs for understanding age-related memory deficits, but relatively few have carried this issue into the domain of memory intervention (see Lachman in this volume). If negative memory beliefs—low self-efficacy, feeling a lack of control, problematic attributions—have some influence on performance, then it follows that altering beliefs in a positive direction should enhance the long-term consequences of any memory intervention. Without intervening actively to change beliefs, a number of studies have measured self-reported memory to determine whether or not it varies as a function of training. Interestingly, those who have measured memory complaints or self-reported memory before and after interventions have seen a mixture of results, with memory scores improving without self-reported change in some cases (Hill, Sheikh, & Yesavage, 1988; Rebok & Balcerak, 1989; Scogin et al., 1985; Zarit, Cole, & Guider, 1981; Zarit, Gallagher, & Kramer, 1981). In other cases, self-reported memory showed improvement, whereas test scores showed mixed improvement or no change (Dittmann-Kohli, Lachman, Kliegl, & Baltes, 1991; Lachman & Dick, 1987; Lachman et al., 1992; Turner & Pinkston, 1993). In a recent meta-analysis, Floyd and Scogin (1997) examined the effectiveness of memory training on what they called "subjective memory functioning." They examined 27 studies with older adults using a wide range of assessments of subjective memory functioning. In their meta-analysis, Floyd and Scogin concluded that the effect size for subjective memory measures is considerably lower than the effect size for objective memory measures (as reported by Verhaeghen et al., 1992). They suggested that subjective memory evaluations may be more difficult to change, and/or that the interventions developed to date are not sufficiently strong. Subjective memory was improved more when participants received mnemonic training combined with "expectancy modification" (an intervention targeting the development of more adaptive attitudes toward memory).

Rationale for This Innovation

Scholars in aging approach the issue of beliefs from a variety of different perspectives (Berry & West, 1994; Cavanaugh & Green, 1990; Erber, Prager, Williams, & Caiola, 1996; Lachman, this volume). In our laboratory, efforts have focused on raising self-efficacy as the central construct in the memory beliefs system. In fact, self-efficacy theory provides a theoretical rationale for beliefs-oriented training for older adults.

Self-efficacy is the domain-specific belief that one can successfully engage in a particular activity. Its importance is manifested in the finding that efficacy translates into action: Many studies have shown that increases in self-efficacy predict future attempts at coping during a difficult task or in a formerly threatening situation (Bandura, 1986, 1997), and that self-efficacy predicts future cognitive success (e.g., Seeman, McAvay, Merrill, Albert, & Rodin, 1996). The initial testing grounds for the theory were phobia interventions, using young adults as participants (e.g., Bandura, Adams, Hardy, & Howells, 1980; Biran & Wilson, 1981; Williams, Turner, & Peer, 1985). These studies and others have shown that self-efficacy predicts coping behavior. Participants with higher self-efficacy persisted longer and increased their effort in anxiety-provoking or difficult task situations (Bandura et al., 1980; Biran & Wilson, 1981; Williams et al., 1985). Self-efficacy has been increased through inactive mastery experiences—experiences that allowed participants to see that they have mastered a feared activity (Bandura et al., 1980; Biran & Wilson, 1981; Gist et al., 1989; Williams et al., 1985; Williams & Zane, 1989). These inactive mastery experiences involved hands-on activities, not just discussions of thoughts or feelings. Mastery experiences were important for building the perception that action can lead to successful outcomes, so that the person has attributional "ownership" of successes (Bandura, 1986).

Although not yet widely applied to older adult populations, self-efficacy theory may be especially important for examining memory beliefs in older adults (Berry & West, 1994; Cavanaugh, 1996; Hultsch, Hertzog, Dixon, & Davidson, 1988; Welch & West, 1995). Real and imagined memory failures (one's own and those of age peers) associated with the aging process—compounded by prevalent negative stereotypes about memory aging—can lead older adults to believe that it is not worthwhile to expend the effort required to learn memory strategies. Older adults are less certain about their memory abilities than are younger adults (Berry, West, & Dennehy, 1989), and their lowered self-efficacy could translate into problematic behavior. For example, the inability to locate personal articles in one's home could create more anxiety in an older adult than in a younger adult, given the elder's worries about memory aging. The behavioral consequences of this anxiety might include avoidance of situations in which object locations must be recalled or a lack of perseverance during search. For instance, an older woman who frequently loses her hearing aids might experience lowered memory self-efficacy for object locations. She might subsequently terminate or fail to search for the hearing aids, despite their obvious importance to her independence and comfort. Thus, everyday functioning and independence may be impaired by a low sense of memory self-efficacy in older adults (Welch & West, 1995). Lachman (this volume) expands on these constructs and the interrelationship between different types of beliefs and memory performance.

Application for Cognitive Rehabilitation

At present, it is not known whether altering low self-evaluations and negative beliefs about memory can boost the effectiveness of memory training, although theories about efficacy and attributions suggest that it should. Previous studies that specifically attempted to provide an efficacy- or attribution-based intervention have yielded mixed findings. In our laboratory, for instance, self-efficacy showed significant positive change following memory training in two conditions, one that intended specifically to raise efficacy along with memory change, and a second that provided only strategy training (West, Bramblett, Welch, & Bellott, 1992). For the efficacy condition, the memory training included evaluation and rejection of memory-aging stereotypes, strategy training, and mastery experiences for recalling prose and grocery lists. Training emphasized the malleable nature of memory skills at any age and attempted to dispel the notion that memory is unchangeable and inevitably worsens with age. In the strategy condition, participants received strategy training and extensive practice in recalling prose and grocery lists. Both interventions led to increased self-efficacy after training and improved prose memory scores, but to no change in list recall. The improvements were maintained at a 1-month follow-up test. Interestingly, prose memory scores improved even more between posttest and follow-up, during a period when no training was given, a strong indication of maintenance of training.

Lachman and colleagues (1992) combined cognitive restructuring with memory training. The cognitive restructuring consisted of educating older adults about adaptive and maladaptive conceptions of memory. This study demonstrated pre-to-posttest increases in general memory control beliefs whether or not cognitive restructuring was a feature of training. However, Lachman et al. did find that the combined approach was the most effective in altering maladaptive conceptions of memory. Unfortunately, the combined approach did not lead to higher performance increases relative to the groups receiving cognitive restructuring or memory training only.

Best, Hamlett, and Davis (1992) compared memory training (MT) to an "expectancy change" condition (EC) in which popular negative stereotypes about aging were challenged, and they also included a no-treatment control and an art discussion group (to control for the more general benefits of group participation). A variety of measures of memory, memory beliefs, and affect were administered. Significant training effects occurred only for memory complaints and some memory tests; reduced complaints occurred for EC only, and higher scores on some tests occurred for MT only. This pattern makes sense, showing the targeted change in beliefs for EC and the targeted change in performance for MT. At the 2-week follow-up, there was strong evidence for maintenance: MT memory scores were higher on most tests, and MT and EC showed comparable levels of memory complaints (the MT complaints had decreased over the delay interval). Memory beliefs measures, however, were not correlated with performance, as hoped (Best et al., 1992; also see Zarit, Gallagher, & Kramer, 1981).

A Canadian study by Caprio-Prevette and Fry (1996) provided the strongest evidence, thus far, that changing beliefs are critical to memory change. These authors compared a cognitive restructuring approach with a memory-training approach and incorporated a variety of assessments of memory beliefs, performance, and affect (depression and anxiety). Their cognitive restructuring group (CRG) was based on cognitive behavioral principles and included the following activities: identifying and replacing irrational thoughts about memory problems with rational views, role playing of positive and negative perspectives on memory, emphasis on a learning-oriented approach (memory can be improved with effort and practice), and verbalizing of positive beliefs. A second group, identified as the traditional memory-training group (TMG), received training and skills practice for more than 10 memory techniques (this is, actually, not a traditional program because most traditional programs emphasize only 1 or 2 strategies). Significant posttest changes in memory and beliefs were apparent for CRG, and not for TMG, but there were no significant changes on the affective measures. Most CRG gains were maintained, and group differences were stronger at the 9-week follow-up assessment (Caprio-Prevette & Fry, 1996). The strength of these results may have been due to the extended time of the intervention (20 hours over 10 weeks) or to the relatively large study sample (approximately 60 per group). The authors' conclusions, like those of Best and colleagues (1992), emphasized the potential value of combining beliefs retraining with memory retraining, rather than keeping these two approaches separate.

While not definitive, this evidence is suggestive, supporting the potential value of beliefs-oriented interventions in late life. The theoretical framework and empirical results for cognitive interventions with other populations, such as phobic adults or children (e.g., Bandura & Schunk, 1981), show that an emphasis on changing beliefs (in addition to teaching strategies) results in greater change and more maintenance of intervention effects. But the limited beliefs-intervention data in the aging literature do not allow us to determine whether memory trainees must change their mindset about memory to maximally benefit from training. Objective memory improvement may occur independently of changes in memory beliefs. Nor do previous studies prove that beliefs retraining necessarily enhances training effects. At the same time, it remains possible that most previous interventions did not alter beliefs enough to effect a change in memory performance.

Keeping in mind the mixed nature of the available evidence, a recent pilot study designed by Welch and West was intended to alter self-efficacy beliefs and memory. The participants were 40 older women identified as "at risk" because they scored 1 standard deviation below their peers on a test of object location recall (the computerized Misplaced Objects Task—MOT; Crook, Youngjohn, & Larrabee, 1990) and/or self-efficacy (Spatial Self-Efficacy Questionnaire—SSEQ; Welch, West, Thorn, & Clark, 1996). A control group was compared with a training group that was offered both strategy training and efficacy retraining. The 5-week intervention program began approximately 9 months after the initial individual test session. This was the schedule for the training group: group pretest and homework (Week 1), homework (Week 2), group practice session and homework (Week 3), homework (Week 4), and group posttest (Week 5), followed by an individual posttest approximately 1 week later. An individual follow-up test took place 6 weeks after the group posttest. The homework included studying an imagery-training video and a strategy manual. The control group completed all individual assessments on the same schedule, but they received the video and manual, to complete at their own pace, after the individual posttest. By assessing beliefs, performance, and strategy usage at all test sessions, this intervention hoped to examine the mechanisms for performance change.

The group tests utilized a "board game" version of the MOT, and the individual tests utilized the computerized MOT. The training materials consisted of board game versions of the MOT that were used for practice or testing in the group sessions, an imagery videotape (see West & Crook, 1992), and a written manual describing a variety of strategies for remembering object locations, including external strategies (e.g., writing notes and using a "memory place") and internal strategies (e.g., verbal association, organization, and imagery). The manual provided examples and sample exercises for each strategy. The video and/or the manual was assigned as homework. The experimenter called each participant at home to answer questions and to ensure that the homework was completed. (Participants in a wait-list control group received the materials and assignments, without telephone follow-up, after the posttest was completed). The trainees, but not the control group, also attended one group practice session in which they practiced with the MOT board games to remember locations. As in the Canadian study described earlier (Caprio-Prevette & Fry, 1996), many different elements were incorporated into the training program to enhance efficacy: goal setting, attributional reframing, personal control, and mastery-ordered practice.

Attributional Reframing

Verbal statements were made to trained individuals during the practice session and during weekly phone calls. These statements deflected negative attributions for failure and reinforced positive attributions for success (see Lachman, this volume). One of the reasons that attributional reframing can be effective is that it emphasizes the process of learning rather than performance outcome (Elliott & Lachman, 1989). When the goal is learning, rather than success per se, anxiety is reduced, and participants are more likely to utilize learned strategies after the completion of training.

Goal Setting

Both experimenters and participants set goals. The experimenter set a goal for participants to complete at least eight exercises during the group practice session. The participants set goals for the number of times they would watch the video, read the chapter, and/or do homework exercises. The setting of reachable, concrete goals has been shown to enhance self-efficacy in children (Schunk, 1985; Schunk & Rice, 1989). When participants reach a goal, they may appropriately infer that they are on their way to task mastery.

Personal Control

The importance of control is explained in the Lachman chapter (this volume). In this research, training-group participants chose how often to watch the video, read the manual, and do the exercises. The manual also enhanced self-efficacy by placing control for strategy selection in the participants' hands. A wide variety of alternative techniques were explained in the manual, and training-group members were encouraged to choose which strategy to use, if any. If they chose to do so, they could avoid using interactive imagery or other strategies high in processing-resources demands. In the practice session, individuals also controlled their own pace and difficulty of the exercises.

Mastery Order

In group sessions for trainees, the practice exercises were structured so that easy tasks were completed first, followed by increasingly difficult tasks (referred to here as "mastery order" of task presentation). Mastery order allows participants to readily see that they are mastering increasingly difficult tasks, and to infer that their skills are improving. Trainees worked at their own pace and decided, on their own, when they had mastered a given level of the task.

Based on self-efficacy theory, it was expected that both self-efficacy and memory performance would show increases in the training group. The reason is that efficacy-based interventions have been shown, in other domains and with other populations, to increase efficacy as well as performance. The control group was not expected to show significant performance improvements until the follow-up test. The results were encouraging, although with a small-N pilot study the findings were not definitive. The trainees showed greater changes in self-efficacy and significant changes in strategy usage (especially increased use of imaginal strategies) that were not apparent in the control group. Surprisingly, both the control and the training groups showed significant improvements in performance from pretest to posttest and maintained these gains at follow-up (after the control group had received the manual and video). These results may shed some light on mechanisms. In this case, the changes in strategy use by the trained group did not result in greater performance change in that group, a finding indicating that strategy increases were not the reason for performance change. Rather, practice effects explained performance change. Interestingly, there is considerable evidence in the child literature concerning strategy utilization deficiencies (SUDs) that may be relevant here (Bjorklund, Miller, Coyle, & Slawinski, 1997). SUDs occur when people spontaneously produce a strategy but do not benefit from it because strategy use, by itself, taxes working memory, and/or because the strategies are not fully mastered. This finding suggests that our "at-risk" trained group needed more practice with high-difficulty location recall exercises (they received only one practice session, with self-paced learning). At the same time, the greater efficacy increases for trainees indicated that we succeeded in making the trainees feel better about themselves—probably because they were accomplishing some of their goals, by learning and utilizing new strategies. Future work should continue to delve into strategies and beliefs in relation to rehabilitation outcomes.

Nondidactic Interventions: The Study Group Methodology

Another potentially valuable approach is based on the notion that learning, especially for older adults, may be more lasting when it is presented in a nondidactic, study group format. With this methodology, each person invests or contributes to her or his own learning, as well as the learning of others in the group. This approach should, theoretically, lead to a greater positive self-evaluation after training because of individuals' greater involvement in their own learning. Study group formats provide for learning at the pace of the older person, a feature that may aid older trainees. Trainees can ask questions or lead discussions that provide for restatement and review of any information that is unclear. Training might be more effective if a particular mnemonic strategy is "advertised" by a same-age peer, who reports successfully using the new technique, rather than by a younger experimenter, especially if older participants have doubts about their potential as learners. This approach, therefore, could obviate the impact of working-memory deficits, slower learning requirements, or negative self-evaluations characteristic of older adults that could limit learning from didactic formats. Although the study group approach has created a great deal of interest in educational circles, its effectiveness has not been examined for memory intervention.

Rationale for This Innovation

An extensive body of literature coming from the field of educational gerontology suggests that group discussions with same-age peers are conducive to learning (e.g., Chene, 1994; Clough, 1992). Group discussions foster the sharing of personal experience and make learning more meaningful. For instance, Chene interviewed 28 older adults who were involved in group learning activities to find out their reason for joining these activities. The participants reportedly attached value to being with peers in a learning context. For them, the group made learning more fulfilling (Chene, 1994). Chene concluded that older learners seek recognition beyond that provided by friends and family. They join groups where affinity is found and prefer homogeneous groups that offer opportunities for self-confirmation.

Group discussion is used extensively for adult learning in Sweden. Study circles are the main form of adult education (one out of three adults participates in a study circle every year). Discussions are democratic and draw on participants' experiences. Study circles encourage learning through the exchange of ideas, critical thinking, and the application of knowledge to everyday life. Participants learn to speak and listen, a process that leads to increased self-worth and confidence (Kurland, 1982; Oliver, 1987). In the United States, study circles have been used since 1981 by the National Issues Forum (sponsored by the Kettering Foundation) to promote the discussion of public issues (Oliver, 1990).

The American equivalent of this learning format may also be found in many Elderhostel classes. Studies with Elderhostel participants have shown that seniors feel quite favorable to learning through discussions, and to learning from and with peers (Buchanan, 1988; Kaplan, 1981; Mills, 1993). Elderhostel classes (study-travel programs for seniors) are age-segregated, and group discussion is the main learning format. In the Elderhostel context, education specialists (Mills, 1993) have suggested that discussions with peers lead to increased self-discovery, self-confidence, and effective learning.

Although there is no direct evidence on the advantage of study group formats over traditional teaching in a memory intervention, scholars in the cognitive aging field have provided some evidence that group discussion may be a promising learning format for older adults. In a chapter on cooperative learning, Millis, Davidson, and Cottell (1994) stated that comprehension is enhanced by sharing ideas and responding to others. According to Millis and associates, cooperative learning leads to higher levels of achievement as well as to higher motivation to learn. Thompson (1992) also suggested that methods involving social interaction are most advantageous to older learners. In an experimental study, Zandri and Charness (1989) trained younger and older adults to use computers and found that small-group training was more effective than individual training. Participants working in pairs received half the hands-on training obtained by those who were given individual training; however, partnered participants achieved equal or higher test scores. Zandri and Charness (1989) reported that the small-group context provided opportunity for group problem solving and social reinforcement, which led to increased learning.

In the domain of memory, Flynn and Storandt (1990) examined the importance of group discussions for memory training with older adults. They compared the effectiveness of self-instructional "bibliotherapy" memory training (participants worked with a manual for 16 hours at home), supplemented by group discussions, to bibliotherapy by itself. The supplemental group discussions covered topics such as concerns about aging, ideas for coping with the aging process, and relaxation, as well as the materials in the manual. The group participating in discussion sessions showed significant memory improvement on two recall tasks, whereas the bibliotherapy group did not improve on any of the measures. Although the training gains were modest, these results suggested that memory training involving group interaction may be more effective than bibliotherapy alone.

The Caprio-Prevette and Fry (1996) study described earlier also contained many elements of the study circle approach. The cognitive restructuring group was involved in

> small group activity, role playing, index card prompts, and oral point-counterpoint (i.e., verbalizing, between two participants, positive responses in place of negative statements). Participants were encouraged to discuss their views on memory as related to aging and they received feedback from the trainer and other participants. (Caprio-Prevette & Fry, 1996, p. 287)

As indicated earlier, this approach was highly effective in changing memory performance and memory beliefs. It should be noted, however, that these authors reported using a similar small-group approach for their traditional memory-training group, which did not show much change. It is clear, however, that the traditional group must have involved considerable didactic instruction, given that more than 10 memory strategies were presented (Caprio-Prevette & Fry, 1996).

Thus, both theoretical and limited empirical evidence supports the view that group discussion is an appropriate format for learning in later life. At the same time, there is little or no evidence that the group discussion format is more effective than traditional teaching formats for older adults. Memory "classes" utilizing group training have typically offered only the didactic approach for strategy training.

Application for Cognitive Rehabilitation

In light of the limited evidence for the effectiveness of the method, a nondidactic study-circle approach was employed in a memory-training program developed in 1997 by Yassuda and West. The goal was to demonstrate that this kind of intervention methodology could lead to significant training effects, relative to a control group. The program compared (a) a waiting-list control group, (b) a mnemonic training group (with placebo pretraining), and (c) a beliefs pretraining group that received informational pretraining about memory and aging as well as mnemonic training. We expected the guided-group-discussion format to promote positive views about memory in later life in the beliefs group, and to lead to mastery and 1-month maintenance of the trained mnemonic techniques. Although the data collection for this research has just been completed, and few results are available, a detailed description of the training program can serve as an example of the study group format. The primary hypothesis of this research was that teaching older adults about memory and aging in a study group would reduce stereotypical memory beliefs and raise memory self-efficacy. Thus, this program combined beliefs retraining (already discussed in detail) with group learning. There were no explicit comparisons of didactic and nondidactic approaches in this research. Instead, the beliefs-pretraining condition, combined with strategy training, was compared to a placebo-pretraining condition combined with strategy training, and both were compared to a wait-list control condition. The study circle approach was utilized for pretraining and strategy training in all conditions so that we could determine whether the study circle approach would be effective for memory rehabilitation for older adults.

Participants in the placebo-pretraining condition had two pretraining sessions focused on grandparenting and driving (presented as "getting-to-know-you" sessions), whereas the beliefs-pretraining sessions explored the memory system, aspects of memory that change and do not change with age, and factors other than age that affect memory, such as depression, medications, and nutrition. Subsequently, both groups had three sessions of strategy training in which they practiced active observation (an attentional intervention), the Preview-Question-Read-Summarize-Test (PQRST method for prose recall, and the name sentence method for remembering names (West, 1985). The control group had no pretraining or strategy training until after the third test session, but all groups completed assessments on the same schedule—before and after pretraining, after strategy training, and at 1-month follow-up. The assessments evaluated memory beliefs, knowledge about memory, strategy utilization, and memory test performance on four tasks, two of which were targeted by training (name recall and prose recall).

The pretraining and strategy sessions were structured in such a way that the information was elicited from participants, rather than presented in lecture. All participants had reading assignments on the session topics (Fogler & Stern, 1994; West, 1985) and knew, in advance, that they would be involved in group discussion. To encourage participants to read and deeply process the information, the homework assignment sheet included questions and indicated to participants that they were going to discuss the answers with peers. The objective was to make participants accountable for the reading. At the beginning of each session, trainees were asked to outline their answers to the preassigned questions and to discuss them with a partner. This method tends to prevent group contamination by opinions contrary to the readings (see Boninger, Brock, Cook, & Gruder, 1990)—in this case, to discourage individual statements that might reinforce age stereotypes about memory.

The experimenter followed a predetermined script, which included a list of session topics. In the first beliefs-pretraining session, for example, trainees needed to learn about the memory system. The experimenter elicited the information from the homework by asking:

> "In your readings you read about the three stages of memory. What are they? Does anyone remember?"

After someone volunteered an answer, the experimenter continued asking questions such as:

> "How long does information stay in sensory, short-term, and long-term memory? Can anyone give me an example of a situation when information is kept in short-term memory and is soon discarded? When the McDonald's clerk tells you the price of your meal, in what memory store do you keep that information?"

When exploring age-related memory changes, the experimenter probed:

> "So you have read about some things that seem to change in memory as we get older. Does anyone remember some of the things that change with age? Have you noticed any of these changes?"

Trainees would volunteer:

> "Well, I have learned that I can't remember it all. I have to choose the things that are most important to me and pay close attention to those."

Another trainee would react to that idea:

> "I think attention is the most important thing for a good memory, and it is our biggest problem. Many times we just don't pay enough attention. That is why we can't remember things."

The experimenter would then help the group to expand productively on this point:

> "So what have you learned about attention and aging in the reading? Is it easier or more difficult for us to focus our full attention as we get older?"

When a topic had been fully explored, the experimenter would summarize:

> "So we have learned that it is very important to avoid distractions when we are learning something new. It is critical to make a conscious effort to pay close attention to the things that we may want to remember later."

After summarizing, the experiment moved to another topic:

> "What else changes as we get older?"

If no one volunteered an answer, the experimenter continued questioning, providing more specific guidance in the question, to lead the trainees to the answers they knew from their reading:

> "How about remembering names and words on demand? Has anyone been in a situation when you knew someone's name but just could not remember it on the spot? What is happening in the memory system when that happens?"

The discussion continued for approximately 2 hours per session until all preassigned topics for that session had been explored. Although the topics were different, the same methodology was used for the placebo discussion sessions on grandparenting and driving, to ensure that the group experience was comparable for these two conditions. It was expected that the questions assessing knowledge about memory would show more accurate responses for those individuals who had beliefs pretraining than for those in the placebo-pretraining or control conditions. Initial analyses indicated that the beliefs group did have more knowledge about memory at the first posttest but that all groups had gained in knowledge by the time of the delayed follow-up, after all groups had obtained training.

Study circles were also used for strategy training. Instead of lecturing about the mnemonic techniques, the experimenter elicited the information from participants who had already read assigned strategy materials. For example, when participants reviewed the name sentence method, they were encouraged to create short sentences to remember each others' names. Participants suggested some possibilities; the group elaborated on them and then reached consensus on the best sentence for a particular name. All participants (with rare exceptions) reported doing the homework reading, and the sessions were quite lively. The reading materials were brought to life when trainees volunteered examples and personal anecdotes.

In sum, current literature suggests that study circle or group learning approaches are appropriate and often successful for older adults, and that older adults subjectively enjoy group learning. A detailed example of the methodology was provided. It is important to recognize, however, that there are no known tests examining the power of this approach, as compared to didactic memory training, with older adults. The potential is clearly there, but empirical evidence is necessary to establish the objective benefits of this type of intervention format.

Conclusions

This chapter has presented three possible approaches to memory rehabilitation for older adults that have not been sufficiently tested, even though all three hold great promise for helping older adults to reverse some memory deficits and maintain memory ability as they age. In each case, we provided a rationale for the value of the methodology, as well as at least one example of the method, although sometimes without empirical results. By presenting each of these possible techniques separately—videotape, self-efficacy enhancement, and nondidactic study groups—we did not intend to suggest that they must always be used separately. In fact, both of the current studies presented in detail here have employed more than one innovation: The Welch project has combined the use of videotape with an intervention focused on enhanced efficacy and mastery, and the Yassuda project has focused on changing beliefs, at the same time testing the effectiveness of a nondidactic group-study intervention. Both studies have measured strategy usage and short-term maintenance. Thus, both studies have simultaneously built on the intervention ideas discussed here while trying to address some of the limitations of earlier research.

As researchers begin to examine these and other innovations, tests of the impact of combinations of techniques may have heuristic value. Herrmann and Searleman (1992) recommended multifactorial training that takes into account a wider variety of factors that influence memory "by optimizing the psychological and physiological systems in which the memory system itself is embedded" (p. 13). Thus, an intervention that is multifactorial should take into account as many processes as possible that could impact successful memory: emotional state (general anxiety or depression, specific memory fears), attitudes or beliefs (self-efficacy, control, stereotyping with respect to age decline), social context (social needs that enhance or impede memory ability), sensory-perceptual processing (wearing glasses and hearing aid, focusing attention), and physiological state (rest, good nutrition, cardiovascular function). Researchers who have already developed successful memory intervention methodologies may find that the addition of videotapes, self-efficacy manipulations, or nondidactic discussions enhances training impact or maintenance of newly learned skills. Recent comparisons of a multifactorial approach (strategy training, attentional retraining, and relaxation) with strategy training or "cognitive activation" by itself showed greater effects and better maintenance after multifactorial training (Stigsdotter & Bäckman, 1989; Stigsdotter Neely & Bäckman, 1993a).

Scholars of memory training and aging have left a number of questions partially answered or unanswered. What is the impact of training over and above the effects of practice alone? Can training effects (performance improvement and/or strategic processing changes) be maintained over long intervals of time? What are the mechanisms for memory improvement? As we move in new directions, testing out new approaches and combining approaches to offer multifactorial interventions, these questions should not continue to be ignored. Whatever innovative directions are taken in terms of offering new types of training, it behooves us as scholars to become more sophisticated about examining these critical issues.

References

Anschutz, L., Camp, C., Markley, R. P., & Kramer, J. J. (1987). Remembering mnemonics: A three-year followup on the effects of mnemonics training in elderly adults. *Experimental Aging Research, 13,* 141–144.

Ayersman, D. J., & von Minden, A. (1995). Individual differences, computers, and instruction. *Computers in Human Behavior, 11,* 371–390.

Baldi, R., Plude, D. J., & Schwartz, L. (1996). New technologies for memory training with older adults. *Cognitive Technology, 1,* 25–35.

Bandura, A. (1986). Self-efficacy. In A. Bandura (Ed.), *Social foundations of thought and action: A social cognitive theory* (pp. 390–453). Englewood Cliffs, NJ: Prentice-Hall.

Bandura, A. (1997). *Self-efficacy: The exercise of control.* New York: W. H. Freeman.

Bandura, A., Adams, N. E., Hardy, A. B., & Howells, G. N. (1980). Tests of the generality of self-efficacy theory. *Cognitive Therapy and Research, 4,* 39–66.

Bandura, A., & Schunk, D. H. (1981). Cultivating confidence, self-efficacy, and intrinsic interest through proximal self-motivation. *Journal of Personality and Social Psychology, 41,* 586–598.

Banyan, C. D., & Stein, D. M. (1990). Voice synthesis supplement to a computerized interviewing training program: Retention effects. *Teaching of Psychology, 17,* 260–263.

Bashman, J. G., & Treadwell, T. W. (1995). Assessing the effectiveness of a psychodrama training video. *Journal of Group Psychotherapy, Psychodrama and Sociometry, 48,* 61–68.

Begg, I. (1983). Imagery instructions and the organization of memory. In J. C. Yuille (Ed.), *Imagery, memory, and cognition: Essays in honor of Allan Paivio* (pp. 91–115). Hillsdale, NJ: Erlbaum.

Berry, J. M., & West, R. L. (1994). Cognitive self-efficacy in relation to mastery and goal setting across the life span. In M. E. Lachman (Ed.), *The development of planning and control processes across the life span.* Hillsdale, NJ: Erlbaum.

Berry, J. M., West, R. L., & Dennehy, D. M. (1989). Reliability and validity of the self-efficacy questionnaire. *Developmental Psychology,, 25,* 701–713.

Best, D. L., Hamlett, K. W., & Davis, S. W. (1992). Memory complaint and memory performance in the elderly: The effects of memory-skills training and expectancy change. *Applied Cognitive Psychology, 6,* 405–416.

Biran, M., & Wilson, T. G. (1981). Treatment of phobic disorders using cognitive and exposure methods: A self-efficacy analysis. *Journal of Consulting and Clinical Psychology, 49,* 886–899.

Bjorklund, D. F., Miller, P. H., Coyle, T. R., & Slawinski, J. L. (1997). Instructing children to use memory strategies: Evidence of utilization deficiencies in memory training studies. *Developmental Review, 17,* 411–441.

Boninger, D. S., Brock, T. C., Cook, T. D., & Gruder, C. L. (1990). Discovery of reliable attitude change persistence resulting from a transmitter tuning set. *Psychological Science, 1,* 268–271.

Buchanan, A. (1988). An emerging new group on the campus. *Lifelong Learning, 11*(5), 4–6.

Caprio-Prevette, M. D., & Fry, P. S. (1996). Memory enhancement program for community-based older adults: Development and evaluation. *Experimental Aging Research, 22,* 281–304.

Carrol, A., Bain, A., & Houghton, S. (1994). The effects of interactive versus linear video on the levels of attention and comprehension of social behavior by children with attention disorders. *School Psychology Review, 23,* 29–43.

Cavanaugh, J. C. (1996). Memory self-efficacy as a moderator of memory change. In F. Blanchard-Fields & T. M. Hess (Eds.), *Perspectives on cognitive change in adulthood and aging* (pp. 488–507). New York: McGraw-Hill.

Cavanaugh, J. C., & Green, E. E. (1990). I believe, therefore I can: Self-efficacy beliefs in memory aging. In E. A. Lovelace (Ed.), *Aging and cognition: Mental processes, self-awareness and interventions* (pp. 189–230). Amsterdam: North-Holland.

Chene, A. (1994). Community based older learners: Being with others. *Educational Gerontology, 20,* 765–781.

Christel, M. G. (1994). The role of visual fidelity in computer-based instruction. *Human-Computer Interaction, 9,* 183–22.

Clough, B. S. (1992). Broadening perspectives on learning activities in later life. *Educational Gerontology, 18,* 447–459.

Craik, F. I. M. (1986). A functional account of age differences in memory. In F. Klix & H. Hagendorf (Eds.), *Human memory and cognitive capabilities, mechanisms, and performance* (pp. 409–422). Amesterdam: Elsevier Science.

Crook, T. H., Youngjohn, J. R., & Larrabee, G. J. (1990). The Misplaced Objects Test: A measure of everyday visual memory. *Journal of Clinical and Experimental Neuropsychology, 12,* 819–833.

Dittmann-Kohli, F., Lachman, M. E., Kliegl, R., & Baltes, P. B. (1991). Effects of cognitive training and testing on intellectual efficacy beliefs in elderly adults. *Journal of Gerontology: Psychological Sciences, 46,* P162–P164.

Dowrick, P. W., & Raeburn, J. M. (1995). Self-modeling: Rapid skill training for children with physical disabilities. *Journal of Developmental and Physical Disabilities, 7,* 25–37.

Dunlosky, J., & Hertzog, C. (1998). Training programs to improve learning in later adulthood: Helping older adults educate themselves. In D. J. Hacker, J. Dunlosky, & A. C. Graesser (Eds.), *Metacognition in educational theory and practice* (pp. 249–276). Mahwah, NJ: Erlbaum.

Elliott, E., & Lachman, M. E. (1989). Enhancing memory by modifying control beliefs, attributions, and performance goals in the elderly. In P. S. Fry (Ed.), *Psychological perspectives of helplessness and control in the elderly* (pp. 339–367). Amsterdam: Elsevier Science.

Erber, J. T., Prager, I. G., Williams, M., & Caiola, M. A. (1996). Age and forgetfulness: Confidence in ability and attribution for memory failures. *Psychology and Aging, 11,* 310–315.

Fitzgerald, G. (1995). The effects of an interactive videodisc training program. *Computers in Human Behavior, 11,* 459–480.

Floyd, M., & Scogin, F. (1997). Effects of memory training on the subjective memory functioning and mental health of older adults: A meta-analysis. *Psychology and Aging, 12*(1), 150–161.

Flynn, T. M., & Storandt, M. (1990). Supplemental group discussions in memory training for older adults. *Psychology and Aging, 5,*(2) 178–181.

Fogler, J., & Stern, L. (1994). *Improving your memory: How to remember what you're starting to forget.* Baltimore: Johns Hopkins University Press.

Follette, W. C., & Callaghan, G. M. (1995). Do as I do, not as I say: A behavior-analytic approach to supervision. *Professional Psychology Research and Practice, 26,* 413–421.

Gehring, R. E., & Toglia, M. P. (1988). Relative retention of verbal and audiovisual information in a national training programme. *Applied Cognitive Psychology, 2,* 213–221.

Gist, M. E., Rosen, B., & Schwoerer, C. (1988). The influence of training method and trainee age on the acquisition of computer skills. *Personnel Psychology, 41,* 255–265.

Gist, M. E., Schwoerer, C., & Rosen, B. (1989). Effects of alternative training methods on self-efficacy and performance in computer software training. *Journal of Applied Psychology, 74,* 884–891.

Henry, M. J. (1995). Remedial math students' navigation patterns through hypermedia software. *Computers in Human Behavior, 11,* 481–493.

Herrmann, D., & Searleman, A. (1992). Memory improvement and memory theory in historical perspective. In D. J. Herrmann, H. Weingartner, A. Searleman, & C. McEvoy (Eds.), *Memory improvement: Implications for memory theory* (pp. 8–20). New York: Springer-Verlag.

Hertzog, C. (1992). Improving memory: The possible roles of metamemory. In D. J. Herrmann, H. Weingartner, A. Searleman, & C. McEvoy (Eds.), *Memory improvement: Implications for memory theory* (pp. 61–78). New York: Springer-Verlag.

Hill, R. D., Sheikh, J. I., & Yesavage, J. A. (1988). Pretraining enhances mnemonic training in elderly adults. *Experimental Aging Research, 14,* 207–211.

Holaday, M., & Smith, A. (1995). Coping skills training: Evaluating a training model. *Journal of Mental Health Counseling, 17,* 360–367.

Hulicka, I. M., & Grossman, J. L. (1967). Age group comparisons for the use of mediators in paired-associate learning. *Journal of Gerontology, 22,* 46–51.

Hultsch, D. F., Hertzog, C., Dixon, R. A., & Davidson, H. (1988). Memory self-knowledge and self-efficacy in the aged. In M. L. Howe & C. J. Brainerd (Eds.), *Cognitive development in adulthood* (pp. 65–92). New York: Springer-Verlag.

Juhnke, G. A. (1994). Teaching suicide risk assessment to counselor education students. *Counselor Education and Supervision, 34,* 53–57.

Kaplan, M. (1981). Elderhostel: Using a lifetime of learning and experience. *Change, 13*(1), 38–41.

Kausler, D. H. (1991). *Experimental psychology, cognition, and human aging* (2nd ed.) New York: Springer-Verlag.

Kliegl, R., Smith, J., & Baltes, P. B. (1989). Testing-the-limits and the study of adult age differences in cognitive plasticity of a mnemonic skill. *Developmental Psychology, 25,* 247–256.

Kotler-Cope, S., & Camp, C. J. (1990). Memory interventions in aging populations. In E. A. Lovelace (Ed.), *Aging and cognition: Mental processes, self-awareness and interventions* (pp. 231–261). Amsterdam: Elsevier Science.

Kurland, N. D. (1982, February). The Scandinavian study circle: An idea for the US. *Lifelong Learning: The Adult Years,* pp. 25–27, 30.

Lachman, M. E., & Dick, L. (1987). *Does memory training influence self-conceptions of memory aging?* Paper presented at the Gerontological Society of America, Washington, DC.

Lachman, M. E., Weaver, S. L., Bandura, M., Elliott, E., & Lewkowicz, C. J. (1992). Improving memory and control beliefs through cognitive restructuring and self-generated strategies. *Journal of Gerontology, 47*(5), P293–299.

Lee, A. Y., Gillan, D. J., & Harrison, C. L. (1996). Assessing the effectiveness of a multimedia-based lab for upper division psychology students. *Behavior Research Methods, Instruments, and Computers, 28,* 295–299.

Le Grice, B., & Blampied, N. M. (1994). Training pupils with intellectual disability to operate educational technology using video prompting. *Education and Training in Mental Retardation and Developmental Disabilities, 29,* 321–330.

Mayer, R. E. (1989). Models for understanding. *Review of Educational Research, 59,* 43–64.

Mayer, R. E., & Anderson, R. B. (1992). The instructive animation: Helping students build connections between words and pictures in multimedia learning. *Journal of Educational Psychology, 84,* 444–452.

McDaniel, M. A., & Pressley, M. (1987). *Imagery and related mnemonic processes.* New York: Springer-Verlag.

McEvoy, C. L. (1992). Memory improvement in context: Implications for the development of memory improvement theory. In D. J. Herrmann, H. Weingartner, A. Searleman, & C. McEvoy (Eds.), *Memory improvement: Implications for memory theory* (pp. 210–231). New York: Springer-Verlag.

Millis, B., Davidson, N., & Cottell, P. (1994). Enhancing adult critical thinking skills through cooperative learning. In J. D. Sinnott (Ed.), *Interdisciplinary handbook of adult lifespan learning* (pp. 270–282). Westport, CT: Greenwood Press.

Mills, E. S. (1993). *The story of elderhostel.* Hanover, NH: University Press of New England.

Murphy, M. D., Schmitt, F. A., Caruso, M. J., & Sanders, R. E. (1987). Metamemory in older adults: The role of monitoring in serial recall. *Psychology and Aging, 2,* 331–339.

Neef, N. A., Trachtenberg, S., Loeb, J., & Sterner, K. (1991). A video-based training of respite care providers: An interactional analysis of presentation format. *Journal of Applied Behavior Analysis, 24,* 473–486.

Oliver, L. P. (1987). *To understand is to act: Study circles.* Cabin John, MD: Seven Locks Press.

Oliver, L. P. (1990). Study circles: New life for an old idea. *Adult Learning, 2*(3), 20–23.

Paivio, A. (1986). *Mental representations: A dual coding approach.* New York: Oxford University Press.

Plude, D. J., & Schwartz, L. K. (1996). Compact disc-interactive memory training with the elderly. *Educational Gerontology, 22,* 507–521.

Rankin, J. L., Karol, R., & Tuten, C. (1984). Strategy use, recall, and recall organization in young, middle-aged, and elderly adults. *Experimental Aging Research, 10,* 193–196.

Rebok, G. W., & Balcerak, L. J. (1989) Memory self-efficacy and performance differences in young and old adults: The effect of mnemonic training. *Developmental Psychology, 25,* 714–721.

Riding, R., Buckle, C., Thompson, S., & Hagger, E. (1989). The computer determination of learning styles as an aid to individualized computer-based training. *Educational and Training Technology International, 26,* 393–398.

Rieber, L. P. (1990). Using computer animated graphics in science instruction with children. *Journal of Educational Psychology, 82,* 135–140.

Rieber, L. P. (1991). Effects of visual grouping strategies of computer-animated presentations on selective attention in science. *Educational Technology Research and Development, 39,* 5–15.

Rubinstein, A., Cherry, R., & Small, S. (1993). Effect of interactive video versus noninteractive video training on speech recognition by hearing-impaired adults. *Volta Review, 95,* 135–141.

Rusted, J., & Hodgson, S. (1985). Evaluating the picture facilitation effect in children's recall of written texts. *British Journal of Educational Psychology, 55,* 288–294.

Salthouse, T. A. (1990). Working memory as a processing resource in cognitive aging. *Developmental Review, 10,* 101–124.

Sanders, R. E., Murphy, M. D., Schmitt, F. A., & Walsh, K. K. (1980). Age differences in free recall rehearsal strategies. *Journal of Gerontology, 35,* 550–558.

Schmitt, F. A., Murphy, M. D., & Sanders, R. E. (1981). Training older adult free recall rehearsal strategies. *Journal of Gerontology, 36,* 329–337.

Schunk, D. H. (1985). Enhancing self-efficacy and achievement through rewards and goals: Motivational and informational effects. *Journal of Educational Research, 78,* 29–34.

Schunk, D. H., & Rice, M. J. (1989). Learning goals and children's reading comprehension. *Journal of Reading Behavior, 21,* 279–293.

Scogin, F., Storandt, M., & Lott, L. (1985). Memory-skills training, memory complaints, and depression in older adults. *Journal of Gerontology, 40,* 562–568.

Seabury, B. A. (1993). Interactive video programs: Crisis counseling and organizational assessment. *Computers in Human Services, 9,* 301–310.

Seeman, T., McAvay, G., Merrill, S., Albert, M., & Rodin, J. (1996). Self-efficacy beliefs and change in cognitive performance: MacArthur studies of successful aging. *Psychology and Aging, 11,* 538–551.

Seymour, G. O., Stahl, J. M., Levine, S. L., & Ingram, J. L. (1994). Modifying law enforcement training simulators for use in basic research. *Behavior Research Methods, Instruments, and Computers, 26,* 266–268.

Sheikh, J. I., Hill, R. D., & Yesavage, J. A. (1986). Long-term efficacy of cognitive training for age-associated memory impairment: A six-month follow-up study. *Developmental Neuropsychology, 2,* 413–421.

Sinnott, J. D. (Ed.). (1994). *Interdisciplinary handbook of adult lifespan learning.* Westport, CT: Greenwood Press.

Slotnick, R. S. (1990). Academic computing in psychology: Trends and issues. *Social Science Computer Review, 8,* 558–591.

Stigsdotter, A., & Bäckman, L. (1989). Multifactorial memory training with older adults: How to foster maintenance of improved performance. *Gerontology, 35,* 260–267.

Stigsdotter Neely, A. S., & Bäckman, L. (1993a). Maintenance of gains following multifactorial and unifactorial memory training in late adulthood. *Educational Gerontology, 19,* 105–117.

Stigsdotter Neely, A., & Bäckman, L. (1993b). Long-term maintenance of gains from memory training in older adults: Two 3 1/2 year followup studies. *Journal of Gerontology, 48,* 233–37.

Thompson, D. N. (1992). Applications of psychological research for the instruction of elderly adults. In R. L. West & J. D. Sinnott (Eds.), *Everyday memory and aging* (pp. 173–181). New York: Springer-Verlag.

Tiong, S. J., Blampied, N. M., & Le Grice, B. (1992). Training community-living, intellectually handicapped people in fire safety using video prompting. *Behaviour Change, 9,* 65–72.

Treat, N. J., Poon, L. W., & Fozard, J. L. (1981). Age, imagery, and practice in paired associate learning. *Experimental Aging Research, 7,* 337–342.

Turner, M., & Pinkston, R. (1993). Effects of a memory and aging workshop on negative beliefs of memory loss in the elderly. *Educational Gerontology, 19,* 359–373.

Verhaeghen, P., & Marcoen, A. (1996). On the mechanisms of plasticity in young and older adults after instruction in the method of loci: Evidence for an amplification model. *Psychology and Aging, 11,* 164–178.

Verhaeghen, P., Marcoen, A., & Goossens, L. (1992). Improving memory performance in the aged through mnemonic training: A meta-analytic study. *Psychology and Aging, 7(2),* 242–251.

Weiner, A., Kuppermintz, H., & Guttmann, D. (1994). Video home training (the Orion project): A short-term preventive and treatment intervention for families with young children. *Family Process, 33,* 441–453.

Welch, D. C., & West, R. L. (1995). Self-efficacy and mastery: Its application to issues of environmental control, cognition, and aging. *Developmental Review, 15,* 150–171.

Welch, D. C., West, R. L., Thorn, R. M., & Clark, N. P. (1996, April). *Self-efficacy, gender, and aging: Spatial self-efficacy in relation to location recall.* Paper presented at the meeting of the Cognitive Aging Conference, Atlanta.

West, R. L. (1985). *Memory fitness over 40.* Gainesville, FL: Triad.

West, R. L. (1995). Compensatory strategies for age-associated memory impairment. In A. D. Baddeley, B. A. Wilson, & F. N. Watts (Eds.), *Handbook of memory disorders* (pp. 481–500). New York: Wiley.

West, R. L., Bramblett, J. P., Welch, D. C., & Bellott, B. (1992, April). *Memory training for the elderly: An intervention designed to improve memory skills and memory self-evaluation.* Paper presented at the meeting of the Cognitive Aging Conference, Atlanta.

West, R. L., & Crook, T. H. (1992). Video training of imagery for mature adults. *Applied Cognitive Psychology, 6,* 307–320.

West, R. L., & Tomer, A. (1989). Everyday memory problems of healthy older adults: Characteristics of a successful intervention. In G. C. Gilmore, P. J. Whitehouse, & M. L. Wykle (Eds.), *Memory, aging, and dementia: Theory, assessment, and treatment* (pp. 74–98). New York: Springer.

West, R. L., Yassuda, M. S., & Welch, D. C. (1997). Imagery training via videotape: Progress and potential for older adults. *Cognitive Technology, 2,* 16–21.

Williams, S. L., Turner, S. M., & Peer, D. F. (1985). Guided mastery and performance desensitization treatments for severe acrophobia. *Journal of Consulting and Clinical Psychology, 53,* 237–247.

Williams, S. L., & Zane, G. (1989). Guided mastery and stimulus exposure treatments for severe performance anxiety in agoraphobics. *Behavior Research and Therapy, 27,* 237–245.

Wood, L. E., & Pratt, J. D. (1987). Pegword mnemonic as an aid to memory in the elderly: A comparison of four age groups. *Educational Gerontology, 13,* 325–339.

Yesavage, J. A., Lapp, D., & Sheikh, J. I. (1989). Mnemonics as modified for use by the elderly. In L. W. Poon, D. Rubin, & B. Wilson (Eds.), *Everyday cognition in adulthood and late life* (pp. 598–614). Cambridge: Cambridge University Press.

Yesavage, J. A., Sheikh, J., Tanke, E. D., & Hill, R. (1988). Response to memory training and individual differences in verbal intelligence and state anxiety. *American Journal of Psychiatry, 145,* 636–639.

Yoder, M. E. (1993). Transfer of cognitive learning to a clinical skill: Linear versus interactive video. *Western Journal of Nursing Research, 15,* 115–117.

Yuille, J. C. (Ed.). (1983). *Imagery, memory, and cognition: Essays in honor of Allan Paivio.* Hillsdale, NJ: Erlbaum.

Zandri, E., & Charness, N. (1989). Training older and younger adults to use software. *Educational Gerontology, 15,* 615–631.

Zarit, S. H., Cole, K. D., & Guider, R. L. (1981). Memory training strategies and subjective complaints of memory in the aged. *Gerontologist, 21,* 158–164.

Zarit, S. H., Gallagher, D., & Kramer, N. (1981). Memory training in the community aged: Effects on depression, memory complaint, and memory performance. *Educational Gerontology, 6,* 11–27.

6

Promoting a Sense of Control Over Memory Aging

MARGIE E. LACHMAN

The goal of this chapter is to present a rationale and framework for targeting beliefs about self-efficacy and control in memory improvement and rehabilitation programs. Negative beliefs about memory aging are widespread, and they are related to memory performance as well as to level of motivation for participating in memory training and rehabilitation programs. A conceptual model for guiding multifaceted interventions is presented. Evidence that self-defeating beliefs can be successfully modified through cognitive behavioral interventions programs is reviewed. Strategies are recommended for enhancing memory self-efficacy and control beliefs among older adults.

Beliefs About Memory Aging

Popular conceptions of aging portray memory loss as inevitable, universal, and irreversible (Lachman, 1991). Many middle-aged and elderly adults begin to report problems remembering important information as they get older. In a recent survey of 300 randomly sampled men and women aged 25–75 from the Greater Boston Area, 39% reported they had memory problems at least once a week or more, and 29% found these problems somewhat or very stressful (Lachman, Maier, & Budner, in preparation). When considered in relation to problems in 25 other domains, problems with memory were first most frequent for older adults, second most frequent for middle-aged adults, and third most frequent for young adults. These memory problems were rated among the top 5 out of 26 stressors for both middle-aged and older adults. These results are consistent with earlier surveys that showed that memory problems are frequently reported by adults over 40 years of age (see Aldwin, 1990; Cutler & Grams,

1988; Lachman, 1991). Thus, a view of aging in which memory problems increase is widespread.

There is some indication that reports of memory problems do not always correspond to actual difficulties (Zarit, Cole, & Guider, 1981; Gilewski, Zelinski, & Schaie, 1990). Thus, to a certain extent, memory complaints may reflect a kind of hypochondriasis of aging. Nevertheless, the prevailing view of aging includes a constellation of beliefs about the perceived change (decline) in abilities, lack of control over the decline, and limited potential for improvement. Indeed, one of the circumstances that may contribute to memory problems being stressful is that memory loss is often seen as a natural part of the aging process, with the accompanying belief that nothing can be done to control it. Beliefs about memory and aging, whether accurate or not, can have important implications for functioning and behavior.

Research on memory performance shows that there are declines with aging (Smith, 1996). However, not all aspects of memory change, not all individuals show decrements, and there is evidence that memory can be improved. Thus, the view of memory aging as inevitable, universal, and irreversible is erroneous. Nevertheless, many older adults believe there is little that can be done to improve their memory. The focus of this chapter is on the enhancement of beliefs about memory self-efficacy and control. These beliefs are considered an important foundation for successful memory improvement or rehabilitation (Elliott & Lachman, 1989; Lachman, Bandura, Weaver, & Elliott, 1995).

Relationship Between Memory Performance and Memory Beliefs

The relationship between memory beliefs and memory performance in later life has been of great interest since the early 1980s (Dixon & Hultsch, 1983; Grover & Hertzog, 1991; Hertzog, Dixon, & Hultsch, 1990; Lachman, Baltes, Nesselroade, & Willis, 1982; Lachman, 1991; Zarit et al., 1981). The nature of this relationship appears to vary as a function of the type of belief or aspect of memory that is studied.

A number of correlational studies have shown that beliefs about efficacy and controllability are related to cognitive performance. Those who have higher efficacy and a more internal sense of control have better performance on a wide variety of intellectual and memory tests (Grover & Hertzog, 1991; Lachman, 1986; Lachman et al., 1982; Stine, Lachman & Wingfield, 1993). Of interest is whether the beliefs develop in response to memory performance or whether the beliefs lead to changes in memory. There is some evidence that performance predicts changes in beliefs (Cornelius & Caspi, 1986; Grover & Hertzog, 1991; Lachman, 1983; Lachman & Leff, 1989). On the other hand, self-efficacy has been identified as an important predictor of cognitive change, along with education and lung function (Albert et al., 1995). Self-efficacy also was found to predict degree of improvement in memory training (Rebok & Balcerak, 1989). These data provide support for the interactive, reciprocal nature of change in cognition and attitudes during the aging process.

Mechanisms

One unanswered question is what the mechanisms are that link control beliefs and performance. There is some evidence that effort is a key mediator. In one study, Berry

(1987) found that those who had higher self-efficacy spent more time studying memory materials. In another study, Stine et al. (1993) found that working memory was a likely mediator between control beliefs and performance. Riggs, Lachman, and Wingfield (1997) found that adults with more external control beliefs were less efficient in memory strategy use for processing text materials and benefited less from performance experience. Those who had greater self-efficacy and more internal control beliefs were more likely to engage in effortful processing, which resulted in better performance.

Another possible mediator is attributions. If performance is attributed to ability, this attribution is likely to affect efficacy. Bandura (1977) found that when internal stable attributions were made for performance outcomes, self-efficacy was more likely to be affected than if external attributions were made. If older adults have trouble remembering something and attribute this trouble to poor ability, this attribution could negatively affect their efficacy. In contrast, if they attribute the trouble to lack of effort, they may try harder the next time, and efficacy may not be lowered. On the other hand, making adaptive attributions in the face of good performance may have positive effects. In support of this contention, Lachman, Steinberg, and Trotter (1987) found that those who attributed successful memory performance to internal and stable factors improved more over two trials. These findings illustrate the processes whereby beliefs can both affect and be affected by memory. Stress is also a potential mediator of the relationship between control beliefs and memory performance. There is evidence that low levels of perceived control are associated with increased anxiety and stress (Bandura, 1997). Recent studies of stress reactivity measured with cortisol have shown links between high levels of stress hormone and impaired memory performance (Seeman, McEwen, Singer, Albert, & Rowe, 1997). McEwen and Sapolsky (1995) have evidence from animals that prolonged stress does damage to hippocampal functioning. The finding that lowering stress can have a beneficial impact on memory performance in later life (Lupien, Lecours, Lussier, Schwartz, Nair, & Meaney, 1994) is encouraging and suggests the promise of interventions focused on control beliefs and stress reduction for improving memory.

Memory Training

Memory training often involves the teaching of mnemonic strategies such as the method of loci (Lapp, 1986; Poon, 1984; West, 1985; Yesavage, 1985). Although this approach has been useful in establishing the plasticity of memory in later life, it has not always been successful in providing a practical means for sustained memory improvement. In some cases, the results have been test-specific, subjects did not adopt the techniques outside the laboratory, and the effects dissipated after a short time (Anschutz, Camp, Markley, & Kramer, 1987). Moreover, memory researchers have not endorsed the use of formal mnemonics (Park, Smith, & Cavanaugh, 1990) because they are cumbersome and limited in their application to everyday tasks.

Multifactorial training programs that focus on training multiple skills have been the most effective (Floyd & Scogin, 1997; Verhaeghen, Marcoen, & Goossens, 1992). For example, Yesavage (1985) and his colleagues used pretraining of visualization techniques in conjunction with mnemonic strategy training and found significant improvement. Others have included anxiety reduction, relaxation, or stress inoculation techniques in conjunction with ability training, the result being enhanced effects (Hayslip, Maloy, & Kohl, 1995; Labouvie-Vief & Gonda, 1976; Neely & Bäckman, 1993). For example, successful memory improvement was found when encoding and attentional training were combined with relaxation (Neely & Bäckman, 1993).

Floyd and Scogin (1997) conducted a meta-analysis to examine the effects of memory training on subjective beliefs about memory functioning. Their general conclusion was that mnemonic training alone had little effect on beliefs about memory. They also found that in cases where memory training was supplemented with pretraining or included direct attention to beliefs, there were greater effects on beliefs.

The Role of Control Beliefs

One possible explanation for the limited impact of some previous cognitive training efforts (e.g., limited transfer or maintenance) is that many older adults believe that cognitive decrement is inevitable and that nothing can be done to control or change cognitive functioning (especially memory) in later life (Bandura, 1989; Elliott & Lachman, 1989). If older adults believe their memory is not as good as it used to be and there is nothing they can do to improve, they are unlikely to use effort to learn or implement new strategies.

Indeed, past work has shown that older adults hold more self-defeating attitudes about memory and other cognitive dimensions than the young, and that these beliefs become less adaptive over time (Cavanaugh, 1989; Cavanaugh & Green, 1990; Lachman, 1991; Lachman & Leff, 1989). Older adults are more likely than the young to believe that their memory is not as good as it used to be (Hertzog et al., 1990). The elderly are also less likely than the young to believe that they can control their memory and intellectual functioning. Finally, older adults are more likely than the young to explain memory failures with internal and stable attributions, such as poor ability (Erber, Szuchman, & Rothberg, 1990; Lachman & McArthur, 1986). The young are more likely to blame failures on lack of effort, which is a more malleable factor (Lachman, 1990).

Negative beliefs about memory competence and controllability, whether they are accurate or not, can have far-reaching consequences. These consequences include increased dependency on others, avoidance of cognitive challenges, seeking unnecessary medical attention, reliance on medication, anxiety, reduced effort, and decreased motivation to use one's cognitive skills (Bandura, 1989; Lachman, 1991). Previous research has shown that confidence in memory ability is related to performance (Bandura, 1989). It is possible that those who lack confidence but who see memory as controllable will be inoculated against a syndrome involving helplessness and dependency as they age (Lachman et al., 1995). The reason is that they see memory problems as surmountable with effort and engage in problem solving in the face of difficulty. In contrast, those who lack confidence and view memory loss as inevitable are likely to become helpless and reliant on others to cope with memory problems. They view difficulties as signs of deterioration over which they have no control. Thus, they will not invest effort in problem solving. The result is poor performance, which perpetuates a downward spiral of ability estimates, decreased motivation, and withdrawal from tasks involving memory.

This set of circumstances provides the basis for a rationale for why it is important to target beliefs about efficacy and control when designing memory-training programs. Negative beliefs are a problem in their own right because they can lead to anxiety, depression, lack of involvement, and avoidance of situations that demand skills and thus can impact quality of life. Moreover, these beliefs may be related to the effectiveness of memory interventions. Those who hold negative beliefs refrain from attempting to improve their memories. Thus, it may be necessary to change negative beliefs prior to recruiting participants for a training program. Without such changes, even participants who do start out with the intention of improving are at higher risk of terminating the program.

There is some evidence that beliefs about efficacy, control, and attributions can be changed (Lachman et al., 1992; Rodin, 1983). However, unless rehabilitation efforts directly target beliefs, there seems to be little effect (Dunlosky & Hertzog, in press; Floyd & Scogin, 1997). Bandura (1997) suggested that older adults' self-efficacy beliefs are especially resistant to change. A number of researchers have used cognitive behavioral techniques such as attributional retraining, increasing motivation through rewards, manipulating control contingencies (Forsterling, 1985; Langer, Rodin, Beck, Weinman, & Spitzer, 1979; Rodin, 1983; Rodin, Cashman, & Desiderato, 1987), and cognitive restructuring (Duke, Haley, & Bergquist, 1991; Lachman et al., 1992) to enhance older adults' control beliefs and attributions. These studies have shown not only that it is possible to change attributions and control beliefs in the elderly, but also that these changes have positive effects on many types of performance and well-being.

Negative cognitions about memory capabilities can cause anxiety and interfere with task-related attention, the result being performance and motivational deficits. Therefore, directly addressing these maladaptive beliefs can result in higher levels of motivation and persistence for cognitive tasks by reducing anxiety and increasing self-confidence and providing motivation for memory improvement.

Importance of Cognitive-Behavioral Interventions in Enhancing Cognitive Training Effects

Research shows that optimal performance requires not only skills but also adaptive beliefs about one's abilities (Bandura, 1989). Those who have lower confidence and those who believe they have little control over their memory show poorer performance (Berry, West, & Dennehey, 1989; Hertzog et al.,1990; Lachman et al., 1987).

Few cognitive training studies have targeted or even assessed self-efficacy or control beliefs. In those that have looked at efficacy or control, there was no evidence that these beliefs changed without additional training focused on attitudes about memory (Floyd & Scogin, 1997; Hill, Sheikh, & Yesavage, 1987; Rebok & Balcerak, 1989). The one exception is test-specific beliefs: Older adults are good at monitoring changes in their test performance after training (Devolder, Brigham, & Pressley, 1990; Dittmann-Kohli, Lachman, Kliegl, & Baltes, 1991).

Anxiety and depression can also affect performance through distraction and interference with sustained attention. What is important is that underlying these affective dimensions there is often a low sense of efficacy and control (Bandura, 1997). Although some training programs have chosen to target anxiety directly with relaxation training (e.g., Labouvie-Vief & Gonda, 1976), it may be more effective to directly address the underlying cognitions that fuel the anxiety—that is, low efficacy and control—rather than to eliminate just the symptoms. Anxiety and stress often occur in response to beliefs about incompetence (efficacy) and lack of ability to change or prevent decline (control).

According to cognitive behavioral models, beliefs in efficacy and control are important for several aspects of the training: to ensure attention to and motivation for the training, to foster an adaptive learning environment (e.g., reduced anxiety, increase effort, focused attention), and to facilitate transfer and maintenance of the skills beyond the initial training by instilling self-confidence in handling challenging situations.

However, the elderly seem to be more resistant than the young to changes in efficacy and control beliefs (Bandura, 1997). Whereas the young boost their efficacy after successful performance experiences, the elderly appear to need multiple inputs to promote efficacy change, such as persuasion, vicarious reinforcement (modeling), and direct performance feedback. This need may be due, in large part, to ingrained societal views about the irreversibility of aging-related changes and implicit views of memory aging (Elliott & Lachman, 1989; McDonald-Miszczak, Hertzog, & Hultsch, 1995). Thus, it is critical to build cognitive-behavioral strategies directly into cognitive training programs to promote beliefs that foster effective learning.

It is unlikely that a focus only on changing beliefs would lead to effective memory enhancement. Ideally, beliefs can be targeted in conjunction with skills training. Confidence and control beliefs provide a resource for dealing with anxiety and failure, the tools needed for persistence, and the motivation to engage in cognitive improvement and challenges in daily life. Instruction and application of skills to daily cognitive tasks can be facilitated by cognitive restructuring.

Self-Guided Practice Versus Instructor-Guided Training

There has been a great deal of debate about the role of experience in memory deficits associated with aging (Baron & Mattila, 1989; Salthouse, 1987, 1991). The current status of this work is that age differences in memory may be minimized, but not completely eliminated, with extended practice. Nevertheless, a number of studies have demonstrated that self-guided practice with cognitive materials results in improved performance, and in many cases, those in testing-only or self-guided practice conditions have done as well as those in instructor-guided training groups, particularly in skills that are already in the repertoire (Baltes, Sowarka, & Kliegl, 1989; Blackburn, Papalia-Finlay, Foyce, & Serlin, 1988; Camp, Markley, & Kramer, 1983; Hofland, Willis, & Baltes, 1981; Kotler-Cope & Camp, 1990; Lachman et al., 1992; Willis, 1990). These results suggest, in part, that performance may improve because of increased experience and familiarity with testing materials as well as reductions in anxiety or other noncognitive beliefs (Salthouse, 1991; Willis, 1990). It is also possible that generating one's own strategies can foster a sense of competence and control. Although practice affects performance, there is less evidence that it has an impact on beliefs (Floyd & Scogin, 1997). Blackburn et al. (1988) found that self-guided practice effects were more durable over time than tutor-guided effects. These studies, however, have typically included highly educated and healthy samples. It will be important to determine whether self-guided practice is equally effective for less positively selected, more diverse samples. Dunlosky and Hertzog (1998) recommended the use of self-regulatory skills to teach older adults to monitor their own learning. This approach is consistent with a cognitive-behavioral one and is likely to foster a sense of efficacy and control, as participants see they can improve through their own efforts.

Conceptual Model of Age-Related Loss, Control, and Motivation

The conceptual model presented in figure 6.1 illustrates the interplay of aging-related losses and changes in attitudes and motivation, and captures the cyclical nature of aging (Lachman, Ziff, & Spiro, 1994). Similar to the social breakdown syndrome proposed by Kuypers and Bengtson (1973), this model examines the relationship between internalized negative expectations and aging-related declines.

As illustrated in Figure 6.1, aging-related loss such as decline in cognitive functioning can lead to a lowered sense of control. This may involve a low sense of efficacy (lack of confidence in abilities to change), external beliefs (feeling one cannot do something about it because it is not under one's own control), and/or attributions to internal stable causes (it is due to aging or poor ability). This lowered control in turn affects motivation to change and results in reduced effort and persistence in the face of difficulties; it may also result in affective changes such as depression and/or anxiety. This process is cyclical in that the lowered effort can result in further mental or physical deterioration through disuse, deconditioning, or atrophy.

Cognitive changes such as memory loss or physical changes such as functional limitations are typically associated with the aging process. These changes, however,

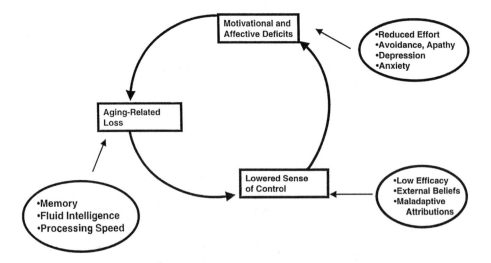

Figure 6.1. Conceptual model of cognitive aging, control, and motivation.

may be modified or even reversed (Evans, 1995; Schaie & Willis, 1986). However, as illustrated in Figure 6.1, experiencing increased forgetfulness or slowing may bring with it a lowered sense of control. There is the feeling that one is less capable of doing things (low efficacy), that these changes are due to unchangeable aspects of the aging process (maladaptive attributions), and, therefore, that nothing can be done (poor outcome expectancies) (Lachman et al., 1994). These lowered control beliefs may be associated with decreased motivation to engage in daily activities with cognitive demands, and to increased distress about one's limitations and the potential downward course of aging. The cyclical nature of the model indicates that regardless of where one begins, this is an ongoing process. Thus, for example, it is just as plausible that motivational deficits trigger memory decrement as it is that memory decline triggers lowered sense of control. What is critical is that once the process is in motion, unless there is some intervention it is likely to continue in a downward path.

In the model of age-related loss, the sense-of-control, motivational, and affective factors are considered antecedents and consequences of aging-related losses. Attention to these components of the model is expected to be useful for interventions designed to encourage older adults not only to begin memory improvement programs, but also to facilitate long-term maintenance of memory skills.

Multifaceted Interventions

Whereas most interventions focus on only one target, the conceptual model presented in Figure 6.1 provides a framework for a multifaceted approach to memory rehabilitation. As shown in Figure 6.2, the intervention strategy involves teaching skills to compensate for or prevent loss (e.g., mnemonics, use of external aids) and changing beliefs in efficacy and control, which are tied to motivational factors—such as setting

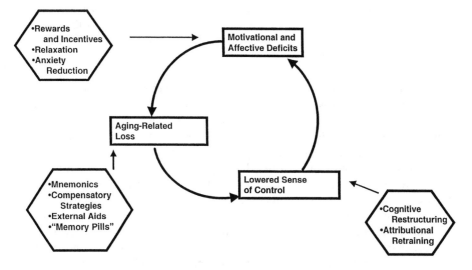

Figure 6.2. Intervention strategies: Multiple targets.

realistic expectations and goals—needed for behavioral changes. There is some evidence from past research that efficacy and control beliefs can be enhanced in older adults (Lachman et al., 1992; Rodin, 1983).

Cognitive Rehabilitation and Cognitive-Behavioral Interventions

Cognitive behavioral strategies, long used for clinical purposes (Bandura, 1989; Beck et al., 1979; Meichenbaum, 1977; Seligman, 1991), instill adaptive beliefs such as greater perceived control and more realistic assessment of cognitive failures and abilities. Rodin et al. (1987) concluded that more generalized and long-term effects would be found in cognitive interventions that affect subjects' feelings of control. Instilling and strengthening the belief that memory can be improved with effort should enhance the elderly's motivation to try new memory challenges and to persist even in the face of difficulties. Desire to try to remember is low if one believes one does not have the necessary skills or that one's efforts will not pay off.

According to Bandura (1977), behavior change is also determined by self-efficacy beliefs and outcome expectations (represented as external control beliefs in Figure 6.1), that is, whether one expects a desirable response to one's actions. One may have high self-efficacy for memory, but if one believes that there is nothing he or she can do to prevent or remediate aging-related losses, there would be little motivation to learn new strategies. The benefits of practice and strategy use are often not immediate, and one needs to stick with them for some time in order to feel the rewards. Thus, one must have a high degree of motivation. The belief that practice will help to improve one's memory and that one has some control over the memory aging process is an important source of motivation.

Given that one may encounter some difficulties as one tries to improve one's memory, another important attitudinal ingredient is the attributions one makes in the face of failure (Abramson, Seligman, & Teasdale, 1978). If one makes adaptive attributions (i.e., sees failures as due to changeable factors), one is more likely to persist and exert effort in difficult circumstances. In contrast if one uses maladaptive attributions (i.e., sees poor outcomes as due to stable, unchangeable factors such as old age), one is more likely to become discouraged and to curtail efforts.

We have developed a cognitive-behavioral intervention that targets efficacy, control, and attributions related to cognitive aging (Lachman et al., 1992). In our program, the cognitive restructuring treatment was administered by two clinical psychologists in two 1.5-hour sessions. There were four components to the program: (a) developing awareness of negative beliefs about memory, (b) promoting the view of memory as controllable through effort, (c) modeling adaptive attributions for memory successes and failures, and (d) practicing positive thinking about memory. Videotapes were used in which actors portrayed different approaches to interpreting memory successes and failures in laboratory and real-world tasks. Some of the actors conveyed positive views by responding to difficult memory tasks with statements about how they could succeed through the use of strategies or extra effort. They also modeled the use of adaptive attributions for memory problems. In contrast, other actors demonstrated negative views by responding to memory loss with maladaptive attributions (e.g., due to getting older) and a sense of hopelessness about memory improvement. The group leader led discussions about the films to highlight the differences between the positive and negative views. These discussions were effective in helping the participants to become aware of their misconceptions and negative, self-defeating beliefs about memory and aging, many of which were similar to those portrayed by the actors.

A homework assignment was designed to help participants develop more adaptive attitudes by thinking of an example where a positive attitude had helped them deal with circumstances that were seemingly insurmountable. The discussion of the homework was then applied to the area of memory to illustrate the point that there are ways to improve memory and that memory is controllable.

The study design for the multifaceted intervention (Lachman et al., 1992) included several conditions with different combinations of the treatments (cognitive restructuring, self-generated memory strategies training, and combined) and two control groups (practice and no-contact). It was predicted that the greatest improvement in self-conceptions of memory would occur for those who received both self-generated memory strategies training and cognitive restructuring, followed by those who received only cognitive restructuring. Similarly, the greatest improvement in memory performance was expected for those in the combined-training group, followed by the strategy-training group. As predicted, the combined-treatment group showed the greatest change on the following memory control beliefs: improvement, effort, and inevitable decrement. The strategy generation group showed the greatest improvement in capacity. For test-specific predictions, the practice group increased the most in the text and working-memory tasks, perhaps because the practice group had more experience with these tasks than the other groups. All groups had equal amounts of practice on list recall and name-face recall and showed similar increases in predictions for these tasks.

Through the use of a cognitive-behavioral intervention, older adults' beliefs about memory controllability and efficacy were improved. The cognitive restructuring was most effective in changing self-conceptions of memory when it was combined with the self-generated memory strategy training.

When combined with cognitive training for encoding and attention, the cognitive-behavioral treatment was effective in changing beliefs about memory efficacy and control (Lachman et al., 1992). We found that beliefs about control changed more when specific information was provided about the relationship between effort and memory improvement and the diversity (rather than universality) of memory aging across persons and different aspects of memory (Lachman et al., 1992).

The training effects were strongest at the first posttest, however, and the effects were weaker by 3 months. These findings highlight the need to concentrate on how to maintain these changes in beliefs to achieve long-term effects. We also found that self-guided practice and retesting were as effective as tutor-guided training for memory improvement. Although practice was as effective as strategy generation for improving memory, this was not the case for changing beliefs about memory.

The cognitive restructuring program was broadly based on cognitive-behavioral theory and clinical methods (Beck & Emery, 1985), with a combined focus on changing attitudes and behaviors (skills). In addition to using this two-pronged intervention approach with memory, we have also applied it in the realm of exercise with a strength (resistance) training program. The cognitive-behavioral technique was effective in promoting regular exercise among sedentary older adults (Lachman et al., 1997; Jette et al., 1999). We found greater adherence to the exercise program and more extensive progression across resistance levels for those who received the cognitive-behavioral training than those reported in previous studies.

A key feature of cognitive-behavioral interventions is individualized goal setting. Programs should be tailored to the individual needs and capacities of the participants, allowing for gradual progress. This approach enables participants to identify their weaknesses and to select areas of desired improvement. Many training studies have shown individual differences among the elderly in their responsiveness to training. Typically, those who are younger and healthier and have higher initial levels of functioning, show greater increments (Bäckman, 1989; Lachman et al., 1992; Schaffer & Poon, 1982; Yesavage, Sheikh, Friedman, & Tanke, 1990). Thus, memory-training programs may need to be modified to ensure their effectiveness for particular target groups.

A customized program can also be beneficial in reducing anxiety levels because the participants know that the program has been designed for them. Otherwise, they may assume the program is too difficult for them or does not address their particular needs. Other behavioral techniques may include a signed commitment or contract, keeping track of work with a diary or log, and incentives or rewards for progress or reaching goals. Periodic feedback from the trainer serves both to check on skill attainment and to provide helpful social support. Cognitive restructuring strategies teach adults how to address their concerns and how to generate alternatives to their negative, self-defeating thoughts. These strategies serve to instill mastery and a sense of control, which are valuable for sustaining newly acquired strategies and skills because they help the individual to overcome challenges and obstacles that interfere with progress.

Within the model (see Figure 6.2), cognitive restructuring, along with memory training, is expected to increase the sense of control because it promotes a view of memory aging as controllable through effort rather than as the result of uncontrollable aging. One important lesson for older adults to learn is that what used to be relatively effortless (e.g., remembering phone numbers, recalling names, remembering the details of a movie) now may require more effort. The cognitive restructuring intervention informs them that they do have some control and that the investment of effort pays off.

Conclusion

Beliefs about memory have been found to become more negative with aging (Lachman, 1991). The assumptions that memory performance declines and that this decline is difficult to prevent or change is pervasive. These beliefs about memory self-efficacy and controllability are related to performance as both antecedents and consequences, as depicted in Figure 6.1. These beliefs can have damaging consequences for performance and the effectiveness of memory-training programs. Memory-training programs that do not include a specific focus on beliefs about memory efficacy and control are typically not effective in changing these beliefs. Thus, a focus on changing memory-related beliefs is important for enhancing the motivation to engage in memory training, as well as for optimizing the degree of effort invested in making memory improvements. Older adults who firmly believe that they have the potential to effect change in their memories are likely to be favorably predisposed to benefit from memory rehabilitation programs.

References

Abramson, L. Y., Seligman, M. E. P., & Teasdale, J. D. (1978). Learned helplessness: Critique and reformulation. *Journal of Abnormal Psychology, 87,* 49–74.

Albert, M. S., Jones, K., Savage, C. R., Berkman, L., Seeman, T., Blazer, D., & Rowe, J. W. (1995). Predictors of cognitive change in older persons: MacArthur studies of successful aging. *Psychology and Aging, 10,* 578–589.

Aldwin, C. (1990). The Elder's Life Stress Inventory: Egocentric and nonegocentric stress. In M. A. P. Stephens, S. E. Hobfoll, J. H. Crowther, & D. L. Tennenbaum (Eds.), *Stress and coping in late life families* (pp. 49–69). New York: Hemisphere.

Anschutz, L., Camp, C. J., Markley, R. P., & Kramer, J. J. (1987). Remembering mnemonics: A three-year follow-up on the effects of mnemonics training in elderly adults. *Experimental Aging Research, 13,* 141–143.

Bäckman, L. (1989). Varieties of memory compensation by older adults in episodic remembering. In L. W. Poon, D. C. Rubin, & B. A. Wilson (Eds.), *Everyday cognition in adulthood and late life* (pp. 509–544). New York: Cambridge University Press.

Baltes, P. B., Sowarka, D., & Kliegl, R. (1989). Cognitive training research on fluid intelligence in old age: What can older adults achieve by themselves? *Psychology and Aging, 4,* 217–221.

Bandura, A. (1977). Self-efficacy: Toward a unifying theory of behavioral change. *Psychological Review, 84,* 191–215.

Bandura, A. (1989). Regulation of cognitive processes through perceived self-efficacy. *Developmental Psychology, 25,* 729–735.

Bandura, A. (1997). *Self-efficacy: The exercise of control.*New York: W. H. Freeman.

Baron, A., & Mattila, W. R. (1989). Response slowing of older adults: Effects of time-limit contingencies on single- and dual-task performances. *Psychology and Aging, 4,* 66–72.

Beck, A. T., & Emery, G. (1985). *Anxiety disorders and phobias: A cognitive perspective.* New York: Basic Books.

Beck, A. T., et al. (1979). *Cognitive therapy of depression.* New York: Guilford Press.

Berry, J. M. (1987, September). *A self-efficacy model of memory performance.* Paper presented at the 95th annual convention of the American Psychological Association, New York.

Berry, J. M., West, R. L., & Dennehey, D. M. (1989). Reliability and validity of the memory self-efficacy questionnaire. *Developmental Psychology, 25,* 701–713.

Blackburn, J. A., Papalia-Finlay, D., Foyce, B. F., & Serlin, R. C. (1988). Modifiability of figural relations performance among elderly adults. *Journal of Gerontology: Psychological Sciences, 43,* 87–89.

Camp, C. J., Markley, R. P., & Kramer, J. J. (1983). Spontaneous use of mnemonics by elderly individuals. *Educational Gerontology, 9,* 57–71.

Cavanaugh, J. C. (1989). The importance of awareness in memory aging. In L. W. Poon, D. C. Rubin, & B. A. Wilson (Eds.), *Everyday cognition in adulthood and late life* (pp. 416–436). New York: Cambridge University Press.

Cavanaugh, J. C., & Green, E. E. (1990). I believe, therefore I can: Self-efficacy beliefs in memory aging. In E. A. Lovelace (Ed.), *Aging and cognition: Mental processes, self-awareness, and interventions* (pp. 189–230). Amsterdam: Elsevier.

Cornelius, S. W., & Caspi, A. (1986). Self-perceptions of intellectual control and aging. *Educational Gerontology, 12,* 345–357.

Cutler, S. J., & Grams, A. E. (1988). Correlates of self-reported everyday memory problems. *Journal of Gerontology, 43,* 582–590.

Devolder, P. A., Brigham, M. C., & Pressley, M. (1990). Memory performance awareness in younger and older adults. *Psychology and Aging, 5,* 291–303.

Dittman-Kohli, F., Lachman, M., Kliegl, R., & Baltes, P. B. (1991). Effects of cognitive training on intellectual efficacy beliefs in elderly adults. *Journals of Gerontology: Psychological Sciences, 46,* 162–164.

Dixon, R. A., & Hultsch, D. F. (1983). Metamemory and memory for text relationships in adulthood: A cross validation study. *Journal of Gerontology, 38,* 687–694.

Duke, L. W., Haley, W. E., & Bergquist, T. F. (1991). Cognitive-behavioral interventions for age-related memory impairment. In P. A. Wisocki (Ed.), *Handbook of clinical behavior therapy with the elderly client* (pp. 245–272). New York: Plenum Press.

Dunlosky, J., & Hertzog, C. (1998). Training programs to improve learning in later adulthood: Helping older adults educate themselves. In D. J. Hacker, J. Dunlosky, & A. C. Graesser (Eds.), *Metacognition in educational theory and practice* (pp. 249–275). Hillsdale, NJ: Erlbaum.

Elliott, E., & Lachman, M. E. (1989). Enhancing memory by modifying control beliefs, attributions, and performance goals in the elderly. In P. S. Fry (Ed.), *Psychology of helplessness and control and attributions in the aged* (pp. 339–367). Amsterdam: North-Holland.

Erber, J. T., Szuchman, L. T., & Rothberg, S. T. (1990). Everyday memory failure: Age differences in appraisal and attribution. *Psychology and Aging, 5,* 236–241.

Evans, W. J. (1995). Effects of exercise on body composition and functional capacity in the elderly. *Journal of Gerontology: Biological and Medical Sciences, 50,* 147–151.

Floyd, M., & Scogin, F. (1997). Effects of memory training on the subjective memory functioning and mental health of older adults: A meta-analysis. *Psychology and Aging, 12,* 150–161.

Forsterling, F. (1985). Attributional retraining: A review. *Psychology Bulletin, 98,* 495–512.

Gilewski, M. J., Zelinski, E. M., & Schaie, K. W. (1990). The memory functioning questionnaire for assessment of memory complaints in adulthood and old age. *Psychology and Aging, 5,* 215–233.

Grover, D. R., & Hertzog, C. (1991). Relationships between intellectual control beliefs and psychometric intelligence in adulthood. *Journal of Gerontology: Psychological Sciences, 46,* 109–115.

Hayslip, B., Jr., Maloy, R. M., & Kohl, R. (1995). Long-term efficacy of fluid ability interventions with older adults. *Journal of Gerontology: Psychological Sciences, 50,* 141–149.

Hertzog, C., Dixon, R. A., & Hultsch, D. F. (1990). Relationships between metamemory, memory predictions, and memory task performance in adults. *Psychology and Aging, 5,* 215–227.

Hill, R. D., Sheikh, J. I., & Yesavage, J. A. (1987). The effect of mnemonic training on perceived recall confidence in the elderly. *Experimental Aging Research, 13,* 185–188.

Hofland, B. F., Willis, S. L., & Baltes, P. B. (1981). Fluid intelligence performance in the elderly: Intraindividual variability and conditions of assessment. *Journal of Educational Psychology, 73,* 573–586.

Jette, A., Lachman, M. E., Giorgetti, M. M., Assmann, S. F., Harris, B. A., Levenson, C., Wernick, M., & Krebs, D. (1999). Exercise: It's never too late. *American Journal of Public Health, 89,* 66–72.

Kotler-Cope, S., & Camp, C. (1990). Memory interventions in aging populations. In E. A. Lovelace (Ed.), *Aging and cognition: Mental processes, self-awareness and interventions* (pp. 231–261). Amsterdam: North-Holland.

Kuypers, J. A., & Bengtson, V. L. (1973). Social breakdown and competence: A model of normal aging. *Human Development, 16,* 181–201.

Labouvie-Vief, G., & Gonda, J. N. (1976). Cognitive strategy training and intellectual performance in the elderly. *Journal of Gerontology, 31,* 372–382.

Lachman, M. E. (1983). Perceptions of intellectual aging: Antecedent or consequence of intellectual functioning? *Developmental Psychology, 19,* 482–498.

Lachman, M. E. (1986). Locus of control in aging research: A case for multidimensional and domain specific assessment. *Psychology and Aging, 1,* 34–40.

Lachman, M. E. (1990). When bad things happen to older people: Age differences in attributional style. *Psychology and Aging, 5,* 607–609.

Lachman, M. E. (1991). Perceived control over memory aging: Developmental and intervention perspectives. *Journal of Social Issues, 47,* 159–175.

Lachman, M. E., Baltes, P. B., Nesselroade, J. R., & Willis, S. L. (1982). Examination of personality-ability relationships in the elderly: The role of the contextual (interface) assessment mode. *Journal of Research in Personality, 16,* 485–501.

Lachman, M. E., Bandura, M., Weaver, S. L., & Elliott, E. (1995). Assessing memory control beliefs: The Memory Controllability Inventory. *Aging and Cognition, 2,* 67–84.

Lachman, M. E., Jette, A., Tennstedt, S., Howland, J., Harris, B. A., & Peterson, E. (1997). A cognitive-behavioral model for promoting regular physical activity in older adults. *Psychology, Health, and Medicine, 2,* 251–261.

Lachman, M. E., & Leff, R. (1989). Beliefs about intellectual efficacy and control in the elderly: A five-year longitudinal study. *Developmental Psychology, 25,* 722–728.

Lachman, M. E., Maier, H., & Budner, R. (in preparation).When and what is midlife? Not just problems and crises.

Lachman, M. E., & McArthur, L. Z. (1986). Adulthood age differences in causal attributions for cognitive, physical, and social performance. *Psychology and Aging, 1,* 127–132.

Lachman, M. E., Steinberg, E. S., & Trotter, S. D. (1987). The effects of control beliefs and attributions on memory self-assessments and performance, *Psychology and Aging, 2,* 266–271.

Lachman, M. E., Weaver, S. L., Bandura, M., Elliott, E., & Lewkowicz, C. (1992). Improving memory and control beliefs through cognitive restructuring and self-generated strategies. *Journals of Gerontology: Psychological Sciences, 47,* 293–299.

Lachman, M. E., Ziff, M. A., & Spiro, A. (1994). Maintaining a sense of control in later life. In R. Abeles, H. Gift, & M. Ory (Eds.), *Aging and quality of life* (pp. 216–232). New York: Sage.

Langer, E. J., Rodin, J., Beck, P., Weinman, C., & Spitzer, L. (1979). Environmental determinants of memory improvement in late adulthood. *Journal of Personality and Social Psychology, 37,* 2003–2013.

Lapp, D. (1986). *Don't forget.* New York: McGraw-Hill.

Lupien, S., Lecours, A. R., Lussier, I., Schwartz, G., Nair, N. P. V., & Meaney, M. J. (1994). Basal cortisol levels and cognitive deficits in human aging. *The Journal of Neuroscience, 14,* 2893–2903.

McDonald-Miszczak, L., Hertzog, C., & Hultsch, D. F. (1995). Stability and accuracy of metamemory in adulthood and aging: A longitudinal analysis. *Psychology and Aging, 10,* 553–564.

McEwen, B. S., & Sapolsky, R. M. (1995). Stress and cognitive function. *Current Opinion in Neurobiology, 5,* 205–216.

Meichenbaum, D. (1977). *Cognitive behavioral modification: An integrative approach.* New York: Plenum Press.

Neely, A. S.,& Bäckman, L. (1993). Long-term maintenance of gains from memory training in older adults: Two 3 1/2 year followup studies. *Journal of Gerontology: Psychological Sciences, 48,* 233–237.

Park, D. C., Smith, A. D., & Cavanaugh, J. C. (1990). Metamemories of memory researchers. *Memory and Cognition, 18,* 321–327.

Poon, L. W. (1984). Memory training for older adults. In J. P. Abrams & V. J. Crooks (Eds.), *Geriatric mental health* (pp. 136–150). New York: Grune & Stratton.

Rebok, G. W., & Balcerak, L. J. (1989). Memory self-efficacy and performance differences in young and old adults: The effect of mnemonic training. *Developmental Psychology, 25,* 714–721.

Riggs, K. M., Lachman, M. E., & Wingfield. A. (1997). Taking charge of remembering: Locus of control and older adults' memory for speech. *Experimental Aging Research, 23,* 237–256.

Rodin, J. (1983). Behavioral medicine: Beneficial effects of self-control training in aging. *International Review of Applied Psychology, 32,* 153–181.

Rodin, J., Cashman, C., & Desiderato, L. (1987). Intervention and aging: Enrichment and prevention. In M. W. Riley, J. D. Matarazzo, & A. Baum (Eds.), *Perspectives in behavioral medicine: The aging dimension* (pp. 149–172). Hillsdale, NJ: Erlbaum.

Salthouse, T. A. (1987). The role of experience in cognitive aging. In K. Warner Schaie & C. Eisdorfer (Eds.), *Annual review of gerontology and geriatrics* (pp. 135–158). New York: Springer.

Salthouse, T. A. (1991). *Theoretical perspectives on cognitive aging.* Hillsdale, NJ: Erlbaum.

Schaffer, G., & Poon, L. W. (1982). Individual variability in memory training with the elderly. *Educational Gerontologist, 8,* 217–229.

Schaie, K. W., & Willis, S. L. (1986). Can decline in adult intellectual functioning be reversed? *Developmental Psychology, 22,* 223–232.

Seeman, T. E., McEwen, B. S., Singer, B. H., Albert, M. S., & Rowe, J. W. (1997). Increase in urinary cortisol excretion and memory declines: MacArthur Studies of Successful Aging. *Journal of Clinical Endocrinology and Metabolism, 82,* 2458–2465.

Seligman, M. E. P. (1991). *Learned optimism.* New York: Knopf.

Smith, A. (1996). Memory. In J. E. Birren & K. W. Schaie (Eds.), *Handbook of the psychology of aging* (4th ed., pp. 236–250). San Diego: Academic Press.

Stine, E. L., Lachman, M. E., & Wingfield, A. (1993). The roles of perceived and actual control in memory for spoken language. *Educational Gerontologist, 19,* 331–349.

Verhaeghen, P., Marcoen, A., & Goossens, L. (1992). Improving memory performance in the aged through mnemonic training: A meta-analytic study. *Psychology and Aging, 7,* 242–251.

West, R. L. (1985). *Memory fitness over 40.* Gainesville, FL: Triad.

Willis, S. L. (1990). Current issues in cognitive training research. In E. A. Lovelace (Ed.), *Aging and cognition: Mental processes, self-awareness and interventions.* Amsterdam: Elsevier.

Yesavage, J. A. (1985). Nonpharmacologic treatments for memory losses with normal aging. *American Journal of Psychiatry, 142,* 600–605.

Yesavage, J., Sheikh, J. I., Friedman, L., & Tanke, E. (1990). Learning mnemonics: Roles of aging and subtle cognitive impairment. *Psychology and Aging, 5,* 133–137.

Zarit, S., Cole, K., & Guider, R. (1981). Memory training strategies and subjective complaints of memory in the aged.*The Gerontologist, 21,* 158–164.

PART III

THE INFLUENCE OF HEALTH AND HEALTH BEHAVIORS ON THE REHABILITATION OF COGNITIVE PROCESSES IN LATE LIFE

7

The Role of Physical Exercise as a Rehabilitative Aid for Cognitive Loss in Healthy and Chronically Ill Older Adults

CHARLES F. EMERY

Older adults are frequently encouraged to participate in physical exercise due to the cumulative evidence indicating physiological benefits of exercise such as enhanced cardiovascular function, physical stamina, and muscle strength (Aniansson, Grimby, Rundgren, Svanborg, & Orlander, 1980; Pyka, Lindenberger, Charette, & Marcus, 1994), weight loss (Evans & Cyr-Campbell, 1997), prevention of osteoporosis (Bachmann & Grill, 1987), and enhanced glucose metabolism (Raz, Hauser, & Bursztyn, 1994). In addition, data suggest that exercise among older adults may be associated with improved quality of life (Singh, Clements, & Fiatarone, 1997), reduced psychological distress (McMurdo & Rennie, 1994), and improved neuropsychological or cognitive performance (Dustman et al., 1984). The potential for exercise-related improvements in cognitive functioning is of particular interest due to the increased prevalence of cognitive deficits among older adults and the widespread inclusion of exercise programs for older adults in a variety of settings (e.g., senior centers, assisted-care living facilities, hospital inpatient units, rehabilitation settings). The purpose of this chapter is (a) to describe briefly the age-related physical and cognitive changes that have been a focus of research in this area, (b) to discuss the physical and cognitive changes associated with exercise among older adults, and (c) to describe the relevance of these research findings for cognitive rehabilitation among older adults.

Age-Related Changes in Physical and Cognitive Functioning

Physical Functioning

Cross-sectional data indicate numerous age-related changes in physical functioning such as decreases in cardiac output and heart rate (Strandell, 1976), and reduced maximal oxygen consumption (VO$_2$max; Buskirk & Hodgson, 1987; Ehsani, 1987). VO$_2$max has been shown to decline approximately 10% each decade after age 25, and the decline may increase to nearly 20% in the seventh decade. Other physiological changes include reduced lung volume and poorer clearance of mucus from the lungs (Mahler, Rosiello, & Loke, 1986), as well as changes with age in the protein and mineral balance of the skeleton, increasing the risk of osteoporosis and bone fractures (DiGiovanna, 1994). Hormonal changes include diminished growth hormone production and decreased sensitivity to insulin (Rudman et al., 1981).

It has been suggested that at least some of the physiological changes associated with age may contribute to the well-documented decreases in cognitive performance associated with age and with disease among older adults. In particular, diseases of the cardiovascular and pulmonary systems may be associated with inadequate circulation and hypoxia, contributing to neuronal degeneration and, ultimately, diminished cognitive function (Spirduso, 1980).

Cognitive Functioning

Cognitive changes in markers of so-called fluid intelligence, such as reaction time and problem-solving ability, have been widely investigated. Age-related slowing of information-processing speed (Salthouse, 1991) and decreased memory performance (Craik & Jennings, 1992) are reflected in impaired performance among older adults on neuropsychological tests of reaction time, psychomotor/sensorimotor performance, visuospatial problem solving, attention and concentration, memory, and executive function (Lezak, 1995). In addition, neurophysiological indicators such as event-related potentials (ERPs) and electroencephalograms (EEGs) reflect slowing of brain signal processing with age (Prinz, Dustman, & Emmerson, 1990).

Physiological Changes Associated With Long-Term Exercise

The benefits of long-term exercise for physiological functioning include slower decline in muscle cell thickness, number of muscle cells, and muscle strength (Pyka et al., 1994). Also, exercise inhibits the gradual increase in fat accumulation, and older adults with a long-standing pattern of exercise may maintain higher levels of high-density lipoproteins (HDL) than sedentary older adults (Nieman et al., 1993; Tamai et al., 1988). These blood lipid factors contribute to exercise being associated with decreased risk of hypertension, atherosclerosis, coronary heart disease (CHD), and stroke. The most widely accepted standard for evaluating exercise capacity is VO$_2$max. Although VO$_2$max is known to decline with age, longitudinal studies suggest that regular physical exercise may attenuate this decline (Bruce, 1984; Kasch, Wallace, & Van Camp, 1985), with exercise training programs among older adults often reporting increases in VO$_2$max of from 15% to 25%. In turn, exercise may contribute to decreases in maximum heart rate required for maximal activity, as well as increases in stroke volume and cardiac efficiency (Tate, Hyek, & Taffet, 1994). Because measurement of VO$_2$max is the gold standard for determining cardiovascular fitness during a standardized exercise stress test, usually either a treadmill or a bicycle ergometer, studies in which fitness levels are assessed with VO$_2$max can more readily be used to evaluate the association of physical exercise with cognitive function. In the absence of VO$_2$max data, it is difficult to ascribe changes in cognitive performance to physical fitness levels.

Physical exercise has been investigated as a means of addressing age-related changes in physiological and cognitive functioning. Although the mechanisms by which exercise affects physiological functioning are well documented (Bouchard, Shephard, Stephens, Sutton, & McPherson, 1990), the mechanism of exercise effects on cognitive function is controversial. Several theories have been proposed to explain the mechanism by which exercise may affect cognitive performance. Most theorists suggest that exercise benefits cognitive functioning via improvements in cardiovascular efficiency, although central nervous system changes and reduced affective distress also are implicated.

Theoretical Bases for the Influence of Exercise on Cognitive Function

There are four dominant theories in the literature pertaining to exercise effects and cognitive function. First, early theorists suggested that exercise contributes to aerobic capacity and cerebral circulation and enhances functioning of the neurons that activate muscle fibers (Spirduso, 1980). It has been thought that diseases of aging, such as cardiovascular disease, contribute to inefficient cerebral circulation and reduced oxygenation of the brain. According to this model, decreased blood flow in the brain is associated with diminished oxygenation of the brain, which, in turn, is associated with diminished brain function. The mechanism responsible for diminished brain function is not total cerebral blood flow, which would not be expected to change, but regional cerebral blood flow. In theory, exercise would be likely to increase regional cerebral blood flow to specific brain areas, including prefrontal, somatosensory, and primary motor cortex (Spirduso, 1980). Exercise would thus be expected to attenuate the naturally occurring reductions in blood flow to specific brain areas. Consistent with this theory, it has been suggested that increased availability of oxygen in the brain with exercise contributes to metabolism of neurotransmitters, especially acetylcholine, dopamine, norepinephrine, and serotonin, which, in turn, are associated with changes in neurophysiological and neuropsychological functioning (Dustman et al., 1984, 1990). Availability of circulating glucose in the bloodstream would be associated with fitness level and would enhance higher level cognitive processes (Elsayed, Ismail, & Young, 1980). In support of this general hypothesis, it has been found that treatment with pure oxygen is associated with significant improvement in neuropsychological functioning among older adults with memory problems (Jacobs, Winter, Alvis, & Small, 1969) and among hypoxemic patients with chronic obstructive pulmonary disease (Heaton, Grant, McSweeny, Adams, & Petty, 1983).

A second broad theory suggests that physical exercise increases physical and mental arousal, which, in turn, contributes to attentional processes that are central to cognitive performance. In this model, it is suggested that exercise may facilitate attentional processes initially by enhancing central nervous system function. The nervous system arousal required for engaging in physical exercise is thought to facilitate other brain functions as well (Powell, 1974). However, as the intensity or duration of the exercise increases, muscular fatigue then may eliminate the facilitative effects of the early arousal (Tomporowski & Ellis, 1986).

A third theory posits that because cognitive functioning may be impaired in individuals who are depressed or anxious (Horn, Donaldson, & Engstrom, 1981; Kennelly, Hayslip, & Richardson, 1985), improved cognitive functioning may result from enhanced psychological well-being following exercise.

Fourth, it has been suggested that because sympathetic hyperarousal is associated with impaired performance on tests of cognitive functioning, the reduction in sympathetic tone accompanying chronic exercise may contribute to improved cognitive performance (Eisdorfer, Nowlin, & Wilkie, 1970).

Emanating from this theoretical background and from the applied interest in exercise interventions, numerous studies and clinical programs have been developed to evaluate physical exercise training among older adults.

Types of Exercise Studies

Past studies of exercise among older adults can be categorized in four ways:

1. Early cross-sectional studies evaluated cognitive performance among existing groups of self-reported exercising or nonexercising older adults. These studies are limited by a selection bias, since exercise patterns in such studies can not be manipulated experimentally.
2. Most studies in the literature have evaluated outcomes of exercise interventions lasting anywhere from several weeks to 1 year or more. Such studies of chronic exercise outcomes can address the extent to which exercise contributes to cumulative outcomes over time, as may be found with a parameter such as VO_2max during exercise, which would be expected to improve gradually over time. These studies address the issue of whether cognitive benefits of exercise accrue over time.
3. A small number of studies have been conducted evaluating outcomes of a single bout of exercise. These studies of acute exercise effects are useful for examining responsiveness to exercise on a parameter such as blood pressure, which would be expected to respond immediately to exercise activity. Studies of this type indicate the extent to which cognitive changes occur immediately following a single bout of exercise.
4. Although most of the past research has been conducted with samples of healthy older adults, recent studies have also evaluated cognitive outcomes of exercise among older adults with chronic illness.

These four broad categories of studies will be used as a framework for discussing the effects of exercise on cognitive performance among older adults.

Cross-Sectional Studies of Exercise and Cognitive Performance

Early studies of exercise and cognitive function among older adults evaluated reaction time speed as an indicator of cognitive performance. A classic study in this area was conducted by Spirduso (1975), who categorized adult men by age (younger = 20–30 years vs. older = 50–70 years) and by physical activity level (active vs. inactive, according to self-reported regular racket-sport involvement at least three times a week). Results indicated that older inactive subjects were significantly slower in simple reaction time and movement time than were inactive younger subjects or than active subjects of either age group. Using a similar methodology among women, Rikli and Busch (1986) found that older inactive women (age = 68.9 years) had slower choice reaction time performance than did older active women (age = 68.7 years; defined as those who participated in aerobic exercise at least three times a week), but that activity level did not distinguish performance among younger women (age = 21–22 years). More recent cross-sectional data suggest that older active men (as defined by self-reported exercise activity) demonstrate significantly better performance than older sedentary men in performance on a coding task requiring visuospatial processing (Stones & Kozma, 1989), and that visuospatial performance is associated with fitness level (as measured by predicted VO_2max) among older men, but not among middle-aged or younger men (Shay & Roth, 1992). The latter study found no fitness effects for performance on cognitive tasks measuring attention and concentration, verbal memory, or sensorimotor performance. However, Clarkson-Smith and Hartley (1989) found that older adults (mean age = 67 years) categorized as high exercisers (based on self-report of overall activity level) performed better than low exercisers (mean age = 72 years) on measures of reasoning, working memory, and reaction time. Dustman and colleagues (1990) evaluated neurophysiological endpoints (e.g., electroencephalogram, event-related potential, visual sensitivity) among young (20–31 years) and old (50–62 years) men, who were categorized as high fit or low fit (by use of VO_2max from an exercise test). Results indicated that high-fit subjects had better neurocognitive performance, enhanced visual sensitivity, and shorter ERP latency regardless of age.

Summary

The data from these cross-sectional studies strongly support the notion that self-reported exercise behavior and/or physical fitness is associated with enhanced performance on cognitive tasks assessing psychomotor performance, visuospatial performance, and reasoning. These fitness differences are generally supported by the data from neurophysiological brain studies, although results on visual sensitivity (as assessed by Critical Flicker Fusion threshold) were equivocal, with one study finding a fitness effect (Dustman et al., 1990) and one study finding no effect (Shay & Roth, 1992). There is no support for the notion that exercise activity is associated with enhanced performance on cognitive tasks requiring attention and concentration, and there is only limited support for an association of exercise with memory. The results are limited by self-selection factors, since subjects were not randomly assigned to conditions. In addition, most of these studies relied on self-report of exercise activity level, without more objective documentation of fitness level. Only Dustman et al. (1990) utilized a maximal exercise stress test to categorize subjects into fitness groups, and Shay and Roth (1992) used predicted VO_2max for categorizing subjects. Although self-reported exercise activity is appealing from a practical standpoint, it presents a confound for determining the relationship between physical fitness and cognitive performance, since self-reports may be biased by many factors including social desirability, education, and socioeconomic status.

Effects of Chronic Exercise on Neuropsychological Functioning

Physical Exercise Interventions

Exercise conditioning programs for older adults typically include aerobic exercise as a foundation. Aerobic exercise requires oxygenation of the muscle cells for metabolism of free fatty acids into energy for muscle contractions and is characterized by the rhythmic movement of large muscle groups, as occurs in activities such as walking, running, bicycling, and swimming. Exercise interventions for older adults also may include anaerobic exercise, such as strength training with weights or elastic bands. Anaerobic exercise requires a high physical work level, which leads to muscular fatigue and limits the duration of the activity. Most researchers and clinicians agree that the cardiorespiratory benefits of exercise will be achieved with a program of exercise lasting at least 8 weeks, with 1-hour exercise sessions two to three times per week. Exercise sessions typically begin with a brief 5- to 10-minute warm-up period, during which participants engage in muscle-stretching exercises to enhance range of motion and prepare the muscles for more intensive exercise. This warm-up is followed by 20–40 minutes of aerobic exercise (or 20–30 minutes of anaerobic exercise), and exercise is completed with a 5- to 10-minute cool-down period during which participants engage in further muscle-stretching exercises while allowing heart rate to return to resting levels.

Cognitive Outcomes of Exercise

Previous studies examining the effects of physical exercise interventions on neuropsychological functioning have produced conflicting results. Early studies suggested a positive association of exercise with enhanced cognitive functioning. Powell (1974) found enhanced performance on the Progressive Matrices Test and Wechsler Memory Scale associated with exercise in a study of 30 institutionalized older adults (mean age = 69.3 years) randomly assigned to exercise, social activity, or a waiting-list control group for 12 weeks. In addition, three observational studies (i.e., with nonrandomized groups) have examined exercise outcomes and cognitive performance. Elsayed et al. (1980) examined the effects of exercise on fluid intelligence (i.e., concept formation, reasoning, and abstract thinking) and crystallized intelligence (i.e., learned information), as measured by the Culture Fair Intelligence Test, among subjects who were initially divided into four groups: high-fit/young, high-fit/old, low-fit/young, and low-fit/old. All subjects attended three sessions of exercise (90 minutes per session) for 4 months. At the end of 4 months, all groups scored higher on the fluid intelligence measures. Across groups, younger subjects scored better than older subjects, and high-fit subjects scored better than the low-fit subjects. In a study of older adult (mean age of two groups = 58 and 62 years) exercise participants at a fitness club (Stacey, Kozma, & Stones, 1985), 6-month follow-up data indicated enhanced performance on a reaction time task and on the Digit Symbol test of the WAIS-R. However, neither of the latter studies included nonexercise controls; thus, improved performance may have reflected practice effects. Perri and Templer (1984–1985) compared memory performance (as measured by the Rey Auditory Verbal Learning Test) of a nonrandomized control group of 19 nonexercising subjects (mean age = 65.3) with that of 23 subjects participating in a 14-week exercise program (mean age = 65.6). Results indicated no effect of exercise on short-term or long-term memory.

Several larger scale randomized studies have been conducted evaluating psychological well-being and neuropsychological functioning of older adults, as shown in Table 7.1. Dustman and colleagues (1984) conducted one of the first randomized studies of community-residing older adults, with documented exercise training effects, demonstrating significant cognitive improvement associated with aerobic exercise. They observed an impressive 27% increase in VO$_2$max among exercise subjects. A recent study by Williams and Lord (1997) found significant benefits of exercise for reaction time and short-term memory. Although this study was impressive in its inclusion of a large sample of women followed over a 12-month period, the study did not evaluate VO$_2$max, and there was a high degree of variability in adherence to the exercise program. Thus, it is difficult to attribute cognitive changes directly to exercise conditioning.

In addition, two large-scale, randomized studies have revealed negative results. Blumenthal and colleagues (1989) found relatively few changes associated with aerobic exercise among 101 older men and women, despite a 12% increase in VO$_2$max. Because experimental and control groups improved on several of the neuropsychological measures, results were attributed to practice effects rather than to the exercise intervention. Exercise also was not associated with improved reaction time performance in this study (Madden, Blumenthal, Allen, & Emery, 1989), and after a 14-month follow-up, improvement in neuropsychological functioning was attributed to practice effects rather than to exercise effects (Blumenthal et al., 1991). Similarly, a 12-month exercise intervention conducted by Hill, Storandt, and Malley (1993) failed to find improvement on cognitive measures assessing memory, psychomotor speed, and attention, despite a significant 23% improvement in fitness level in the exercise group.

Six additional studies suggest that exercise interventions have minimal influence on cognitive performance among healthy older adults (Emery & Gatz, 1990; Hassmen, Ceci, & Backman, 1992; Molloy, Richardson, & Crilly, 1988; Okumiya et al., 1996; Panton, Graves, Pollock, Hagberg, & Chen, 1990; Stevenson & Topp, 1990), as shown in Table 7.1. Five of these studies were conducted with community-residing healthy older adults, and only the Molloy et al. study was conducted with institutionalized women. Although the study by Okumiya et al. indicated significant improvement on two of the neurobehavioral measures, neither test reflected specific cognitive functions (i.e., one test reflected physical mobility; the other, balance).

Summary

Early studies indicated improved cognitive performance associated with exercise interventions, but more recent studies have indicated minimal effects of exercise on cognitive function. Two exceptions are the studies by Dustman et al. (1984) and Williams and Lord (1997). The positive results of the Dustman et al. study may stem from inclusion of a relatively younger sample and a very large increase in VO$_2$max. The Williams and Lord results are countered by those of Hill et al. (1993), who studied subjects over a similar (12-month) time frame and found no cognitive effects. Al-

Table 7.1. Selected Randomized Intervention Studies of Exercise Effects on Cognitive Function Among Older Adults

Author	Sample	Exercise/duration	Results
Dustman et al. (1984)	Health men ($n = 27$) and women ($n = 16$) Mean age = 60.1	AE, stength/flex., nonrandom NEC, 4-month follow-up	+Critical Flicker Fusion +Digit symbol +RT, Stroop
Williams and Lord (1997)	187 community-residing women. Mean age = 72	AE, NEC, 442-week follow-up	+RT, Digit Span −Picture arrangement −Cattell's Matrices
Blumenthal et al. (1989)	Health men ($n = 50$) and women ($n = 51$) Mean age = 67	AE, yoga, NEC, 16-week follow-up	−Tapping, Story Memory −Digit Span, visual retention −Selective Reminding, Digit Symbol, Trail Making, 2 and 7 Test, Verbal Fluency, Non-Verbal Fluency, Stroop
Hill, Storandt, and Malley (1993)	121 men (50%) and women Mean age = 64	AE, NEC, 12-month follow-up	−Digit Symbol −Logical memory −Crossing-off
Molloy, Richardson, and Crilly (1988)	50 institutionalized women Mean age = 82–83	AE, NEC, 3-month follow-up	−Color slide test −Digit Symbol, Digit Span −Logical memory, word fluency
Emery and Gatz (1990)	48 community-residing women (83%) and men Mean age = 72	AE, social control, NEC, 12-week follow-up	−Digit Symbol, Digit Span, −Writing speed
Panton, Graves, Pollock, Hagberg, and Chen (1990)	49 men (47%) and women Age range: 70–79	Walk/jog vs. strength training, 6-month follow-up	−Total RT, premotor time, movement time, speed of movement
Stevenson and Topp (1990)	72 community-residing men and women (55%) Mean age = 64	AE hi-intensity, AE lo-intensity, 9-month follow-up	+Strub and Black Test (attention, memory, higher cognitive skills) −Intensity effect
Hassmen, Ceci, and Backman (1992)	32 older women, two age groups (55–65, 66–75)	AE, NEC, 3-month follow-up	−SRT, CRT, Digit Span, face recognition
Okumiya et al. (1996)	42 community-residing men (43%) and women Mean age = 79	Home walking, NEC, 6-month follow-up	−Mini-Mental State Exam −Hasegawa Dementia Scale −Visuospatial cognitive performance +Up and Go Test, functional reach

Note. AE = aerobic exercise; NEC = nonexercise control; + = significant improvement on this outcome associated with exercise only; − = no improvement associated with exercise; CRT = choice reaction time; SRT = simple reaction time; RT = reaction time.

though the Williams and Lord results are limited by the absence of VO_2max data, the inclusion of only women in their study may suggest gender effects that could warrant further exploration.

Acute Exercise Outcomes

It has been suggested that acute bouts of exercise initially may facilitate attentional processes by directly stimulating the central nervous system (Tomporowski & Ellis, 1986). However, this facilitative effect then may be counteracted by muscular fatigue. Thus, in theory, an individual's level of physical fitness would have an impact on neuropsychological changes following an acute bout of exercise (Tomporowski & Ellis, 1986). An interaction effect has been observed among younger subjects, wherein physically fit individuals improve more than less fit individuals on cognitive measures following acute exercise (Gutin, 1966; Gutin & DiGennaro, 1968). Few studies have examined the acute effects of exercise, and most of the extant studies have been conducted with college-age subjects. However, two relatively recent studies of older adults help illustrate both the strengths and the weaknesses of research in this area. Molloy, Beerschoten, Borrie, Crilly, and Cape (1988) examined acute effects of a 45-minute exercise session on mood and cognitive functioning of 15 older adults (mean age 66) who had complained of memory loss or cognitive impairment. The exercise condition consisted of a 5-minute warm-up, 20 minutes of light aerobic exercise (walking or playing games), and 15 minutes of stretching exercises. The control condition consisted of watching another subject participate in the exercise condition. The study was counterbalanced, with all subjects participating in both the exercise and the control conditions, and a period of 1 week separated each testing session. Assessments included measures of memory, problem solving, and verbal fluency, and results indicated improvement in logical memory (from the Wechsler Memory Scale) and in scores on the Mini-Mental State Examination.

Emery, Honn, Becker, and Frid (1996) conducted a study of acute exercise effects and cognitive function among 24 older (mean age = 68.6) men and women. Each subject participated in 20 minutes of exercise on a stationary bicycle and 20 minutes of watching a videotape about exercise, with assessments of cognitive function (psychomotor speed, memory, executive function) before and after each condition. Order of conditions was randomly assigned to subjects, and participation in each condition was separated by 1 week. Results indicated improved cognitive performance associated with both conditions, suggesting practice effects rather than exercise effects.

Summary

No additional published studies have examined acute effects of exercise on cognitive function, although several other studies have evaluated emotional changes associated with acute bouts of exercise. The methodological limitations of studies in this area (e.g., small sample size, confounding practice effect due to repeated measures occurring in short time interval, potential for regression to the mean when subjects enter the study complaining of memory problems) may restrict the conclusions that can be drawn. However, this methodology may be promising for further evaluation of mechanisms by which exercise is associated with cognitive function. Cognitive changes occurring acutely would be more likely to support an arousal model of exercise effects, but changes occurring following an intervention would be more likely to support a model of cardiovascular fitness as a critical factor.

Exercise Effects Among Chronically Ill Older Adults

Increased life expectancy in recent decades has meant that greater numbers of older adults are afflicted with chronic, physically debilitating illnesses, including chronic obstructive pulmonary disease (COPD), arthritis, hypertension, and Alzheimer's disease. Often exercise is an integral aspect of rehabilitation programs for such individuals, and the data available from exercise rehabilitation programs, although limited, suggest positive cognitive outcomes.

Lung Disease

Patients with COPD generally suffer from long-lasting reductions of blood oxygen (PaO_2), and it has been suggested that chronic reduction of PaO_2 also significantly contributes to cognitive deficits (Fishman & Petty, 1971). In studies of hypoxemic patients, deficits in simple motor skills and concentration were found (Grant, Heaton, McSweeny, Adams, & Timms, 1982), although language and memory were relatively unaffected, and neuropsychological impairment was associated with low levels of blood oxygen. Prigatano, Parsons, Wright, Levin, and Hawryluk (1983) concluded that the most likely explanation for impaired cognitive functioning in COPD patients is either (a) lower levels of blood oxygenation, leading to inefficiencies in neural functioning, or (b) COPD contributing to increased vascular disease, which, in turn, leads to reductions in cerebral blood flow and oxygen consumption. In either case, among COPD patients, the primary source of cognitive deficits appears to be directly related to blood oxygen levels. Further support for this hypothesis comes from studies in which continuous oxygen treatment reversed impairments among COPD patients on measures of visuospatial function and simple motor movement (Krop, Block, & Cohen, 1973).

In a recent study, Emery, Schein, Hauck, and MacIntyre (1998) evaluated the effects of exercise on psychological well-being and cognitive functioning among 79 older adults (mean age = 66.6 ± 6.5) with COPD. Subjects were randomly assigned to an exercise condition (exercise, education, and social support), an education condition (education and social support), or a waiting-list group during a 10-week intervention period. The exercise component included walking, strength training, and bicycle ergometry training. The cognitive assessments (attention, motor speed, mental efficiency, and verbal processing) conducted before and after the intervention period indicated that subjects in the exercise condition improved significantly on the measure of verbal processing showing self-control and self-monitoring characteristic of executive cognitive functions. Subjects in the two control groups manifested no change on this measure. Thus, the study offers preliminary evidence of cognitive benefit of exercise among COPD patients participating in exercise rehabilitation and suggests that improvement in executive cognitive function resulted from changes in neural processing.

Heart Disease

Age-related increases in the incidence of cardiovascular disease have been attributed, in part, to deconditioning and inactivity (Bortz, 1982). In turn, patients with coronary heart disease (CHD) may be at risk for cerebral infarction or hemorrhage. Deterioration of the cardiovascular system associated with arteriosclerosis and heart disease may reduce cerebral blood flow and thus result in decreased cerebral oxygen consumption. A relatively high incidence of cognitive deficits has been observed in one past study of medically stable cardiac inpatients (approximately 20% of the sample) despite the absence of neurological deficits (Garcia, Tweedy, & Blass, 1984), and cognitive deficits have been observed among cardiac rehabilitation patients following cardiac surgery (Robinson, Blumenthal, Burker, Hlatky, & Reves, 1990). Although the nature and extent of postsurgical cognitive deficits varies widely across studies, the deficits are thought to result from intraoperative microemboli or hypoperfusion, and they may resolve spontaneously over a period ranging from several days to several months. However, in a cardiac rehabilitation setting, Barclay, Weiss, Mattis, Bond, and Blass (1988) observed mild to moderate cognitive impairment among 70% of 20 clinically stable older (mean age $= 72.5 \pm 2.1$ years) patients. A large proportion of the sample (35%) was impaired to such a degree that they were unable to self-administer medications appropriately. Thus, cognitive impairment among cardiac patients may range from mild difficulty on standardized tests of attention and concentration, to more significant memory deficits, to very significant difficulty with activities of daily living (ADLs) such as medication use.

Exercise studies of patients with coronary artery disease (CAD) have also been conducted, but only one study has been conducted with older cardiac patients. Satoh, Sakurai, Miyagi, and Hohshaku (1995) studied walking behavior among 46 mostly female (76%) older (age > 70 years) Japanese cardiac patients. All subjects had a history of myocardial infarction (MI) or arrhythmia, but none had cerebrovascular disease. Subjects were evaluated with a standard Japanese cognitive assessment of memory and general knowledge, which indicated that the largest proportion of subjects performed in the normal range at baseline (43%), but a significant proportion were demented (9%), and the remainder were either subnormal (30%) or predementia (17%). Results of repeated testing at 1-year follow-up indicated that greater walking was associated with a reduction in cognitive deficits (i.e., subjects categorized at a less impaired level at one-year testing). One strength of this study was its use of a community-based sample of older cardiac patients, although it was limited by the absence of a control group, minimal cognitive outcomes, and no objective measurement of fitness level.

Alzheimer's Disease

Only one published study has examined the impact of exercise on cognitive function among patients with Alzheimer's disease. Palleschi, Vetta, De Gennaro, and Idone (1996) evaluated the effects of a 3-month stationary-bicycle-riding intervention among 15 men (mean age 74 years) with dementia of the Alzheimer type. Cognitive assessment evaluated attention, verbal span, and the Mini-Mental State Exam. Results indicated improved performance on all cognitive tests. Although no control group was included to account for practice effects, this study is an important first step in evaluating exercise effects among demented older adults. The paucity of research studies in this area may reflect, in part, the difficulty of conducting a systematic evaluation of patients with Alzheimer's disease. It also reflects the relative novelty of assessing exercise effects among patients with dementia, although exercise is often included in treatment programs for Alzheimer's patients in nursing-home or day-treatment settings.

Summary

Few studies have been conducted evaluating cognitive effects of exercise among chronically ill older adults. However, the limited data suggest that exercise may have beneficial effects for tasks reflecting attention, verbal capacity, and self-monitoring. Further, the data may indicate that subjects with cognitive impairment at baseline may be more likely to achieve cognitive gains with exercise. However, the data in this area are minimal, and only preliminary conclusions are possible at present.

Conclusions

Research studies of exercise among healthy older adults have become increasingly sophisticated in recent years. Studies now commonly utilize randomized control groups, including exercise controls as well as nonexercise controls, and objective indicators of cardiovascular fitness, such as VO_2max. Studies have successfully recruited larger samples to increase the power of statistical analyses, and most studies of chronic exercise effects now routinely provide an exercise intervention of at least three 1-hour sessions per week over a 3- to 4-month period. Several studies have achieved more ambitious interventions of 12-month duration. However, there remains a lack of consistency in the data. While cross-sectional studies comparing long-term exercisers with sedentary older adults indicate an association of exercise with aspects of cognitive performance, these studies are severely limited by a self-selection bias. Intervention studies tend to suggest that exercise does not have a beneficial effect on cognitive functioning. One potential problem with past intervention studies documenting minimal improvements in neuropsychological functioning is that participation criteria for studies of healthy older adults may eliminate subjects exhibiting cognitive impairment, who could most benefit from exercise. Studies of impaired or chronically ill older adults are commonly conducted with small numbers of subjects, in part, because of the additional resources required to maintain adequate exercise adherence in these subjects. Although the small samples and unique characteristics of the subjects restrict generalizability, there is need for further study of exercise among chronically ill older adults (e.g., those with cardiovascular disease, pulmonary disease, dementing illnesses). Indeed, because changes in nondiseased older adults may, in fact, reflect early cognitive signs of occult disease, studies of older adults with chronic illness may have greater generalizability than it would appear.

One methodological limitation of data in this area is that the neuropsychological measures used to assess cognitive functioning may not be sensitive to the kinds of changes occurring during exercise among older adults. Data indicate that older adults perceive significant improvements in cognitive function following regular exercise despite the absence of objective evidence of change (Emery & Blumenthal, 1990). Although self-reports of cognitive improvement may reflect a demand effect of exercise studies or a secondary result of enhanced mood following exercise, it is also possible that alternate measures of cognitive performance should be considered, assessing the types of everyday problem solving that older adults would be most likely to confront.

The research literature does not clearly support any single model to explain the association of cognitive functioning and exercise. The limited data from studies of acute exercise would support the notion that exercise increases mental arousal via enhanced central nervous system function or, perhaps, via reduction in sympathetic tone. Intervention studies, overall, do not provide support for cardiovascular fitness as a central factor in cognitive outcomes. Although the cross-sectional data provide support for the importance of cardiovascular fitness, these data are limited by self-selection factors. The data also do not support mood changes as a likely moderator of cognitive improvement in exercise intervention studies. Of the two studies in table 7.1 that demonstrated positive effects of aerobic exercise on cognitive function (Dustman et al., 1984; Williams & Lord, 1997), only the Williams and Lord study reported enhanced psychological well-being as well. Studies of acute exercise effects suggest positive effects on mood, although this may be true only for subgroups of subjects (Emery, Honn, Becker, & Frid, 1996). Any improvement in mood resulting from individual exercise sessions would be likely to contribute to exercise adherence and thus could be indirectly associated with enhanced cognitive performance. From this perspective, cognitive change in exercise programs may reflect several different processes associated with exercise. Further elaboration of acute exercise effects versus chronic effects may help to elucidate further the mechanisms by which exercise may affect cognitive functioning.

One practical goal for future research in this area would be to develop data-based guidelines for the use of exercise in prevention and rehabilitation of older adults with cognitive deficits or at risk for cognitive deficits. At present, there is no hard evidence to support the use of exercise for cognitive rehabilitation, and there are not clear guidelines for determining a correct "dose" of exercise. Thus, the research problem must be approached directly, and clinical applications must be instituted cautiously. Studies of physiological outcomes indicate guidelines for ensuring an exercise training effect (e.g., three times a week over a 3- to 4-month period). Presumably this would be a minimal criterion for interventions designed to increase cognitive performance, but positive results from the Dustman et al. (1984) study and Williams and Lord (1997) suggest that intensity level or duration may need to be considered further, since Dustman et al. observed a 27% increase in VO_2max, and Williams and Lord evaluated a 42-week program of exercise. Thus, although cardiovascular improvements may occur within several months, cognitive changes may not occur without a very sizable increase in fitness or a long-term intervention. To the extent that the cross-sectional data indicate benefits of long-term exercise for cognitive performance, exercise may be important in preventing cognitive decline. From a prevention perspective, it may be more appropriate to hypothesize that exercise will prevent cognitive decline rather than that exercise will augment cognitive functioning. Longitudinal studies would help address the utility of a prevention model in research on cognitive function.

Indeed, the data overall suggest a need for methodologically strong longitudinal studies evaluating exercise performance and cognitive functioning. Use of objective markers of cardiovascular fitness would be imperative, as well as providing a consistent exercise stimulus and accounting for important individual differences in health behavior, educational attainment, and cultural differences. Although most exercise interventions are conducted in a group format, several studies have evaluated home exercise programs in which the subject may exercise alone. Such interventions may have greater practical utility among older populations and may facilitate collecting longitudinal data. In addition to studies evaluating longitudinal effects of exercise interventions, there is a need for further research evaluating gender differences in cognitive outcomes of exercise.

References

Aniansson, A., Grimby, G., Rundgren, A., Svanborg, A., & Orlander, J. (1980). Physical training in old men. *Age and Ageing, 9,* 186–187.

Bachmann, G. A., & Grill, J. (1987). Exercise in the postmenopausal woman. *Geriatrics, 42,* 75–77, 81–85.

Barclay, L. L., Weiss, E. M., Mattis, S., Bond, O., & Blass, J. P. (1988). Unrecognized cognitive impairment in cardiac rehabilitation patients. *Journal of the American Geriatrics Society, 36,* 22–28.

Blumenthal, J. A., Emery, C. F., Madden, D. J., George, L. K., Coleman, R. E., Riddle, M. W., McKee, D. C., Reasoner, J., & Williams, R. S. (1989). Cardiovascular and behavioral effects of aerobic exercise training in healthy older men and women. *Journal of Gerontology, 44,* M147–157.

Blumenthal, J. A., Emery, C. F., Madden, D. J., Schniebolk, S., Walsh-Riddle, M., George, L. K., Higginbotham, M. B., McKee, D. C., Sullivan, M. J., & Coleman, R. E. (1991). Long term effects of exercise on psychological functioning in older men and women. *Journal of Gerontology, 46,* P352–361.

Bortz, W. (1982). Disease and aging. *Journal of the American Medical Association, 248,* 1203–1208.

Bouchard, C., Shephard, R. J., Stephens, T., Sutton, J. R., & McPherson, B. D. (1990). Exercise, fitness, and health: The consensus statement. In Bouchard, C., Shephard, R. J., Stephens, T., Sutton, J. R., & McPherson, B. D. (Eds.), *Exercise, fitness, and health* (pp. 3–28). Champaign, IL: Human Kinetics.

Bruce, R.A. (1984). Exercise, functional aerobic capacity, and aging-another viewpoint. *Medicine and Science in Sports and Exercise, 16,* 8–13.

Buskirk, E. R., & Hodgson, J. L. (1987). Age and aerobic power: The rate of change in men and women. *Aging and Exercise: Physiological Interactions. Federation Proceedings, 46,* 1824–1829.

Clarkson-Smith, L., & Hartley, A. A. (1989), Relationships between physical exercise and cognitive abilities in older adults. *Psychology and Aging, 4,*(2), 183–189.

Craik, F. I. M., & Jennings, J. M. (1992). Human memory. In F. I. M. Craik & T. A. Salthouse (Eds.), *Handbook of aging and cognition* (pp. 51–110). Hillsdale, NJ: Erlbaum.

DiGiovanna, A .G. (1994). *Human aging: Biological perspectives.* New York: McGraw-Hill.

Dustman, R. E., Emmerson, R. Y., Ruhling, R. O., Shearer, D. E., Steinhaus, L. A., Johnson,

S. C., Bonekat, H. W., & Shigeoka, J. W. (1990). Age and fitness effects on EEG, ERPs, visual sensitivity, and cognition. *Neurobiology of Aging, 11,* 193–200.

Dustman, R., Ruhling, R., Russell, E., Shearer, D., Bonekat, W., Shigeoka, J., Wood, J., & Bradford, D. (1984). Aerobic exercise training and improved neuropsychological function of older individuals. *Neurobiology of Aging, 5,* 35–42.

Ehsani, A. A. (1987). Cardiovascular adaptations to exercise training in the elderly. *Aging and Exercise: Physiological Interactions. Federation Proceedings, 46,* 1840–1843.

Eisdorfer, C., Nowlin, J., & Wilkie, F. (1970). Improvement of learning in the aged by modification of autonomic nervous system activity. *Science, 170,* 1327–1329.

Elsayed, M., Ismail, A., & Young, R. (1980). Intellectual differences of adult men related to age and physical fitness before and after an exercise program. *Journal of Gerontology, 35,* 383–387.

Emery, C. F., & Blumenthal, J. A. (1990). Perceived change among participants in an exercise program for older adults. *Gerontologist, 30,* 516–521.

Emery, C. F., & Gatz, M. (1990). Psychological and cognitive effects of an exercise program for community-residing older adults. *Gerontologist, 30,* 184–188.

Emery, C. F., Honn, V., Becker, N. L., & Frid, D. J. (1996). Acute effects of exercise on mood and cognitive function of older adults (abstract). *Gerontologist, 36*(1), 53.

Emery, C. F., Schein, R. L., Hauck, E. R., & MacIntyre, N. R. (1998). Psychological and cognitive outcomes of a randomized trial of exercise among patients with chronic obstructive pulmonary disease. *Health Psychology, 17,* 232–240.

Evans, W. J., & Cyr-Campbell, D. (1997). Nutrition, exercise, and healthy aging. *Journal of the American Dietetic Association, 97,* 632–638.

Fishman, D. B., & Petty, T. L. (1971). Physical, symptomatic and psychological improvement in patients receiving comprehensive care for chronic airway obstruction. *Journal of Chronic Diseases, 24,* 775–785.

Garcia, C. A., Tweedy, J. R., & Blass, J. P. (1984). Underdiagnosis of cognitive impairment in a rehabilitation setting. *Journal of the American Geriatrics Society, 32,* 339–342.

Grant, I., Heaton, R. K., McSweeny, A. J., Adams, K. M., & Timms, R. M. (1980). Brain dysfunction in COPD. *Chest, 77*(Suppl.), 308–309.

Grant, I., Heaton, R. K., McSweeny, A. J., Adams, K. M., & Timms, R. M. (1982). Neuropsychologic findings in hypoxemic chronic obstructive pulmonary disease. *Archives of Internal Medicine, 142,* 1470–1476.

Gutin, B. (1966). Effect of increase in physical fitness on mental ability following physical and mental stress. *Research Quarterly, 37:* 211–220.

Gutin, B., & DiGennaro, J. (1968). Effect of one-minute and five-minute step-ups on performance of simple addition. *Research Quarterly, 39,* 81–85.

Hassmen, P., Ceci, R., & Backman, L. (1992). Exercise for older women: A training method and its influences on physical and cognitive performance. *European Journal of Applied Physiology & Occupational Physiology, 64*(5), 460–466.

Heaton, R. K., Grant, I., McSweeny, A. J., Adams, K. M., & Petty, T. L. (1983). Psychologic effects of continuous and nocturnal oxygen therapy in hypoxemic chronic obstructive pulmonary disease. *Archives of Internal Medicine, 143,* 1941–1947.

Hill, R. D., Storandt, M., & Malley, M. (1993). The impact of long-term exercise training on psychological function in older adults. *Journal of Gerontology: Psychological Sciences, 48,*(1),12–17.

Horn, J., Donaldson, G., & Engstrom, R. (1981). Apprehension, memory, and fluid intelligence decline in adulthood. *Research on Aging, 3,* 33–44.

Jacobs, E. A., Winter, P. M., Alvis, H. J., & Small, S. M. (1969). Hyperoxygenation effect on cognitive functioning in the aged. *New England Journal of Medicine, 281,* 753–757.

Kasch, F. W., Wallace, J. P., & Van Camp, S. P. (1985). Effects of 18 years of endurance exercise on the physical work capacity of older men. *Journal of Cardiopulmonary Rehabilitation, 5,* 308–312.

Kennelly, K., Hayslip, B., & Richardson, S. (1985). Depression and helplessness-induced cognitive deficits in the aged. *Experimental Aging Research, 11,*169–173.

Krop, H., Block, A. J., & Cohen, E. (1973). Neuropsychologic effects of continuous oxygen therapy in chronic obstructive pulmonary disease. *Chest, 64,* 317–322.

Lezak, M. D. (1995). *Neuropsychological assessment* (3rd ed.). New York: Oxford University Press.

Madden, D. J., Blumenthal, J. A., Allen, P. A., & Emery, C. F. (1989). Improving aerobic capacity in healthy older adults does not necessarily lead to improved cognitive performance. *Psychology and Aging, 4,* 307–320.

Mahler, D. A., Rosiello, R. A., & Loke, J. (1986). The aging lung. *Geriatrics Clinics of North America, 2,* 215–225.

McMurdo, M. E. T., & Rennie, L. M. (1994). Improvements in quadriceps strength with regular seated exercise in the institutionalized elderly. *Archives of Physical Medicine and Rehabilitation, 75,* 600–603.

Molloy, D., Beerschoten, D., Borrie, M., Crilly, R., & Cape, D. (1988). Acute effects of exercise on neuropsychological function in elderly subjects. *Journal of the American Geriatrics Society, 36,* 29–33.

Molloy, D. W., Richardson, L. D., & Crilly, R. G. (1988). The effects of a three-month exercise programme on neuropsychological function in elderly institutionalized women: A randomized controlled trial. *Age and Ageing, 17,* 303–310.

Nieman, D. C., Warren, B. J., O'Donnell, K. A., Dotson, R. G., Butterworth, D. E., & Henson, D. A. (1993). Physical activity and serum lipids and lipoproteins in elderly women. *Journal of the American Geriatrics Society, 41,* 1339–1344.

Okumiya, K., Matsubayashi, K., Wada, T., Kimura, S., Doi, Y., & Ozawa, T. (1996). Effects of exercise on neurobehavioral function in community-dwelling older people more than 75 years of age. *Journal of American Geriatric Society, 44,* 569–572.

Palleschi, L., Vetta, F., De Gennaro, E., & Idone, G. (1996). Effect of aerobic training on the cognitive performance of elderly patients with senile dementia of Alzheimer type. *Archives of Gerontology and Geriatrics* (Suppl. 5), 47–50.

Panton, L. B., Graves, J. E., Pollock, M. L., Hagberg, J. M., & Chen, W. (1990). Effect of aerobic and resistance training on fractionated reaction time and speed of movement. *Journal of Gerontology, 45,* M26–31.

Perri, S., & Templer, D. (1984–1985). The effects of an aerobic exercise program on psychological variables in older adults. *International Journal of Aging and Human Development, 20,* 167–172.

Powell, R. R. (1974). Psychological effects of exercise therapy upon institutionalized geriatric mental patients. *Journal of Gerontology, 29,* 157–161.

Prigatano, G. P., Parsons, O., Wright, E., Levin, D. C., & Hawryluk, G. (1983). Neuropsychological test performance in mildly hypoxemic patients with chronic obstructive pulmonary disease. *Journal of Consulting and Clinical Psychology, 51,* 108–116.

Prinz, P. N., Dustman, R. E., & Emmerson, R. Y. (1990). Electrophysiology and aging. In J. E. Birren & K. W. Schaie (Eds.), *Handbook of the psychology of aging* (3rd ed.). San Diego: Academic Press.

Pyka, G., Lindenberger, E., Charette, S., & Marcus, R. (1994). Muscle strength and fiber adaptations to a year-long resistance training program in elderly men and women. *Journal of Gerontology, 49,* 22–27.

Raz, I., Hauser, E., & Bursztyn, M. (1994). Moderate exercise improves glucose metabolism in uncontrolled elderly patients with non-insulin-dependent diabetes mellitus. *Israel Journal of Medical Sciences, 30,* 766–770.

Rikli, R., & Busch, S. (1986). Motor performance of women as a function of age and physical activity level. *Journal of Gerontology, 41*(5), 645–649.

Robinson, M., Blumenthal, J. A., Burker, E. J., Hlatky, M., & Reves, J. G. (1990). Coronary artery bypass grafting and cognitive function: A review. *Journal of Cardiopulmonary Rehabilitation, 10,* 180–189.

Rudman, D., Kutner, M. H., Rogers, C. M., Lubin, M. F., Fleming, G. A., & Bain, R. P. (1981). Impaired growth hormone secretion in the adult population relation to age and adiposity. *Journal of Clinical Investigation, 67,* 1361–1369.

Salthouse, T. A. (1991). *Theoretical perspectives on cognitive aging.* Hillsdale, NJ: Erlbaum.

Satoh, T., Sakurai, I., Miyagi, K., & Hohshaku, Y. (1995). Walking exercise and improved neuropsychological functioning in elderly patients with cardiac disease. *Journal of Internal Medicine, 238,* 423–428.

Shay, K. A., & Roth, D. L. (1992). Association between aerobic fitness and visuospatial performance in healthy older adults. *Psychology and Aging, 7,* 15–24.

Singh, N. A., Clements, K. M., & Fiatarone, M. A. (1997). A randomized controlled trial of the effect of exercise on sleep. *Sleep, 20,* 95–101.

Spirduso, W. W. (1975). Reaction and movement time as a function of age and physical activity level. *Journal of Gerontology, 30,* 435–440.

Spirduso, W. W. (1980). Physical fitness, aging, and psychomotor speed: A review. *Journal of Gerontology, 35,* 850–865.

Stacey, C., Kozma, A., & Stones, M. J. (1985). Simple cognitive and behavioural changes resulting from improved physical fitness in persons over 50 years of age. *Canadian Journal on Aging, 4,* 67–74.

Stevenson, J. S., & Topp, R. (1990). Effects of moderate and low intensity long-term exercise by older adults. *Research in Nursing & Health, 13*(4), 209–218.

Stones, M. J., & Kozma, A. (1989). Age, exercise, and coding performance. *Psychology and Aging, 4,* 190–194.

Strandell, T. (1976). Circulatory studies on healthy old men. *Acta Medica Scandinavica, 414,* 1–43.

Tamai, T., Nakai, T., Takai, H., Fujiwara, R., Miyabo, S., Higuchi, M., & Kobayashi, S. (1988). The effects of physical exercise on plasma lipoprotein and apolipoprotein metabolism in elderly men. *Journal of Gerontology, 43,* M75–79.

Tate, C. A., Hyek, M. F., & Taffet, G. E. (1994). Mechanisms for the responses of cardiac muscle to physical activity in old age. *Medicine and Science in Sports and Exercise, 26,* 561–567.

Tomporowski, P. D., & Ellis, N. R. (1986). Effects of exercise on cognitive processes: A review. *Psychological Bulletin, 99,* 338–346.

Williams, P., & Lord, S. R. (1997). Effects of group exercise on cognitive functioning and mood in older women. *Australian and New Zealand Journal of Public Health, 21*(1), 45–52.

8

Smoking and Cognitive Function

Issues in Cognitive Rehabilitation

ROBERT D. HILL

KAREN ROTHBALLER SEELERT

Cigarette smoking is a pervasive high-risk behavior that has been linked to the early emergence and rapid progression of chronic disease in middle and late life. The mechanisms through which smoking impairs healthy functioning and predisposes older adults to chronic illness has been well documented (Fielding, 1985; La-Croix et al., 1991). The vast majority of this research points to the deleterious effects of chronic smoking on both physiological capacity and efficiency as it relates to specific organ systems (Jenkins, Rosenman, & Zyzanski, 1968; Lange et al., 1989; Shinton & Beevers, 1989). What is less well understood about cigarette smoking is its potential to interact with cognitive processes in both normal and diseased aging.

The current chapter explores the mechanisms through which smoking may influence cognitive function across the adult life span as well as examines the impact that smoking behavior may have on rehabilitation efforts in those individuals who smoke into old age and are at risk for cognitive impairment. One goal of this chapter is to develop a conceptual model that outlines specific pathways through which smoking influences cognitive function. Through this model, several important issues are explored: (a) Cigarette smoking exerts both a direct and indirect effect on cognitive performance—direct in that cigarettes themselves contain psychoactive substances that are delivered to the brain via smoke inhalation, and indirect in that chronic use of cigarettes can produce stable changes in systemic efficiency that, in turn, influence brain function; (b) even though smoking has been shown to be hazardous to overall physical health, some aspects of tobacco consumption (e.g., nicotine delivery) may have facilitative effects on cognition. For example, some evidence links cigarette smoking to lowered incidence rates in Alzheimer's disease (AD; Lee, 1994). On the other hand, the role of smoking as an exacerbating agent in vascular and pulmonary disease may magnify the deleterious impact that these exert on cognitive processes (Launer et al., 1996).

This chapter also examines how the connection between cognitive function and chronic smoking may impact cognitive rehabilitation efforts in older adults. Specific sections throughout the chapter highlight these issues and address such questions as: (a) What role might cognitive variables play in smoking cessation and relapse prevention planning? (b) Can efforts to improve cognitive function through compensatory techniques such as physical exercise or memory training benefit older smokers? (c) How does the relationship between cognition and cigarette smoking enhance our understanding of strategies for remediating cognitive loss in diseases of aging such as AD?

An Explanatory Model

Figure 8.1 is an overview of the pathways through which cigarette smoking may mediate cognitive abilities. This figure highlights both (a) the acute and long-term action and (b) the direct and indirect effects of cigarette smoking on cognitive function. By necessity, any model that attempts to capture a phenomenon that involves such a wide array of potential relationships as can be found in cigarette smoking and cognitive function is limiting. However, it can be used as a starting point to organize different bodies of research that have connected cigarette smoking to cognitive performance variables. This model can also facilitate discussion on the possible role that cigarette smoking may play as a mediating variable in late-life cognitive change.

Three pathways are depicted through which cigarette smoking may exert an influence on cognitive function, through (a) nicotine delivery, (b) chronic disease, and (c)

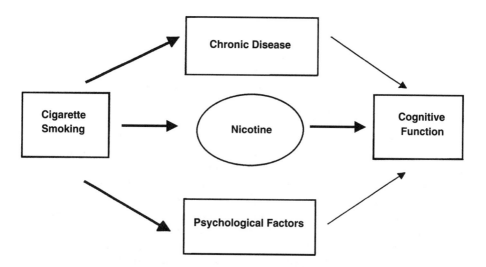

Figure 8.1. Smoking and cognition: An explanatory model.

psychological factors. The nicotine delivery pathway highlights the acute effects of smoking on cognitive function and is based on the notion that cigarette smoke inhalation is an efficient delivery method of nicotine to the brain. The bold arrows characterizing the smoking-nicotine pathway denote the direct effect of cigarette-delivered nicotine on cognitive function. The latter two pathways that show a bold arrow from cigarette smoking to chronic disease and psychological factors denote the direct effect of smoking on these processes. The lighter arrows pointing to cognitive function denote the mediating role that smoking plays on cognitive processes.

It is noteworthy that in most of this research, cognitive function is defined specifically through measures of attention, memory, and psychomotor skills. Measures of attention have included, but are not limited to, alertness and sustained attention (as assessed through vigilance tasks), selectivity (measures of attentional switching and selective attention), and processing capacity (measures of processing speed). With regard to memory, investigations have utilized measures of long- and short-term memory, working memory, and even incidental memory. The measurement of psychomotor skills has included simple and choice reaction time tasks as well as pure psychomotor speed (e.g., tapping). Finally, measures of cognitive impairment have been employed to determine the extent to which smoking can predict the early emergence of organic brain syndromes such as Alzheimer's disease (AD).

Cigarette Smoking, Nicotine, and Short-Term Cognitive Function

There is substantial disagreement as to whether cigarette smoking exerts a short-term deleterious or facilitative effect on cognitive function, particularly with regard to its role as a nicotine delivery mechanism. Of the studies that have investigated acute effects of cigarette smoking, most presume that the active agent is nicotine. Given this assumption, the sections that follow examine (a) the extent to which nicotine itself can influence cognitive performance and (b) the acute effects of cigarette-delivered nicotine on cognitive function.

Nicotine as a Cognitive Enhancer

Nicotine has been described as a tertiary amine that binds with nicotinic cholinergic receptors in the brain (Benowitz, 1996) and, even in relatively low doses, produces a number of predictable physiological and behavioral responses in animals and in humans (Baron, 1996). In humans, nicotine as a central nervous system (CNS) stimulant has been shown to produce a sympathetic nervous system response that is characterized by increased heart and respiratory rate, increased blood pressure, and blood vessel vasoconstriction, as well as changes in body temperature. Nicotine also increases metabolic activity (Perkins et al., 1994), and some research has even suggested that it influences the endocrine system, primarily by stimulating the release of beta endorphins. In this regard, nicotine has been linked to increased levels of ACTH and cortisol (Benowitz, 1996; Newhouse et al., 1990). It has also been documented that nicotine tolerance develops rapidly in humans; that is, increased dosages are needed to maintain stable levels of drug efficacy over time (Perkins et al., 1994).

Nicotine has been linked to a number of behavioral phenomena in animals, including increased locomotor activity and rate of conditioning, and this research has generally supported the hypothesis that nicotine is a cognitive enhancer. The strength of this assertion, however, varies with the concentration of nicotine delivered, the delivery interval, the type of experimental animal used, and the kind of performance tasks employed (Stolerman, Mirza, & Shoaib, 1995).

In humans, studies have examined the relative impact of small amounts of nicotine delivered to nonsmokers (via subcutaneous injection, tablets, nasal sprays, gum, and transdermal patches) on cognitive function. Although research supports its enhancing effects on psychomotor performance (see West & Jarvis; 1986; Perkins et al., 1990), findings are somewhat mixed with regard to nicotine's influence on more complex cognitive tasks, with some studies supporting nicotine as a cognitive enhancer (Provost & Woodward, 1991; Wesnes & Warburton, 1984; Wesnes, Warburton, & Matz, 1983), while others have been unable to reliably establish such an effect (Dunne, MacDonald, & Hartley, 1986; Heishman, Snyder, & Henningfield, 1991). Several generalizable findings have emerged from this research with regard to the impact of nicotine on nonsmokers. First, nicotine administered in sufficient quantities accelerates motor function. Second, nicotine appears to have a short-term enhancing effect on selected indices of cognitive function, given that the dose is optimal and the tasks contain attentional and/or psychomotor properties (e.g., reaction time, vigilance, sustained attention tasks). Whether nicotine enhances memory function or complex cognitive abilities in any reliable way remains an open question.

Based on data that nicotine can have a short-term effect on cognition, its role as an active ingredient in cigarette smoke is examined next. What is critical in this literature is the proposition that if change in smoking behavior can alter cognitive function in the short run in relatively young, nonaddicted smokers, cognitive rehabilitation efforts in older long-term smokers will be influenced by both the length of time that the individual has smoked and the frequency of cigarettes smoked within a given time interval.

Cigarette Smoking and Short-Term Cognitive Function

Although the particulates in cigarette smoke contain potentially several thousand different identifiable compounds, including carbon monoxide (CO), acetaldehyde, and many nonnicotine alkaloids (Dube & Green, 1982), evidence suggests that nicotine is the substance in cigarettes that exerts the greatest psychopharmacological effect on human performance (Stolerman et al., 1995). It is an established fact that cigarettes contain nicotine, although the dosage level varies widely across brands, ranging from less than 0.5 mg to more than 4.0 mg per cigarette. Further, nicotine is rapidly absorbed into the blood from inhaled cigarette smoke and requires less than 20 seconds to pass the blood-brain barrier, so that cigarette smoking can be construed as a highly efficient nicotine delivery mechanism (Benowitz, 1996).

Given the cognitive enhancing properties of nicotine, it should be expected that studies would generally confirm the cognitive enhancing effects of cigarette smoke. Interestingly, this has not been the case. Findings from this literature have varied, with some research demonstrating cognitive advantages associated with cigarette intake (see Wesnes & Warburton, 1984), while others have found no cognitive benefits and even detrimental effects on cognitive performance (Andersson, 1975; Andersson & Hockey, 1977; Gonzales & Harris, 1980; Hill, 1989; Spilich, June, & Renner, 1992). These studies have employed a variety of methodological strategies, including contrasting regular smokers with never-smokers, regular smokers with occasional smokers, nondeprived versus deprived smokers (who vary with regard to the deprivation interval), and even smokers who vary with regard to the time they smoke their first cigarette (early morning versus afternoon). Given this variability in the literature, several reviews have highlighted experimental control problems that make it difficult to interpret these data (see Levin, 1992; Spilich, 1994; Stolerman et al., 1995), including (a) difficulty in accurately assessing smoking history in current and former smokers, (b) individual differences in tissue concentrations of nicotine at the time of testing (which is particularly problematic in long-term smokers), and (c) sampling biases. Further, this research has not made a systematic attempt to disentangle the specific effects of nicotine from those of other substances in cigarette smoke that may offset its nicotine's influence, such as carbon monoxide (CO).

Several theories have been proposed to explain how cognitive performance may be affected by cigarette consumption. The first suggests that cigarette-delivered nicotine should objectively enhance cognition. Thus, those who smoke cigarettes at the time of testing should outperform comparable nonsmokers on selected cognitive tasks that are sensitive to the CNS-arousing properties of nicotine. In support of this contention, West and Hack (1991) examined the effect of cigarette smoking on a memory search task in regular and occasional smokers. Subjects were tested before and after a 24-hour period of abstinence, at which point they smoked cigarettes that either contained nicotine or were nicotine-free. Smoking the nicotine-containing cigarettes resulted in increased search speed in both groups of smokers, and it was concluded that nicotine was responsible for this increase. Several methodological problems are noteworthy, however. First, there was not a nonsmoking control group, and second, although search speed increased when the nicotine-containing cigarette was smoked, search efficiency was not assessed. These issues underscore the difficulty of disentangling the specific effects of nicotine from the overall impact of cigarette smoking on cognitive performance.

The second, and perhaps more compelling, theory postulates that acute cognitive deficits may occur in smokers during nonsmoking intervals between cigarettes. This "withdrawal effect" hypothesis (Levin, 1992; Parrot, 1994) suggests that the resumption of smoking may compensate for this transitory decrement by reinstating nicotine and creating a perception (on the part of the smoker) of cognitive benefits due to smoking. This theory coincides with the known addictive potential of nicotine and is also supported by research that has found that the short-term cognitive enhancing effect of nicotine varies depending on the length of cigarette deprivation (length of time between cigarettes) and baseline levels of cigarette intake (heavy versus light smokers). In support of this theory, studies indicate that tobacco use is associated with improved mood and perceptions of well-being in smokers, but that withdrawal can lead to depressed mood as well as increased anxiety and decrements in perceived cognitive function (e.g., difficulty concentrating, inability to focus attention; Gilbert, 1979; Hughes, Hatsukami, Mitchell, & Dahlgren, 1986; Wesnes & Warburton, 1983). Data are not available, however, that gauge the extent to which such deficits are magnified in long-term smokers or whether a reinstatement of cigarette smoking can reduce such deficits.

Issues in Cognitive Rehabilitation

With few exceptions, research on the short-term effects of cigarette smoking on cognitive performance has been confined to individuals who were relatively young with brief smoking histories (less than 10 years). Thus, it is difficult to generalize these findings to older adults who are chronic smokers (20 or more years) and who may be cognitively impaired or at risk for cognitive impairment. Further, most of the research in this domain has focused on laboratory studies that have examined the extent to which nicotine (delivered with or without cigarettes) impacts performance on experimental tasks, and how such tasks may or may not be relevant in day-to-day functioning.

Two studies specifically address the short-term impact of cigarette smoking on (a) older adults and (b) applied tasks relevant to cognitive rehabilitation program planning. A cross-sectional study conducted by Hill (1989) documented performance decrements in a sample of older self-reported smokers (mean age = 72 years) across cognitive tasks that were dichotomized with regard to the presence or absence of processing speed. Smokers were disadvantaged on tasks that placed heavy demands on speeded processing. The second study involved a series of experiments conducted by Spilich et al. (1992), who examined college students, grouped as smokers or nonsmokers, who performed graded cognitive tasks that increased in complexity with regard to time and performance demands. Smokers were further divided into a deprived and nondeprived subgroup. The nondeprived smokers were given cigarettes containing 1.2 mg of nicotine, and deprived smokers were given nicotine-free cigarettes. Tasks ranged from a simple visual search paradigms to a complex driving-simulation procedure. No differences between groups were found in visual search; however, differences favoring the nonsmokers were found on the simulated driving procedure.

These two studies suggest that chronic smokers may show the greatest deficits in cognitive performance on those tasks that push the limits of information processing resources. Older smokers may be at particularly high risk for these deficits due to the fact that aging itself is associated with diminished cognitive function (see Salthouse, 1991). Further, older smokers, as a group, are at higher risk for chronic disease which, in turn, has been shown to be associated with poorer cognitive performance. Although Hill (1989) reported screening older smokers for disease, he postulated that even in this case subclinical disease processes may have exerted a subtle influence on those cognitive tasks that placed the heaviest demands on processing resources (e.g., speeded verses non-speeded tasks).

In support of this contention, some research has alluded to poorer driving performance in smokers versus nonsmokers (DiFranza, Winters, Goldberg, Cirillo, & Biliouris, 1986; Heimstra, Bancroft, & DeKoch, 1967), although in these studies age and years of smoking were specifically examined as mediating variables. Assessing the frequency of driving-related problems (e.g., traffic violations, minor and major accidents, automobile-related deaths) between older smokers and nonsmokers seems warranted. Should research support this contention in older drivers who smoke cigarettes, changing smoking habits may be an important component in optimizing performance skills, particularly in older drivers who are showing early signs of age-related cognitive impairment. In addition, smoking status may be an important factor in predicting how long older adults in cognitively demanding occupations (airline pilot, air traffic controller, corporate executive, computer programmer) can maintain optimal on-the-job performance. Quitting smoking may be advised to preserve cognitive flexibility that may be critical in such occupations (Strayer & Kramer, 1994).

Cigarette Smoking, Chronic Disease, and Cognitive Function

Population-based longitudinal and cross-sectional research has examined cigarette smoking as one of many "lifestyle" predictors of cognitive stability and/or change in middle to late adulthood. Methods of assessing cognitive function in this context have included brief mental status exams and an array of cognitive tasks selected to track the normal aging process and predict early cognitive impairment. These studies make few claims as to "why" cigarette smoking predicts cognitive function and/or change across the life course; however, the link between cigarette smoking, the emergence of chronic disease in middle and late life, and cognitive functioning is apparent.

Smoking as a Predictor of Cognitive Function in Healthy Aging

Cross-sectional and longitudinal data in community-dwelling middle-aged and late-life adults have produced somewhat mixed results regarding the role that cigarette smoking plays in indices of cognitive performance. In cross-sectional data, Farmer et al. (1987) documented that self-reported smokers performed more poorly than non-smokers in two out of eight of their cognitive tasks, namely, immediate recall and similarities. Hultsch, Hammer, and Small (1993), in a sample of 484 subjects who were all over 55 years of age, found minimal if any relationship between tobacco use and cognitive performance. A unique aspect of this study was the wide array of measures employed, including verbal processing time, working memory, vocabulary, verbal fluency, world knowledge and word and text recall. Emery, Huppert, and Schein (1997), in a population-based study of 4,399 subjects who ranged in age from 19 to 94 years, found that smoking behavior was not related to performance on any of their cognitive tasks, and in several (e.g., choice reaction time and immediate memory), smokers outperformed nonsmokers. Smoking was defined as a categorical variable, namely, never-smoker, past smoker (quit at least 1 year ago), and current smoker. What is interesting in this study is that pulmonary function, as assessed by objective spirometry (forced expiratory velocity in 1 second; FEV_1), was related to diminished cognitive function even after controlling for demographics and smoking status. This finding is surprising in light of strong evidence that smoking diminishes pulmonary efficiency and capacity in old age (Lange et al., 1989). The lack of pulmonary deficits in these smokers was indicative of their overall good health and may have represented a sampling bias favoring the inclusion of disease-free smokers. This study does, however, represent an ambitious attempt to test the hypothesis that pulmonary function is a mechanism through which cigarette smoking may interact with cognitive processes. A more definitive test of this assumption would be to examine whether an interaction between smoking and cognitive performance would emerge in subjects with pulmonary disease.

Several longitudinal studies have also included cigarette smoking as a factor in cognitive decline in older adults. Herbert et al. (1993) examined the relationship between smoking and cognitive function in a sample of 1,201 adults aged 65 years and older from East Boston, Massachusetts. Using a composite variable of tobacco consumption that included self-reported smoking status (never-smoker, former smoker, and current smoker) and pack-years of smoking, the authors noted a decline in performance from baseline in those former smokers who had a relatively long pack-year history. Launer, Feskens, Kalmijn, and Kromhout (1996) reported data from the Zutphen Elderly Study, a large community-based longitudinal sample in the Netherlands consisting of 1,266 men. Subjects were initially categorized as current smokers, never-smokers, and former smokers. Former and never-smokers were further dichotomized by length of time they had engaged in smoking (more or less than 10 years). Cognitive function was assessed by means of the Mini-Mental State Examination (MMSE). Smokers showed MMSE performance declines, which were most marked in those who also had disease symptoms. From these data, the authors argued that smoking may interact with disease processes to accelerate late-life cognitive decline.

Galanis et al. (1997), reporting data from 3,429 middle-aged Japanese-American men who were part of the Honolulu Heart Program, found that age-related cognitive decrements were magnified in those who were continuous smokers. Although this was a subgroup of individuals who were healthier than the overall study sample as demonstrated by their positively skewed test scores, smoking continued to be associated with increased cognitive decline, particularly in those diagnosed with vascular disease. Interestingly, cognitive performance in those who were long-term quitters (more than 5 years) was indistinguishable from that of never-smokers.

In a final study, Prince, Lewis, Bird, Blizard, and Mann (1996) analyzed data from 2,567 hypertensive adults (65–74 years of age) from the Medical Research Council's (MRC) "Trial of the Treatment of Moderate Hypertension in Older Subjects." They selected a paired associate learning task that was administered to all participants at entry, followed by 1-, 9-, 21-, and 54-month retest intervals. Smoking status was dichotomized (smoker or nonsmoker) and included as part of a collection of risk factor variables for cardiovascular disease. Smoking was not a significant predictor of change in cognitive function in the overall sample; however, it did predict change in a subgroup of postmenopausal women who had lower socioeconomic status (SES) and less education and were of lower intelligence. It should be noted that as a group, smokers in this sample were more likely to die at an earlier age, creating a potential bias in favor of healthier smokers, who may have been less likely to experience chronic disease.

From these studies, it could be argued that in community-dwelling adults, cigarette smoking may be most influential as a predictor of performance change over time, rather than of cognitive function at any specific point in time. The effects of long-term smoking on cognitive function, therefore, are likely to become more apparent when multiple assessments are made over increasing time intervals, particularly when indicators of disease are also present. In the section that follows, we examine how cigarette smoking is likely to interact with chronic disease. In this regard, two assumptions are made: (a) that cigarette smoking is a risk factor for many disease states, including cardiovascular and pulmonary disease, and (b) that continued smoking into late life increases the risk of premature disease and disease-related mortality. Both of these assumptions highlight potential sources of bias in research that includes smoking status as an explanatory variable in cognitive decline in diseased aging.

Cigarette Smoking and Cognitive Function in Chronic Disease

Highlighted in this section are cardiovascular disease, pulmonary disease, and Alzheimer's disease (AD). Cardiovascular and pulmonary disease were selected because (1) they have been linked to declines in cognitive performance without respect to smoking per se, and (2) cigarette smoking is a prominent risk factor in the emergence and progression of these disease states. Alzheimer's disease represents a twist in terms of a proposed association between cigarette smoking and decreased incidence rates in AD.

VASCULAR DISEASE   Cigarette smoking is a well-known risk factor for cardiovascular disease (CVD), and this risk has been consistently documented in numerous epidemiological studies (Aronow, 1990; Jajich, Ostfeld, & Freeman, 1986). There are several mechanisms through which cigarette smoking may contribute to the early emergence and more rapid progression of CVD. The first, as described earlier in this chapter, is due primarily to the effect of nicotine on sympathetic nervous system activation. The second is the long-term systemic impact of smoking on overall cardiovascular capacity and efficiency, including (a) repeated episodes of systemic and coronary vasoconstriction; (b) increased concentrations of free fatty acids low density lipoprotein (LDL) cholesterol, and fibrinogen; (c) reduced High Density Lipoprotein (HDL) cholesterol; and (d) increased platelet reactivity (Winniford, 1990). Combined with other particulates in cigarette smoke such as carbon monoxide (CO), these effects gradually compromise cardiac capacity and efficiency. These chronic effects also appear to be dose-related, heavier smoking over longer time intervals further damaging functioning.

The link between CVD and cognitive function has received considerable attention in the research literature, although the findings have been somewhat mixed. Several studies have documented a relationship between CVD and diminished cognitive function (Elias, D'Agostino, Elias, & Wolf, 1995; Elias & Robbins, 1991), while others have found no such relationship (Farmer et al., 1987). A study that attempted to make a causal link between cigarette smoking, CVD, and cognitive function was reported by Frasure-Smith and Rolicz-Woloszyk (1982), who self-reported memory problems in 157 middle-aged males recovering from ischemic heart disease. At the time of the interview, which was approximately 1 year following initial hospitalization for an incident of ischemic heart disease, 39% of their subjects reported experiencing memory difficulties, and cigarette smoking was reported to be a contributing factor. Most intriguing was that those who had quit smoking since the initial hospitalization were twice as likely to complain about memory problems as those who continued to smoke. The authors proposed two seemingly contrasting effects of cigarette smoking on memory complaints, namely, an acute enhancing effect—likely due to the action of nicotine—and a chronic deleterious effect caused primarily by the role of cigarette smoking in speeding the progression of CVD.

It is important to note the potential role that cigarette smoking may play in magnifying the deleterious effects of cerebrovascular disease. For the purpose of this chapter, cerebrovascular disease is defined as a variant of CVD that influences only those aspects of the vascular system responsible for blood-oxygen transfer to the central nervous system. Although the literature that examines the role of cigarette smoking in cognitive decline through cerebrovascular disease is small in comparison to the literature on CVD, cerebrovascular disease may provide the most powerful test of this relationship. For example, hypertension (which is highly influenced by cigarette smoking) has been linked to reduced cerebral blood flow and brain atrophy in middle- and late-life adults (Hatazawa et al., 1984). Cerebrovascular disease is a well-known risk factor in dementia, and it has been consistently documented that chronic smokers have reduced regional cerebral blood flow when compared to nonsmokers (Kubota, Yamaguchi, Fujiwara, & Matsuzawa, 1987). Further, long-term continuous smoking has even been associated with increased brain atrophy due in part to its effects on cerebrovascular disease (Kubota, Matsuzawa, Fujiwara, Yamaguchi, Wantanabe, & Ono, 1987). From this literature, it is possible to specifically implicate cigarette smoking as an exacerbating agent in cerebrovascular disease, which in turn results in documentable changes in brain capacity and function and accelerated cognitive decline. Although this represents a strong argument for predicting that smokers will suffer larger cognitive deficits in the presence of cerebrovascular disease, research has yet to document this logic. For example, Desmond, Tatemichi, Paik, and Stern (1993) were unable to find a significant effect of smoking behavior as a predictor of cognitive decline in their sample of older adults with cerebrovascular disease. This may have been due to their constrained definition of cigarette smoking, as well as to the relative health of their diseased smokers. Nonetheless, more research is needed to more fully explore this assumption.

PULMONARY DISEASE   Extensive literature exists linking (a) cigarette smoking to chronic pulmonary disease and (b) chronic pulmonary disease to impairment in cognitive function. Evidence indicates that cigarette smoking is a major risk factor for chronic lung disease in middle-aged and older adults. The pattern of lung injury due to cigarette smoke involves sustained declines in forced vital capacity (FVC), abnormal increases in mucous production, the excessive accumulation of neutrophils, increased airway obstruction, and declines in the optimal exchange of oxygen and carbon dioxide (Coultas & Samet, 1989). The Framingham Study documented a more rapid decline in FVC and FEV over a 10-year period in smokers versus nonsmokers, with highly accelerated declines in those who continued to smoke into the fifth and sixth decade of life (Ashley, Kannel, Sorlie, & Mason, 1975). Chronic obstructive pulmonary disease (COPD) is an impressive example of the cumulative impact that long-term smoking can have on lung functioning. Within COPD, cigarette smoking magnifies disease processes by blocking small airway passages, reducing gas exchange, and creating hypoxemic effects (Weiss, 1984), and these connections are so well established that the first-line treatment for COPD is mandatory smoking cessation.

The link between pulmonary disease and cognitive functioning has also been well established. In a study examining age-related pulmonary efficiency and cognitive function in 3,812 community-dwelling adults 65 years and older, Cook et al. (1989) found that objective declines in peak expiratory flow were associated with deficit performance in simple measures of immediate memory, attention, and orientation. Two related studies that contrasted pulmonary disease patients with nondiseased subjects on a battery of cognitive tasks found a significant relationship between the degree of hypoxemia in the presence of disease and neuropsychological impairment (Grant et al., 1987; Prigatano, Parsons, Wright, Levin, & Hawryluk, 1983). Grant, Heaton, McSweeney, Adams, and Timms (1980) examined 121 individuals (average age 65.1 years) with hypoxemic COPD on a battery of neuropsychological tests that included measures of attention, language, abstract reasoning, and perceptual motor skills. A positive correlation was reported between measures of lung function and performance across each of these neuropsychological tasks. It is noteworthy that although the smoking status of patients in this study was not assessed, the authors implicated chronic hypoxemia (a common feature of COPD in the presence of cigarette smoking) as the most likely explanation for the poorer cognitive performance in those patients with more severe manifestations of COPD.

In sum, data indicate that cigarette smoking alters pulmonary function through predictable declines in lung efficiency and overall capacity. Decline in pulmonary health is a precursor to pulmonary disease, of which smokers are at very high risk. Smoking in the presence of pulmonary disease places the individual at high risk for acute pulmonary deficits and speeds the overall disease. The role of smoking as an exacerbating agent is likely to be important in gauging the extent to which COPD diminishes cognitive function in old age and may be an important factor to consider in cognitive rehabilitation programming in older adults who have cognitive deficits associated with COPD.

ALZHEIMER'S DISEASE   What has been of primary interest with regard to Alzheimer's disease, cognition, and cigarette smoking is the long-term impact of nicotine on brain neuroanatomy. Briefly, some epidemiological evidence has indicated that cigarette smokers have a lower incidence of Alzheimer's disease, and this has led to the belief that smoking into advanced age may be protective of AD (Graves et al., 1991; Lee, 1994). It should be noted, however, that these findings have not consistently been endorsed by the scientific community (Graves & Mortimer, 1994; Shalat, Seltzer, Pidcock, & Baker, 1987). In either case, such research has important implications in identifying potential pathways that may underlie the linkage between cigarette smoking, AD, and cognitive decline in AD.

The most compelling pathway is underscored by the finding that nicotinic cholinergic receptors in the brain may play a significant role in cognition, and that in AD, such receptors are in very short supply (Stolerman et al., 1995). Given the connection between nicotine, nicotinic receptors, and cognitive functioning in AD, interventions have attempted to capitalize on this relationship by administering nicotine at various dosage levels to early AD patients in the hope of offsetting cognitive losses associated with the disease (see Levin, 1992; Stolerman et al., 1995). The short-term effectiveness of this approach is highlighted by a double-blind placebo-controlled study with six AD patients that involved continuous delivery of nicotine (via a transdermal patch) over a 7-day period (Wilson et al.,1995). Those receiving nicotine showed improved learning in the short run; however, no long-term follow-up was conducted. Thus, whether such a strategy could produce substantial and consistent improvement in cognitive functioning in AD remains an open question. It should be noted that none of the aforementioned interventions employed cigarette smoking as the nicotine delivery mechanism. In fact, subjects in such studies have generally been nonsmoking volunteers. Thus, such data may provide evidence only for the efficacy of nicotine and do not address the role of cigarette smoking (and its modification) in the progression of cognitive deterioration in AD.

Another explanation of the epidemiological data demonstrating fewer smokers with AD is that cigarette smoking may be a marker variable of other, more salient confounding factors. For example, cigarette smokers have a higher morbidity rate than comparable nonsmokers, and if sampling targets older individuals, a bias may exist in favor of younger smokers who are somewhat healthier at baseline than nonsmokers. In other instances, cigarette smokers may be misrepresented in specific disease categories (or in other subgroups) that are screened when healthy volunteers are selected in studies tracing the course of AD. Letenneur, Dartigues, Commenges, Pacale, Tessier, and Orgogozo (1994) found smoking status to be initially highly predictive of AD; however, after controlling for the effects of occupational category and educational level, its predictive power disappeared. Thus, great care should be emphasized in suggesting the beneficial effects of cigarette-delivered nicotine on brain function, particularly as related to the onset of AD. What appears to be absent in this literature is an appreciation of the complex (and predictable) impact that cigarette smoking could exert on AD through reductions in cerebral blood flow, diminished oxygen transfer, and impaired pulmonary and vascular functioning. Disentangling any beneficial effects of cigarette-delivered nicotine from the role that cigarette smoking plays in exacerbating disease processes is warranted in future research.

Issues in Cognitive Rehabilitation

It is not surprising that continued smoking in the presence of chronic disease will have adverse consequences on cognitive function; thus, smoking cessation is a recommended strategy to minimize continued cognitive decline. However, what is less obvious and may have important implications in smoking cessation efforts in older diseased adults is the complex interrelationship between smoking, cognitive processes, and disease, as well as how these may influence the potential success of relapse prevention efforts. This potential interrelationship was proposed by Frazure-Smith and Rolicz-Woloszyk (1982), who suggested that continued smoking in the presence of CVD may mask its effects on cognitive function. Thus, quitting smoking may be perceived as causing more cognitive problems than it alleviates. Given that older adults are likely to make global attributions about even short-term cognitive deficits (Bolla, Lingren, Bonaccorsy, & Bleecker, 1991), addressing these as a part of relapse prevention programming may be critical in helping older quitters maintain abstinence. One way to address such issues is through focused memory-training interventions that could help older quitters learn to compensate for such short-term deficits. Although memory training has, to date, focused primarily on nondiseased, high-functioning older adults, a few strategies—namely, spaced retrieval and simplified mnemonic procedures (see Camp & McKitrick, 1992)—have been used to remediate cognitive loss in impaired groups. It may be useful to incorporate such strategy training in the maintenance of smoking cessation.

From the COPD literature, it is possible to identify impaired oxygen transfer as the specific disease mechanism causing cognitive loss in the late-life smoker. A definitive test of this assumption would be to examine cognitive function in subjects who vary with regard to smoking status and the presence or absence of COPD. Should this relationship be established, not only would it provide evidence for the importance of quitting to preserve cognitive function in COPD, but mechanisms to upregulate oxygen transfer to the brain might also be recommended. One such mechanism may be a regular program of physical exercise, since some research has suggested that exercise training can enhance cognitive function in old age through increased oxygenation to the brain (see Dustman et al., 1984). Thus, the effect of exercise on cognitive variables following smoking cessation in the presence of disease may be a particularly promising cognitive rehabilitation strategy.

Cigarette Smoking, Psychological Variables and Cognitive Function

As noted in Figure 8.1, psychological variables are another pathway through which cigarette smoking may exert an indirect influence on cognitive function. In this regard we highlight two processes: (a) personality style and (b) depression. Although the connection between cigarette smoking and cognitive processes has been investigated in this context, the rationale underlying this research, to date, has been to examine the propensity of individuals with psychological vulnerabilities to utilize cigarette smoking as a compensatory mechanism for suboptimal affective and/or cognitive function.

A few early studies have suggested that cigarette smoking may be used to mediate deficits in information processing as a result of personality style. The central element of this proposal is the stimulating and/or tranquilizing effect of nicotine. Eysenck (1965) first proposed this line of reasoning based on the notion that both introverts and extroverts mediate arousal levels in order to optimize information processing; that is, extroverts attempt to increase a characteristically low baseline level of arousal, whereas introverts work to decrease high baseline arousal levels. The proposition that cigarette smoking could be used to optimize cognitive function in this way is intriguing, and a few studies have examined this hypothesis with mixed results regarding the potential action of cigarette smoking (Revell, Warburton, & Wesnes, 1985; Warburton, Wesnes, & Revell, 1983). Thus, this issue remains open to future research.

Research indicates that depressive symptoms may influence cognitive function, and this finding is highlighted by the observation that in some instances, cognitive decrements inherent in depressive symptomatology have been mistaken for organic brain syndrome (Newhouse & Hughes, 1991). In a series of studies, Forsell, Jorm, and Winblad (1994) examined a large sample of depressed older adults who were participating in a population-based study in Sweden. Among these individuals, depressive symptomatology was found to cluster into two distinct categories reflecting (a) mood (dysphoria, appetite disturbance, feelings of guilt, suicidal ideation) and (b) motivation (lack of interest, psychomotor change, loss of energy, and concentration difficulties). Following this research, Bäckman, Hill, and Forsell (1996) found motivational symptoms were most predictive of deficits in cognitive function. Given that related research suggests that cigarette smoking may be used by some depressed individuals to self-medicate for depressive symptoms (Hughes et al. 1986), it could be argued that depressed older adults may utilize cigarette smoking in a similar way to compensate for cognitive deficits associated with depression. Such a link could provide a possible explanation as to why it is difficult for depressed older adults, who may be at risk for cognitive impairment, to stop smoking and avoid relapse (Hall, Muñoz, & Reus, 1994). Although it is difficult to draw generalizable conclusions on the role that cigarette smoking may play as a mediator of cognitive loss in depression in old age, this may represent an important avenue for future research.

Issues in Cognitive Rehabilitation

The major postulate of this section is that cigarette consumption may be used by smokers to optimize cognitive processes within a particular personality style, or to compensate for cognitive deficiencies associated with an affective state, namely, depression. If cigarette smoking as a form of self-medication does play a role in mediating cognitive loss in this way, two important questions arise: (a) How does it operate? (b) What are its implications in strategy training to remediate cognitive deficits related to psychological factors?

With regard to the first question, nicotine once again appears to be a likely candidate, given its previously described psychopharmacological action. In this case, it may be that nicotine simply acts to relieve cognitive symptoms associated with depression, or it may be that cigarette smoking exerts a more general antidepressant effect, enhancing cognitive function by acting on the disease process itself. What is needed is research that can disentangle the specific effect of nicotine from other components of cigarette smoke that may be influencing depression. With regard to the implications for cognitive rehabilitation, if cigarette smoking is complicating a physical disease (e.g., CVD or COPD) yet is also being used by the individual as a way to mediate cognitive problems associated with depression or personality style, efforts to address and/or replace this role should be made prior to attempting smoking cessation. As more research emerges, it may be that nicotine-like compounds (e.g., nicotine agonists) will become increasingly important in the development of more efficacious pharmacological treatments for psychiatric illnesses such as depression.

Summary and Implications

This chapter has examined the potential short- and long-term roles that cigarette smoking may play in cognitive functioning in late life. An explanatory model was created to provide a framework to organize the empirical literature related to this issue. It is without question that habituation to cigarette smoking occurs even in short-term smokers, and that quitting smoking is a difficult undertaking. It may be that cognitive factors play a mediating role in enhancing the addictive potential of cigarettes by creating a false perception that smoking is critical for optimal cognitive function. Further, the direct impact that cigarette smoking has on cognitive function has been explored in terms of the short- and long-term effects of nicotine on the CNS. Although considerable evidence suggests that nicotine can have cognitive enhancing effects, it remains unclear whether cigarette-delivered nicotine can produce objective (and reliable) short-term gains in cognitive function. In the presence of disease, cigarette smoking exacerbates disease processes as has been shown in CVD and COPD, both of which are linked to diminished cognitive function. Thus, cigarette smoking may play an indirect role in cognitive decline by accelerating disease progression. The cumulative effect of cigarette smoking on cerebral vascular disease provides a potential test of this logic by demonstrating significant functional and structural declines in the brains of older smokers in comparison to nonsmokers.

A major goal of this chapter has been to link research on cognitive processes in old age and cigarette smoking to issues in cognitive rehabilitation. To this end, we have highlighted the following:

1. Short-term losses in cognitive function from nicotine withdrawal as part of the quitting process could put older smokers into a vicious relapse cycle. Rehabilitation counselors could anticipate this issue by providing education and compensatory strategy training. We also examined how everyday activities, such as driving, may be affected by the interaction of cigarette smoking and cognitive functioning and have recommended further research on this issue.
2. Compensatory interventions such as physical exercise and memory training may be useful for older smokers who are experiencing cognitive deficits associated with a chronic disease state. These strategies may also be important components in comprehensive smoking cessation planning to offset cognitive losses associated with smoking cessation in the presence of disease. Such interventions may help the individual to refocus the experience of cognitive loss as a transitory process in improving health through smoking cessation.
3. Research examining nicotine as a cognitive enhancer in AD and, to a lesser extent, in depression introduces the potential use of nicotinic compounds in the treatment of these, as well as other, diseases of aging.

References

Andersson, K. (1975). Effects of cigarette smoking on learning and retention. *Psychopharmacologia, 41*, 1–5.

Andersson, K., & Hockey, G. R. J. (1977). Effects of cigarette smoking on incidental memory. *Psychopharmacology, 52*, 223–226.

Aronow, W. S. (1990). Cardiac risk factors: Still important in the elderly. *Geriatrics, 45*, 71–80.

Ashley, F., Kannel, W. B., Sorlie, P. D., & Masson, R. (1975). Pulmonary function: Relation to aging, cigarette habit, and mortality. *Annals of Internal Medicine, 82*, 739–745.

Bäckman, L., Hassing, L., Forsell, Y., & Viitanen, M. (1996). Episodic remembering in a population-based sample of nonagenarians: Does major depression exacerbate the memory deficits seen in Alzheimer's Disease? *Psychology and Aging, 11*, 649–656.

Bäckman, L., Hill, R. D., & Forsell, Y. (1996). The influence of depressive symptomatology on episodic memory functioning among clinically nondepressed older adults. *Journal of Abnormal Psychology, 105*, 97–105.

Baron, J. A. (1996). Beneficial effects of nicotine and cigarette smoking: The real, the possible and the spurious. *British Medical Journal, 52*, 58–73

Benowitz, N. L. (1996). Pharmacology of nicotine: Addiction and therapeutics. *Annual Review of Pharmacology and Toxicology, 36*, 597–613.

Bolla, K. I., Lindgren, K. N., Bonaccorsy, C., & Bleecker, M. L. (1991). Memory complaints in older adults: Fact or fiction? *Archives of Neurology, 48*, 61–64.

Camp, C. J., & McKitrick, L. A. (1992). Memory interventions in DAT populations: Methodological and theoretical issues. In R. L. West & J. D. Sinnott (Eds.), *Everyday memory and aging: Current research and methodology* (pp. 155–172). New York: Springer-Verlag.

Cook, N. R., Evans, D. A., Scherr, P. A., Speizer, F. E., Vedal, S., Branch, L. G., Huntley,

J. C., Hennekens, C. H., & Taylor, J. O. (1989). Peak expiratory flow rate in and elderly population. *American Journal of Epidemiology, 130,* 66–78.

Coultas, D. B., & Samet, J. M. (1989). Cigarette smoking. In M. J. Hensley & N. A. Saunders (Eds.), *Lung biology in health and disease* (Vol. 43). New York: Marcel Dekker.

Desmond, D. W., Tatemichi, T. K., Paik, M., & Stern, Y. (1993). Risk factors for cerebrovascular disease as correlates of cognitive function in a stroke-free cohort. *Archives of Neurology, 50,* 162–166.

DiFranza, J. R., Winters, T. H., Goldberg, R. J., Cirillo, L., & Biliouris, T. (1986). The relationship of smoking to motor vehicle accidents and traffic violations. *New York State Journal of Medicine, 86,* 464–467.

Dube, M. F., & Green, C. R. (1982). Methods of collection of smoke for analytical purposes. *Recent Advances in Tobacco Science, 8,* 42–102.

Dunne, M. P., MacDonald, D., & Hartley, L. R. (1986). The effects of nicotine on memory and problem solving performance. *Physiology and Behavior, 37,* 849–854.

Dustman, R. E., Ruhling, R. O., Russell, E. M., Shearer, D. E., Bonekat, H. W., Shigeoka, J. W., Wood, J. S., & Bradford, D. C. (1984). Aerobic exercise training and improved neuropsychological function of older individuals. *Neurobiology of Aging, 5,* 35–42.

Elias, M. F., D'Agostino, R. B., Elias, P. K., & Wolf, P. A. (1995). Neuropsychological test performance, cognitive functioning, blood pressure and age: The Framingham Heart Study. *Experimental Aging Research, 21,* 369–391.

Elias, M. F., & Robbins, M. A. (1991). Cardiovascular disease, hypertension, and cognitive function. In A. P. Shapiro & A. Baum (Eds.), *Behavioral aspects of cardiovascular disease* (pp. 249–285). Hillsdale, NJ: Erlbaum.

Emery, C. F., Huppert, F. A., & Schein, R. L. (1997). Do pulmonary function and smoking behavior predict cognitive function? Findings from a British sample. *Psychology and Health, 12,* 265–275.

Eysenck, H. J. (1965). *Smoking, health, and personality.* London: Weidenfeld & Nicolson.

Farmer, M. E., White, L. R., Abbott, R. D., et al. (1987). Blood pressure and cognitive performance: The Framingham Study. *American Journal of Epidemiology, 126,* 1103–1114.

Fielding, J. E. (1985). Smoking: Health effects and control. *New England Journal of Medicine, 313,* 491–498.

Forsell, Y., Jorm, A. F., & Winblad, B. (1994). Association of age, sex, cognitive dysfunction, and disability with major depressive symptoms in an elderly sample. *American Journal of Psychiatry, 151,* 1600–1604.

Frasure-Smith, N., & Rolicz-Woloszyk, E. (1982). Memory problems after ischemic heart disease episodes: effects of stress, benzodiazepines and smoking. *Journal of Psychosomatic Research, 26*(6), 613–622.

Galanis, D. J., Petrovitch, H., Launer, L. J., Harris, T. B., Foley, D. J., & White, L R. (1997). Smoking history in middle age and subsequent cognitive performance in elderly Japanese-American men. *American Journal of Epidemiology, 145,* 507–515.

Gilbert, D. G. (1979). Paradoxical tranquilizing and emotion-reducing effects of nicotine. *Psychological Bulletin, 86,* 643–662.

Gonzales, M. A., & Harris, M. B. (1980). Effects of cigarette smoking in recall and categorization of written material. *Perceptual and Motor Skills, 50,* 407–416.

Grant, I., Heaton, R. K., McSweeney, A. J., Adams, K. M., & Timms, R. M. (1980). Brain dysfunction in COPD. *Chest, 77,* 308–309.

Grant, I., Prigatano, G. P., Heaton, R. K., McSweeny, A. J., Wright, E. C., & Adams, K. M. (1987). Progressive neuropsychological impairment and hypoxemia: Relationship in chronic obstructive pulmonary disease. *Archives of General Psychiatry, 44,* 999–1006.

Graves, A. B., & Mortimer, J. A. (1994). Does smoking reduce the risk of Parkinson's and Alzheimer's diseases? *Journal of Smoking Related Disease, 5,* 79–90.

Graves, A. B., van Duijn, C. M., Chandra, V., et al. (1991). Alcohol and tobacco consumption as risk factors for Alzheimer's disease: A collaborative re-analysis of case-control studies. *International Journal of Epidemiology, 20,* S48–S57.

Hall, S. M., Muños, R. F., & Reus, V. I. (1994). Cognitive-behavioral intervention increases abstinence rates for depressive-history smokers. *Journal of Consulting and Clinical Psychology, 62,* 141–146.

Hatazawa, J., Yamaguchi, T., Ito, M., Yamaura, H., & Matsuzawa, T. (1984). Association of hypertension with increased atrophy of brain matter in the elderly. *Journal of the American Geriatrics Society, 32,* 370–374.

Heimstra, N. W., Bancroft, N. R., & DeKoch, A. R. (1967). Effects of smoking upon sustained performance in a simulated driving task. *Annals of the New York Academy of Sciences, 142,* 295–307.

Heishman, S. J., Snyder, F. R., & Henningfield, J. E. (1991). Effect of repeated nicotine administration in nonsmokers. In L. S. Harris (Ed.), *Problems of Drug Dependence, 1990.* Washington, DC: U. S. Government Printing Office, DHHS Publication No. (ADM) 91–1753.

Herbert, L. E., Scherr, P. A., Beckett, L. A., Albert, M. S., Rosner, B., Taylor, J. O., & Evans, D. A. (1993). Relation of smoking and low-to-moderate alcohol consumption to change in cognitive function: A longitudinal study in a defined community of older persons. *American Journal of Epidemiology, 137,* 881–891.

Hill, R. D. (1989). Residual effects of cigarette smoking on cognitive performance in normal aging. *Psychology and Aging, 4,* 251–254.

Hughes, J. R., Hatsukami, D. K., Mitchell, J. E., & Dahlgren, L. A. (1986). Prevalence of smoking among psychiatric outpatients. *American Journal of Psychiatry, 143,* 993–997.

Hultsch, D. F., Hammer, M., & Small, B. J. (1993). Age differences in cognitive performance in later life: Relationships to self-reported health and activity life style. *Journal of Gerontology: Psychological Sciences, 48,* 1–11.

Jajich, C. L., Ostfeld, A. M., & Freeman, D. H. (1986). Smoking and coronary heart disease mortality in the elderly. *Journal of the American Medical Association, 252,* 2831–2834.

Jenkins, C. D., Rosenman, R. H., & Zyzanski, S. J. (1968). Cigarette smoking: Its relationship to coronary heart disease and related risk factors in the Western Collaborative Group Study. *Circulation, 38,* 1140–1155.

Kubota, K., Matsuzawa, T., Fujiwara, T., Yamaguchi, T., Wantanabe, I. K., & Ono, S. (1987). Age-related brain atrophy enhanced by smoking: A quantitative study with computed tomography. *Tohuku Journal of Experimental Medicine, 153,* 301–311.

Kubota, K., Yamaguchi, T., Fujiwara, T., & Matsuzawa, T. (1987). Effects of smoking on regional cerebral blood flow in cerebral vascular disease patients and normal subjects. *Tohuku Journal of Experimental Medicine, 151,* 261–268.

LaCroix, A. Z., Lang, J., Scherr, P., Wallace, R. B., Coroni-Huntley, J., Berkman, L., Curb, D. J., Evans, D., & Hennekens, C. H. (1991). Smoking mortality among older men and women in three communities. *New England Journal of Medicine, 324,* 1619–1625.

Lange, P., Groth, S., Nyboe, J., Mortensen, M., Appleyard, G., Jensen, P., & Schnohr, S. (1989). Effects of smoking and changes in smoking habits on the decline of FEV1. *European Respiratory Journal, 2,* 811–816.

Launer, L. J., Feskens, E. J. M., Kalmijn S., & Kromhout (1996). Smoking, drinking, and thinking: The Zutphen elderly study. *American Journal of Epidemiology, 143,* 219–227.

Lee, P. N. (1994). Smoking and Alzheimer's disease: A review of the epidemiological evidence. *Neuroepidemiology, 13,* 131–144.

Letenneur, L., Dartigues, J. G., Commenges, D., Pacale, B.-G., Tessier, J.-F., & Orgogozo, J.-M. (1994). Tobacco consumption and cognitive impairment in elderly people: A population-based study. *Annals of Epidemiology, 4,* 449–454.

Levin, E. D. (1992). Nicotinic systems and cognitive function. *Psychopharmacology, 108,* 417–431.

Newhouse, P. A., & Hughes, J. R. (1991). The role of nicotine and nicotinic mechanisms in neuropsychiatric disease. *British Journal of Addiction, 86,* 521–526.

Newhouse, P. A., Sunderland, T., Narang, P. K., Mellow, A. M., Fertig, J. B., Lawlor, B. A., & Murphy, D. L. (1990). Neuroendocrine, physiologic, and behavioral responses following intravenous nicotine in non smoking healthy volunteers and in patients with Alzheimer's disease. *Psychoneuroendocrinology, 15*(5,6), 471–484.

Parrot, A. (1994). Does cigarette smoking increase stress? *Addiction, 89,* 142–144.

Perkins, K. A., Epstein, L. H., Stiller, R. L., Sexton, J. E., Debski, T. D., & Jacob, R. G. (1990). Behavioral effects of nicotine in smokers and non-smokers. *Pharmacology, Biochemistry, and Behavior, 37,* 11–15.

Perkins, K. A., Grobe, J. E., Fonte, C., et al. (1994). Chronic and acute tolerance to subjective, behavioral and cardiovascular effects of nicotine in humans. *Journal of Pharmacology and Experimental Therapeutics, 270,* 628–638.

Prigatano, G. P., Parsons, O., Wright E., Levin, D. C., & Hawryluk, G. (1983). Neuropsychological test performance in mildly hypoxemic patients with chronic obstructive lung disease. *Journal of Consulting and Clinical Psychology, 51,* 108–116.

Prince, M., Lewis, G., Bird, A., Blizard, R., & Mann, A. (1996). A longitudinal study of factors predicting change in cognitive test scores over time, in an older hypertensive population. *Psychological Medicine, 26,* 555–568.

Provost, S. C., & Woodward, R. (1991). Effects of nicotine gum on repeated administration of the Stroop test. *Psychopharmacology, 104,* 536–540.

Revell, A. D., Warburton, D. M., & Wesnes, K. (1985). Smoking as a coping strategy. *Addictive Behaviors, 10,* 209–224.

Salthouse, T. A. (1991). *Theoretical perspectives on cognitive aging.* Hillsdale, NJ: Erlbaum.

Shalat, S., Seltzer, B., Pidcock, C., & Baker, E. (1987). Risk factors of Alzheimer's disease: A case-control study, *Neurology, 37,* 1630–1633.

Shinton, R., & Beevers, G. (1989). Meta-analysis of the relation between cigarette smoking and stroke. *British Medical Journal, 293,* 6–8.

Spilich, G. J. (1994). Cognitive benefits of nicotine: Fact of fiction. *Addiction, 89,* 141–142.

Spilich, G. J., June, L., & Renner, J. (1992). Cigarette smoking and cognitive performance. *British Journal of Addiction, 87,* 1313–1326.

Stolerman, I. P., Mirza, N. R., & Shoaib, M. (1995). Nicotine psychopharmacology: Addiction, cognition and neuroadaptation. *Medicinal Research Reviews, 15,* 47–72.

Strayer, D. L., & Kramer, A. F. (1994). Aging and skill acquisition: Learning-performance distinctions. *Psychology and Aging, 9,* 589–605.

Warburton, D. M., Wesnes, K., & Revell, A. D. (1983). Personality factors in self-medication by smoking. In W. Janke (Ed.), *Response variability in psychotropic drugs.* London: Pergamon.

Weiss, S. T. (1984). Chronic bronchitis, asthma, and obstructive airways disease: Age, smoking and other risk factors. In R. Bosse and C. L. Rose (Eds.), *Smoking and aging.* Lexington, MA: Lexington Books.

Wesnes, K., & Warburton, D. M. (1983). Smoking, nicotine and human performance. *Pharmacological Therapy, 21,* 189–208.

Wesnes, K., & Warburton, D. M. (1984). The effects of cigarettes of varying yield on rapid information processing performance. *Psychopharmacology, 82,* 338–342.

Wesnes, K., Warburton, D. M., & Matz, B. (1983). Effects of nicotine on stimulus sensitivity and response bias in a visual vigilance task. *Neuropsychobiology, 9,* 41–44.

West, R., & Hack, S. (1991). Effect of cigarettes on memory search and subjective ratings. *Pharmacology, Biochemistry and Behavior, 38,* 281–286.

West, R. J., & Jarvis, M. J. (1986). Effects of nicotine on finger tapping rate in non-smokers. *Pharmacology, Biochemistry, and Behavior, 25,* 727–731.

Wilson, A. L., Langley, L. K., Monley, J., Bauer, S. R., McFalls, E., Kovera, C., & McCarten, J. R. (1995). Nicotine patches in Alzheimer's disease: Pilot study on learning, memory, and safety. *Pharmacology Biochemistry and Behavior, 51,* 509–514.

Winniford, M. D. (1990). Smoking and cardiovascular function. *Journal of Hypertension, 9,* S17–S23.

9

Executive Function and Cognitive Rehabilitation

JEFFREY W. ELIAS

JULIA E. TRELAND

Researchers and practitioners have become increasingly aware that executive cognitive functions (ECFs) appear to choreograph abilities such as insight, planning, problem solving, and motivation into the goal-directed behavior required for daily living. Deficits in ECFs are common and result in specific behavioral and affective impairments that impact an individual's cognition and ability to participate in rehabilitation. Irritability, mood swings, disorganization, apathy, indifference, and inattention are some of the manifestations of ECF deficits. Impaired ECFs due to head injury, stroke, disease process, or normal aging challenges both physical and cognitive rehabilitation. For effective rehabilitation treatment and discharge planning, it is essential for the practitioner to anticipate and recognize impaired ECFs in the client. In this chapter, we will discuss definitions of ECF, its anatomical correlates, the assessment of ECF, behavior associated with ECF impairment, and issues related to cognitive rehabilitation.

Defining Executive Cognitive Function

Definitions of ECF are influenced by theory, clinical observation, and brain circuitry. As a consequence, the concept of ECF can be elusive and difficult to confine. Lezak (1995) described ECF as "capacities that enable a person to engage successfully in independent, purposive, self-serving behaviors" (p. 42). Royall (1994), citing Lezak (1983), Stuss and Benson (1986), and Shallice (1982) described ECF as "cognitive processes that govern the orchestration of relatively simple ideas, movements, and actions into complex goal-directed behaviors; . . . they help orchestrate and maintain goal-directed behavior in the face of both internal, and external distractions" (p. 75). A succinct definition was offered by Denkla (1996), who suggested that ECF is the manipulation of representational systems and is what goes on during the delay between stimulus and response; for example, ECF is the "working" component of working memory.

To explain the ECF concept to others, we offer the acronym *SOS-MOMMI*, which stands for *s*election, *o*rganization, *s*equencing, *mo*tivation, *m*onitoring, *m*emory (working or event updating), and *i*nhibition. As information-processing systems, individuals are constantly bombarded with stimuli and potential behavioral options. Once a behavioral option is chosen (selected), behavioral organization is an important element in the successful attainment of the final goal. Behavioral patterns must be initiated and maintained (motivation). An evaluative component (self-monitoring) is needed to judge the viability of the organization and behavioral sequence relative to the goal. This evaluative component is necessary for cognitive flexibility when an ineffective strategy needs to be altered. To effectively self-monitor, one must be able to keep track of what has been accomplished (memory), while updating and carrying out the next part of the sequence. This involves what has been called *working memory*, or holding information on-line while adding to it and updating or changing it (Baddeley, 1996). Once a task has been initiated, there are many stimuli competing for attention, including both external and internal distractions. Attention needs to be diverted from these competing distractions, and at times, the competing distractions may have to be actively inhibited from breaking into the primary behavior sequence.

The acronym *SOS-MOMMI* not only represents the elements involved in carrying out goal-directed behavior but is descriptive metaphorically: To be functionally independent, individuals must be able to direct themselves. From a developmental perspective, executive functions should be maturing about the time parental influence on planning and everyday functioning decreases. As ECF develops, the ability to efficiently execute on-line functions in the present also leads to the ability to integrate old and new information. With further cognitive development, this integration process can be used to plan for the future.

The ability to plan for the future is a major benefit of adult-level ECF. One should be cautious, however, in evaluating ECF based on the effectiveness of the plan. That is, with regard to planning, ECF should be defined as the process of planning, not the outcome. In lieu of the ability to develop a new plan, it is possible to achieve a successful outcome by executing a routine based on past knowledge. In measuring ECF, it can be difficult to tease apart planning ability from past knowledge because higher cognitive functioning and effective decisions are not simply the result of ECF; that is, the whole is greater than the sum of the parts.

The issue of definition is important when considering the assessment of ECF. As described above, ECF would seem necessary for performing well on IQ tests. The concept of ECF has been considered analogous to the concept of IQ. Attempts to discriminate between the concepts of IQ and ECF have associated ECF more closely with the "doing" or "fluid" aspects of IQ (Denkla, 1996; Pennington, 1997), and less closely with the "knowing" or "crystallized" aspects of IQ, such as those related to verbal IQ (Pennington, 1997). This does not mean that verbal IQ can be ignored when assessing ECF. Denkla (1996) pointed out that some tests of ECF may be less sensitive in individuals with a high IQ (much of it determined as verbal IQ). In many cases, therefore, changes in ECF need to be evaluated against some estimate of IQ.

The variable sensitivity of instruments designed to assess ECF raises a difficult measurement and definition issue. Correlations between measures of ECF often are lower than would be expected if ECF is to be considered a construct (cf. Baddeley, 1996). This lack of correlation between ECF measures is more likely to be observed in normal young adults. In an older or impaired population, however, the same set of ECF measures may correlate well, perhaps due to the interaction of ECF and various cognitive domains (e.g., memory and attention; cf. Royall, 1994). For example, greater attentional demands may require greater executive control, resulting in increased correlation between measurements of the domains of ECF and attention. Further, the impact of ECF on overall functioning frequently is modulated by interactions between the individual, the environment, and the familiarity or novelty of task requirements. For example, a highly structured setting can reduce the degree of ECF required for task performance, while the same task, carried out in an unstructured environment, places more importance on ECF.

Anatomy of Executive Function

ECF also has functional anatomy correlates. Executive function developmental processes and ECF deficits have been primarily associated with the functions of the frontal lobes or with lesions involving the frontal systems. As an anatomical area, the frontal lobes per se are confined by the central sulcus as the posterior boundary, the lateral fissure as the inferior boundary, and the cingulate sulcus as a medial boundary (Kolb & Whishaw, 1996). Within this anatomical area, the brain is composed of specialized subregions, each contributing to a specific set of behaviors. Five frontal circuits have been identified: a motor circuit originating in the supplementary motor area, an oculomotor circuit starting in the frontal eye fields, and three prefrontal cortex circuits originating in the dorsolateral prefrontal cortex, lateral orbital cortex, and anterior cingulate cortex (Cummings, 1993; Malloy & Richardson, 1994).

The three regions composing the prefrontal cortex are most often referred to with respect to the ECF concept and behavioral syndromes (Krasnegor, Lyon, & Goldman-Rakic (1997). The prefrontal-dorsolateral circuit is involved in the planning, organizational, monitoring, sensory integration, and cognitive flexibility components of ECF. The prefrontal-lateral orbital circuit is involved in inhibition and affective control, and the prefrontal-anterior cingulate circuit in initiation, motivation, and adherence to task (Cummings, 1993; Malloy & Richardson, 1994).[1]

It is important to note that these regions have numerous projections to and from other areas of the cortex, to include the posterior parietal and temporal sulcus areas (Kolb & Whishaw, 1996), as well as the subcortex (Cummings, 1993; Denkla & Reiss, 1997; Malloy & Richardson, 1994). Therefore, a lesion anywhere within a frontal circuit could result in an ECF failure.

All three prefrontal cortical circuits have common structures with the subcortex (striatum, globus pallidus, substantia nigra, and thalamus) (Cummings, 1993; Denkla & Reiss, 1997). The circuits are described as contiguous but are anatomically separated throughout the subcortical structures (Cummings, 1993). This emphasis on the involvement of the basal ganglia in frontal lobe circuitry is very important for understanding the behavioral changes associated with disorders of subcortical origin (e.g., Parkinson's disease, Huntington's disease, and attention deficit/hyperactivity disorders; Denkla & Reiss, 1997), as well as understanding the distinction between dementias that present with cortical features (memory, language, constructions) and dementias that present with prefrontal-subcortical ECF features (Elias, 1995; Lovell & Smith, 1997; Royall & Mahurin, 1996; Royall & Polk, 1998; Usman, 1997).

Cummings (1993) noted that as the projections pass from the cortical structures of the prefrontal cortex to the subcortical structures of the basal ganglia (putamen, globus pallidus, striatum), they are progressively focused into smaller bundles of neurons. Therefore, a focal lesion in the basal ganglion area could have more diffuse effects on frontal functions than a lesion in a frontal area.

While changes in behavior related to the prefrontal cortex area have received the most attention, Malloy and Richardson (1994) noted the importance of evaluating motor functioning due to the prefrontal cortex. They suggested assessing fine motor function and the volitional movements and praxis associated with the premotor and supplementary motor areas.

Assessment of Executive Function

Assessment is a vital part of any rehabilitation plan. The client's current cognitive and ECF abilities are the vehicle for reaching rehabilitation goals; neuropsychological assessment delineates the client's cognitive capacities. Considering the assessment results in terms of "why" particular errors occurred can result in a list of target impairments to be used in rehabilitation treatment planning (Goldstein, 1984). From this perspective, the assessment data are not only diagnostic (knowing), but also prescriptive (doing) (Golden, 1984).

A number of investigators have provided good summary tables of neuropsychological assessment batteries focused on ECF (cf. Chafetz, Friedman, Kevorkian, & Levy, 1996; Lezak, 1995; Lovell & Smith, 1997; Malloy & Richardson, 1994; Royall, 1994). These assessment batteries cover the general areas of planning, organization, set shifting, staying on task, overcoming distraction, visual construction and planning, inhibition, use of strategies, and working memory. There is no one test that assesses all of ECF; a group of tests is usually chosen that will fulfill the particular needs of the examiner.

A number of these measures may be quite arduous for clients and can drain their attentional and motivational reserves (e.g., Wisconsin Card Sort—Heaton, 1981; California Verbal Learning Test—Delis, Kramer, Kaplan, & Ober, 1987). Although it would be difficult to achieve a good score by chance on most tests of ECF, poor motivation or the presence of tiredness or depression can adversely affect test performance. This highlights a problem of most individual measures of ECF: They do not isolate specific aspects of ECF, and most require memory, attention, visual perception, and language, which are separate from, but are to some extent under the control of, ECF.

Only a few of the measures of ECF are easily administered at the bedside. A bedside measure that we highly recommend is the Executive Interview (EXIT) (or

Table 9.1 Symptoms of ECF Failure Elicited by the EXIT

1. Perseveration
2. Imitation behavior: echopraxia, echolalia
3. Intrusions
4. Frontal release signs
5. Lack of spontaneity/prompting required
6. Disinhibited behaviors
7. Utilization behavior

EXIT25), developed by Royall, Mahurin, and Gray (1992). The EXIT consists of 25 items (each scored 0, 1, or 2), administered in a structured interview format that can be completed in about 15 minutes. The interview follows a set format, but the items are not highly structured, so the client must organize and initiate a response. As shown in Table 9.1, the EXIT items cover several symptoms of ECF failure. As a consequence, this brief screening measure covers the general area of ECF about as well as any of the assessment batteries in current use. The EXIT can be given across the life span, beginning with age 6. The interview has demonstrated ECF impairment in several conditions, to include Alzheimer's disease, Pick's disease, subcortical vascular dementia, major depression, and schizophrenia (Royall & Mahurin, 1996).

We have used this assessment extensively in our own research with individuals diagnosed with Parkinson's disease (PD). The EXIT has detected cognitive impairment, while the most commonly used cognitive screen, the Mini-Mental State Exam (MMSE; Folstein, Folstein, & McHugh, 1975), has indicated no impairment (Elias & Treland, 1999).

In one data set consisting of 46 PD patients, 21 patients were within normal limits on the MMSE (scores of 23 and above) but were in the impaired range on the EXIT (scores of 15 and above). Nineteen patients showed impairment on both the MMSE and the EXIT. Six patients showed no impairment on either test. If only MMSE scores had been used to screen these patients, we would have missed 21 cases of ECF impairment (Elias, 1995).

Parkinson's disease is a motor disorder that originates in the basal ganglia-nigrostriatal area. A second data set, shown in Table 9.2, is composed of PD patients who were staged according to the Hoehn and Yahr (1967) system (Elias et al., 1996). Parkinson's disease patients in Stage I have unilateral motor symptoms with little balance difficulty. Stage II represents the appearance of bilateral symptoms and some

Table 9.2 Frequency of EXIT Scores Within Each Hoehn and Yahr Stage for 36 Patients With Parkinson's Disease

I	5, 6, 7, 9, 11, 12
II	7, 7, 9, 8, 1, 10, 12, 12, 13, 14, 14, 14, 14
III	9, 9, 11, 12, 14, 14, 18, 19, 19, 23
IV	14, 17, 19, 21, 21, 22, 22, 25

Note. Scores >15 indicate executive function impairment.

gait and balance difficulty. Stage III represents bilateral symptoms and increased gait and balance difficulty, including loss of the postural righting reflex (retropulsion on the pull test). Stage IV represents advanced motor, gait, and balance difficulties, plus inability to function independently. The progression of the disease is paralleled by declining ECF and increasing EXIT scores. As can be seen in Table 9.2, ECF impairment as measured by the EXIT (scores >15) begins to appear in Stage III PD. All but one individual in Stage IV PD showed ECF impairment. The loss of independent functioning observed in Stage IV PD is not simply due to impaired motor functioning; it also is strongly affected by a cognitive component. Only one of the 38 PD patients had an MMSE score below 24.

Royall (1994) estimated that screening with the MMSE alone misses 40% of serious noncortical dementias in the general population. This does not mean that the MMSE is not a good screening device for cognitive impairment, merely that it is insensitive to ECF impairment in the absence of postcortical dysfunction (Royall & Polk, 1998). The use of both instruments as screening measures is recommended.

As noted above, the issue of IQ assessment is always important with respect to ECF. In the case of rehabilitation, premorbid estimates of IQ often are not available and have to be obtained following a loss of functioning (e.g., stroke, head injury). To separate premorbid IQ from premorbid ECF, the premorbid estimate of IQ should reflect the crystallized (knowing) components of intelligence (i.e., verbal IQ estimates). Tests such as the National Adult Reading Test (NART; Nelson, 1982) estimate crystallized IQ by focusing on the correct pronunciation of words. The automatic, overlearned, and procedural aspect of the pronunciation of well-known words is expected to only minimally tap ECF. The number of words that are correctly pronounced (regional pronunciations considered) would indicate knowledge and/or use of those words and therefore reflect verbal IQ. Such tests generally correlate modestly to moderately with IQ (Lezak, 1995, pp. 102–106).[2]

We suggest the use of the Wide Range Achievement Test Revised (WRAT-R) for North American clients.[3] If premorbid Verbal and Performance IQ scores are available, then some premorbid estimate of crystallized (knowing) and fluid (doing) intelligence could be provided by the Verbal IQ and Performance IQ, respectively.

The Behavioral Sequelae of Impaired ECF

When executive function is impaired, complex goal-directed behavior breaks down (Royall, 1994). Many behavioral routines are habitual, so this breakdown is particularly noticeable in situations that are relatively unstructured or novel (Gillis, 1996; Royall, 1994). Instrumental activities of daily living (e.g., cooking, cleaning, self-care) can become disrupted so that living independently is no longer prudent. The ability to interact socially (e.g., with family or friends) also may be diminished (Eslinger, Grattan, & Geder, 1996).

Executive function impairment (EFI) appears to be accompanied by "active" and "passive" patterns of behavior (Royall, 1994; see Table 9.3). The active pattern is distinguished by behavioral disinhibition, such as environmentally dependent (i.e., stimulus-bound) behavior. For example, an object can elicit spontaneous, yet purpose-

Table 9.3 Active and Passive Behavior Patterns Seen With
Executive Function Impairment

Active behaviors	Passive behaviors
Environmental dependency	Apathy
Utilization behavior	Loss of initiative
Imitation behavior	Loss of spontaneity
Echolalia, echopraxia	Lack of persistence
Disinhibition	Need for prompting
Occupational or other habits	Behavioral stereotypy
Impulsivity	Perseveration (motor and cognitive)
Social awkwardness	
Vulnerability to intrusions	
Distractibility	
Tangentiality	
"Childishness"	

Note. From "Precis of Executive Dyscontrol as a Cause of Problem Behavior in Dementia,"
by D. R. Royall, 1994, *Experimental Aging Research, 20*, p. 74. Copyright 1994 by Taylor
and Francis. Adapted by permission.

less, handling or use (utilization behavior). Active behavior can be seen in individuals
diagnosed with Alzheimer's or Pick's disease.

The passive pattern of behavior is characterized by environmental indifference, or
apathy (Royall, 1994). These clients can show cognitive and motor perseveration, as
is evident in verbal and design fluency tasks (Royall, 1994). Perseveration appears to
be linked with difficulty in shifting attentional focus, so that a particular behavior
continues despite a change in contextual cues (Malec, 1984). These clients may have
deficient abstract thinking and so have difficulty generating alternatives (i.e., concrete
thinking); the result is in perseverative behavior (Jones, Anderson, Cole, & Hathaway-
Nepple, 1996). The passive pattern can be observed in people who have dementia
associated with PD or the pseudodementia of depression.

The family or caregivers of clients with EFI often note "personality" changes in
the client (Jones et al., 1996; Royall, 1994). Disinhibition, social awkwardness, "child-
ishness," impulsivity, and low frustration tolerance are some of the behavioral expres-
sions of these personality changes. Disinhibited behaviors tend to be related to the
client's "life story," that is, her or his habits, occupation, hobbies, and premorbid
personality characteristics (Jones et al., 1996; Royall, 1994).

Eslinger and colleagues (1996) emphasized the distinction between "personality
changes" and "social-emotional executive impairments." Clients can have difficulty
in "prioritizing, organizing, and managing social information as well as their own
emotional reactions in novel and complex social settings" (p. 427; see this reference
for a more detailed description of this concept). The degree to which social functioning may have changed with EFI should not be underestimated. Individuals with EFI
often describe themselves as being at a loss in social encounters, unable to read the
subtleties in human interaction or to apply rules for social interaction (e.g., turn taking
in conversation).

Executive Function and Rehabilitation

Planning for the rehabilitation of ECF reveals a frustrating dilemma: The problem (the failure of ECF) interferes with traditional solutions to the problem (the application of ECF). A clear definition of ECF (as discussed above) and an awareness of the basis of rehabilitation are helpful in resolving the dilemma.

Ability, skill, process, and *function* are terms used in rehabilitation that need clarification relative to ECF. In ECF, *ability* refers to having sufficient resources for orchestrating and executing behaviors. A *skill* can be thought of as a well-learned habit. Well-learned habits appear to remain intact despite ECF impairment and can provide a foundation upon which to build new habits (Royall, 1994). A *process* is a series of operations executed to a specific end; this relates to the way ECF facilitates goal-directed behavior. *Function* refers generally to "natural, required, or expected activity" (Gillis, 1996, p. 142). In ECF, it is necessary to consider function in terms of the individual's context or environment.

The theoretical constructs that fit well with ECF address "restorative" and "compensatory" approaches to cognitive rehabilitation. The restorative approach, rooted in theories of "neuronal plasticity and redundancy of functional neural systems" (Anderson, 1996, p. 458), would employ cognitive retraining to facilitate recovery of functioning. From this perspective, the goal would be to improve ECF, rather than merely to compensate for the impairment. The compensatory approach accepts that cognitive ability may remain impaired, so the goal is to train the client to function by performing tasks using compensatory strategies.

In treatment planning, the distinction between the restorative and compensatory approaches highlights the need to consider the origins of the EFI. If the EFI is the result of a nonprogressive brain disorder (e.g., head injury), the client is "stable" relative to a client who develops EFI in the course of a progressive illness (e.g., Alzheimer's disease, late-stage PD). In the latter case, the expected course of the illness is an important consideration in developing the rehabilitation treatment plan (Goldstein, 1984). In some conditions, like PD, the rehabilitation goal may be restorative in the early stages and compensatory in the later stages.

When working with clients with EFI, augmenting the cognitive rehabilitation with psychosocial perspective is beneficial. Self-concept is likely to be affected by EFI, and depression, low frustration tolerance, and an inability to appropriately express emotions often accompany EFI (Gillis, 1996; Muir & Haffey, 1990). Interactions with the client may be facilitated by sensitivity to these issues.

Family involvement in the rehabilitation program benefits both the family members and the treatment staff in terms of information and support (Anderson, 1996; Gillis, 1996). The family or caregivers probably will wonder why previous means of interacting are no longer effective or why they may have to assume some of the client's ECF responsibilities. Educating the family about the client's EFI helps quell some of the uncertainty about the client's condition. Involving the family in the rehabilitation goal-setting and training techniques allows them to be active, rather than passive, in the treatment process.

The rehabilitation treatment plan for a client with EFI generally focuses on two areas: changes in the environment (contextual variables) and interventions with the client (intrinsic variables). The ideal rehabilitation setting would be highly structured

Table 9.4 Extrinsic and Intrinsic Variables That Affect
Treatment Performance and Daily Functioning

Extrinsic variables	Intrinsic variables
Speed/rate of presentation	State of arousal
Order of presentation	Mood state
Length of each stimulus item	Hunger
Complexity of information	Pain
Single or multiple choice	Medications
Therapist attitude	Alcohol/drugs

Note. From *Traumatic Brain Injury Rehabilitation for Speech-Language Pathologists* (p. 165), by R. J. Gillis, 1996, Boston: Butterworth Heinemann. Copyright 1996 by Butterworth Heinemann. Adapted by permission.

and distraction-free and have ample rest breaks. Home or community settings are not ideal, however, so treatment planning should focus on the contextual and intrinsic variables that can be manipulated to elicit optimal performance and benefit under conditions that more closely mirror reality (Gillis, 1996; see Table 9.4). Interventions in these areas fit with the goals of the compensatory approach.

Environmental stimuli can serve as cues to overlearned subroutines and evoke either compensatory or "problem" behavior (Royall, 1994); altering contextual variables can have a significant impact on the disinhibited client's actions (Gillis, 1996; Royall, 1994). Royall (1994) used an example of a nursing-home resident who "wandered" outside when cued by the sight of the door. Placing a "Stop" sign at the door reduced the problem behavior by providing a cue for the desired behavior (staying indoors). The family or caregiver can work with the rehabilitation specialist to "listen" to what the environment is "telling" the client (Royall, 1994). Once the potential triggers are elucidated, then the stimuli may be changed or disguised. For example, a door knob could be concealed by a shoe box, or elevator buttons could be covered with a picture. Royall's (1994) recommendations for managing problem behavior are provided in Table 9.5.

When uncooperative behavior is the target of treatment, it is important to remember the link between environmental stimuli and behavioral responses. Resistance to care

Table 9.5 Recommendations for the Management of
Problem Behavior in Dementia

1. Establish a daily ritual.
2. Use new routines to break old habits.
3. Build "good" habits through repetition.
4. "Listen" to what the environment is "saying" to the patient.
5. Use social and environmental cues to your advantage.
6. Remove or alter cues that seem to trigger problem behaviors.

Note. From "Precis of Executive Dyscontrol as a Cause of Problem Behavior in Dementia," by D. R. Royall, 1994, *Experimental Aging Research, 20*, p. 86. Copyright 1994 by Taylor and Francis. Reprinted by permission.

can be conceptualized as a conflict between the client's old habits and the demands of a new environment (Royall, 1994). A positive social cue (e.g., a handshake), rather than a stern tone of voice, might disarm the conflict and make it easier to redirect the client's behavior. Verbal or physical force should be avoided in favor of a supportive, clear, gentle, but firm approach.

Clients with EFI may not immediately comprehend or follow instructions. Rushing these clients elicits opposition and can provoke aggressive behavior. If aggressive behavior is present, the situation needs to be carefully evaluated for possible triggers of this behavior (Anderson, 1996). In a highly structured environment, it may help to reinforce prosocial behavior in situations likely to activate aggression. Extinction techniques also could be effective. In cases of persistent or serious disruptive behavior, a psychological consultation may assist in devising interventions (Sufrin, 1984).

Behavior modification techniques (e.g., a token economy) provide structure for clients with EFI and can be used to decrease inappropriate behavior and increase prosocial behavior. This type of intervention works best in a structured inpatient setting and is more difficult to manage on an outpatient basis (Anderson, 1996). Behavior modification procedures are enhanced by family or caregiver participation and exaggerated reinforcement schedules; delayed or variable reinforcement is less effective.

With clients who are able to be self-aware, short-term anger control may be accomplished by teaching the client self-instruction in anger management. This could be enhanced by training the family or caregiver in the use of time-out procedures (Anderson, 1996).

Group rehabilitation settings provide practice for prosocial behavior, as they resemble social situations and supply multiple distractions and increased unpredictability. While the group experience can foster social skills, group social skills training may be needed before other rehabilitation activities can proceed.

If the client has the capacity for recovery of function, interventions at the "client level" facilitate the restorative approach to rehabilitation. Intervention at this level can also help clients function within their environment, the aim of the compensatory approach. What follows is a brief summary of techniques that have been used with clients with EFI.

In order to adapt to the environment, the client requires executive strategy training. This includes training to recognize a problem (requires awareness), select a strategy (requires goal setting and planning), apply the strategy (requires initiation), and monitor the success of the strategy (requires self-monitoring and self-regulation) (Gillis, 1996). Training in metacognitive or verbal self-strategies, along with the use of checklists and schedules, has provided effective compensatory techniques for planning, self-monitoring, and problem-solving.

Cognitive mediation and verbal self-regulation have been effective strategies for planning. These strategies appear to transfer to other circumstances (Eslinger et al., 1996). External aids (e.g., calendars, checklists, flowcharts, programmed strategies) also can facilitate planning (Chafetz et al., 1996). Verbal analysis of the components of a task can be used to encourage sequencing and self-instruction and to correct errors in problem solving (Malec, 1984).

Strategies used in a restorative approach target improving the underlying processing operations. Toward this goal, planning could be trained by beginning with simple sequencing and categorization tasks and gradually progressing to more complex tasks (Gillis, 1996). Another technique is to reduce the task into its component parts, then use time estimation tasks to address the time constraint aspects of completing the task. Additionally, asking clients to appraise their ability to perform the task encourages self-awareness.

Gillis (1996) suggested using self-appraisal (e.g., "How well am I doing?") to improve self-monitoring. Error detection and correction tasks (e.g., spelling, arithmetic problems) also are useful. To be effective, this training requires repetitive practice of self-check strategies together with external signals (e.g., sounds, commands). Improved self-regulation also has been seen with training in self-instruction, self-prediction, and error-monitoring techniques (e.g., notebooks; cf. Burke, Zencius, Wesolowski, & Doubleday, 1991; Cicerone & Giacino, 1992).

Problem-solving models have utility in helping clients systematically analyze a situation. The process of solving a problem is active and changing and may require several repetitions to achieve an effective solution. In some cases, cognitive functions utilized in problem solving (e.g., attention, memory) will need remediation before they can be used in the service of solving problems. The IDEAL problem-solving model, devised by Gillis (1996), is shown in Table 9.6. For additional examples of problem-solving models see Gillis (1996).

Impaired initiation (i.e., passive features of EFI) can be difficult to treat. Clients may have both the motivation and the capacity to perform but may lack the ability to initiate and sustain purposeful activity (Royall, 1994). These individuals should not be labeled "unmotivated." The lack of initiation or apathy may stem from the EFI.

In the case of apathetic clients, modeling and prompting could be helpful in activating the desired behavior. In the absence of naturally occurring environmental cues, external cues can be employed (e.g., watch alarm, timer; Gillis, 1996). Imposing structure (e.g., checklists, schedules) and training in self-instruction provide support in behavior initiation and problem solving (Anderson, 1996; Chafetz et al., 1996) and have been shown to be quite effective (cf. Burke et al., 1991).

In terms of general principles of intervention, Anderson (1996) and Gillis (1996) agreed that the rehabilitation treatment plan should be based on neuropsychological evaluation, client goals, and practical issues. Planned short-term interventions should be directed at specific goals with real-world impact.

Generalizing skills learned in therapy to the client's everyday life can be challeng-

Table 9.6 Gillis IDEAL Problem-Solving Model

*I*dentify the problem
*D*efine the problem
*E*xplore alternative approaches (options)
*A*ct on the plan
*L*ook at the results

Note. From *Traumatic Brain Injury Rehabilitation for Speech-Language Pathologists* (p. 202) by R. J. Gillis, 1996, Boston: Butterworth Heinemann. Copyright 1996 by Butterworth Heinemann. Adapted by permission.

ing. For example, strategy-specific memory techniques have been found useful and appear to be maintained about 3 years, but they tend not to generalize to other tasks or to be used in daily life (Malec, 1996). Suggestions for facilitating the generalization process include (a) addressing real-world problems from the onset of treatment; (b) using homework assignments; (c) choosing activities to simulate work and social environments; and (d) using in vivo experiences (Anderson, 1996). Multimodal rehabilitation approaches (combining ECF strategies with training specific to other cognitive functions) have been effective with the elderly (Malec, 1996) and are recommended to improve skills generalization. Research is needed to establish how treatment gains can be generalized and maintained.

With respect to rehabilitation planning, Sufrin (1984) pointed out that the elderly often do not receive adequate rehabilitation treatment because they are viewed as experiencing the "normal" consequences of aging. The negative bias toward older adults promotes the myth that the elderly are crotchety, stubborn, unmotivated, and unwilling to actively engage in a treatment program. In fact, these behaviors can be indicative of EFI. When these assumptions are operating, diagnosis, treatment, and rehabilitation tend to be nonaggressive. Consider the implications of this bias in the case of head injury. Studies show that initial recovery in uncomplicated cases appears similar for young and old patients (cf. Goldstein, 1984). Advanced age, however, is a risk factor for not returning to premorbid functioning (Fields, 1997). Less aggressive treatment practices with older patients could mediate this age-related risk factor.

Executive cognitive functions are specifically affected by normal aging (Malloy & Richardson, 1994). Raz (1996) reported MRI findings showing shrinkage of the prefrontal cortex as a function of age. Coffey and associates (1992) examined the MRI data of healthy elderly individuals (i.e., those with no vascular disease or hypertension) and found that cortical atrophy of the frontal regions was disproportionately greater than atrophy in temporal, parietal, and hippocampal regions. Likewise, disproportional frontal metabolic deficits have been observed in the healthy elderly (Kuhl, 1984). Royall and Polk (1998) suggested that normal aging can be associated with an ECF dementia syndrome in the absence of Alzheimer's disease or ischemic vascular disease.

These findings with respect to normal aging suggest that assessment of ECF in elderly individuals is advisable even when rehabilitation is not specifically related to cognition. For example, individuals who have knee replacement surgery have to follow directions, motivate themselves for rehabilitation, reorganize their lives, distinguish expected from unexpected pain, and plan to avoid environments that they can no longer easily negotiate. The tiredness, pain, anxiety, and depression following anesthesia and surgery can disrupt ECF for several months. It should not be taken for granted that ECF is intact before initiating physical rehabilitation programs.

A fact often overlooked in the days of managed care is that age is important with respect to speed of rehabilitation, particularly cognitive rehabilitation. For example, studies of stroke patients by Falconer, Naughton, Strasser, and Sinacore (1994) indicate that discharge options for older stroke patients are likely to be limited not only by the frailty and functional status of the patient, but also by the available social support and resources. For the elderly, longer, less intensive rehabilitation programs in many cases promote and maintain optimal functional status and are more cost-effective.

Notes

1. Descriptions of areas of the brain are often accompanied by the Brodmann location. In the early part of this century, Korbinian Brodmann noted that areas of the brain had unique neuronal configurations and organizations, and he described about 50 areas within a now commonly used cytoarchitectonic map. The sequence of numbers in the map relates to Brodmann's sequence of interest and has no value beyond description (Kolb & Whishaw, 1996). The motor cortex is Brodmann area 4. The premotor areas are 6 and 8. Within the premotor area is the supplementary motor area 6. The frontal eye fields are area 8. The dorsolateral prefrontal cortex encompasses areas 9 and 46. The inferior ventral prefrontal cortex encompasses areas 11, 12, 13, 14. The medial frontal cortex Brodmann areas are 25 and 32. Areas 11, 13, and 14 are often referred to as the orbital frontal cortex due to the relationship with the socket of the eye. The medial area is composed of the anterior cingulate gyrus cortex and the supplementary motor area.

2. See Krull, Scott, and Sherer (1995) for discussion of NART and other measures of premorbid intelligence.

3. See Johnstone, Callahan, Kapila, and Bowman (1996) for a comparison of the WRAT-R to the North American Adult Reading Test (NAART).

References

Anderson, S. W. (1996). Cognitive rehabilitation in closed head injury. In M. Rizzo & D. Tranel (Eds.), *Head injury and post concussive syndrome* (pp. 457–468). New York: Churchill-Livingstone.

Baddeley, A. D. (1996). Exploring the central executive. *Quarterly Journal of Experimental Psychology, 49A,* 5–28.

Burke, W. H., Zencius, A. H., Wesolowski, M. D., & Doubleday, F. (1991). Improving executive function disorders in brain-injured clients. *Brain Injury, 5,* 241–252.

Chafetz, M. D., Friedman, A. L., Kevorkian, G. K., & Levy, J. D. (1996). The cerebellum and cognitive function: Implications for rehabilitation. *Archives of Physical Medicine and Rehabilitation, 77,* 1303–1308.

Cicerone, K. D., & Giacino, J. T. (1992). Remediation of executive function deficits after traumatic brain injury. *Journal of Neurologic Rehabilitation, 2,* 12–22.

Coffey, C. E., Wilkinson, W. E., Parashoe, I. A., Soady, S. A. R., Sullivan, R. J., Patterson, L. J., Figel, G. S., Webb, M. C., Spritzer, C. E., & Djang, W. T. (1992). Quantitative cerebral anatomy of the aging human brain: A cross-sectional study using magnetic resonance imaging. *Neurology, 42,* 527–536.

Cummings, J. L. (1993). Frontal-subcortical circuits and human behavior. *Archives of Neurology, 50,* 873–880.

Delis, D. C., Kramer, J. H., Kaplan, E., & Ober, B. A. (1987). *California Verbal Learning Test: Research edition.* New York: Psychological Corporation.

Denkla, M. B. (1996). A theory and model of executive function. In G. R. Lyon & M. A. Krasnegor (Eds.), *Attention, memory, and executive function* (pp. 263–278). Baltimore: Paul Brookes.

Denkla, M. B., & Reiss, A. L. (1997). Prefrontal-subcortical circuits in developmental disorders. In N. Krasnegor, G. R. Lyon, & P. S. Goldman-Rakic (Eds.), *Development of the prefrontal cortex* (pp. 283–293). Baltimore: Paul Brookes.

Elias, J. W. (1995). Normal versus pathological aging: Are we screening adequately for dementia? *Experimental Aging Research, 21,* 97–100.

Elias, J. W., & Treland, J. (1999). Executive function in Parkinson's disease and subcortical disorders. *Seminars in Clinical Neuropsychiatry, 4,* 34–40.

Elias, J., Treland, J., Hutton, J., New, P., Royall, D., & Shroyer, J. (1996, April). *The value of using brief assessment measures for executive function as well as Mini-Mental State type screening measures.* Poster session presented at the Sixth Cognitive Aging Conference, Atlanta, GA.

Eslinger, P. J., Grattan, L. M., & Geder, L. (1996). Neurologic and neuropsychologic aspects of frontal lobe impairments in postconcussive syndrome. In M. Rizzo & D. Tranel (Eds.), *Head injury and post concussive syndrome* (pp. 414–440). New York: Churchill-Livingstone.

Falconer, J. A., Naughton, B. J., Strasser, D. C., & Sinacore, J. M. (1994). Stroke inpatient rehabilitation: A comparison across age groups. *Journal of the American Geriatrics Society, 42,* 39–44.

Fields, R. B. (1997). Geriatric head injury. In P. D. Nussbaum (Ed.), *Handbook of neuropsychology and aging* (pp. 280–297). New York: Plenum Press.

Folstein, M. F., Folstein, S. E., & McHugh, P. R. (1975). "Mini-mental state." *Journal of Psychiatric Research, 12,* 189–198.

Gillis, R. J. (1996). *Traumatic brain injury rehabilitation for speech-language pathologists.* Boston: Butterworth Heinemann.

Golden, C. (1984). Rehabilitation and the Luria-Nebraska neuropsychological battery: Introduction to theory and practice. In B. A. Edelstein & E. T. Couture (Eds.), *Behavioral assessment and rehabilitation of the traumatically brain-damaged* (pp. 83–120). New York: Plenum Press.

Goldstein, G. (1984). Methodological and theoretical issues in neuropsychological assessment. In B. A. Edelstein & R. T. Couture (Eds.), *Behavioral assessment rehabilitation of the traumatically brain-damaged* (pp. 1–21). New York: Plenum Press.

Heaton, R. K. (1981). *Wisconsin Card Sorting Test.* Odess, FL: Psychological Assessment Resources.

Hoehn, M. M., & Yahr, M. D. (1967). Parkinson onset, progression and mortality. *Neurology, 17,* 427–442.

Johnstone, B., Callahan, C., Kapila, & Bowman, D. E. (1996). The comparability of the WRAT-R reading test and NAART as estimates of premorbid intelligence in neurologically impaired patients. *Archives of Clinical Neuropsychology, 11,* 513–519.

Jones, R. D., Anderson, S. W., Cole, T., & Hathaway-Nepple, J. (1996). In M. Rizzo & D. Tranel (Eds.), *Head injury and post concussive syndrome* (pp. 395–414). New York: Churchill-Livingstone.

Kolb, B., & Whishaw, I. Q. (1996). *Fundamentals of human neuropsychology* (4th ed.). New York: Freeman.

Krasnegor, N. A., Lyon, G. R., & Goldman-Rakic, S. (1997). *Development of the prefrontal cortex.* Baltimore: Paul Brookes.

Krull, K. R., Scott, J. G., & Sherer, M. (1995). Estimation of premorbid intelligence from combined performance and demographic variables. *The Clinical Neuropsychologist, 9,* 83–88.

Kuhl, D. E. (1984). The effects of normal aging on patterns of local cerebral glucose utilization. *Annals of Neurology, 15,* S133–137.

Lezak, M. D. (1983). *Neuropsychological assessment* (2nd ed.). New York: Oxford University Press.

Lezak, M. D. (1995). *Neuropsychological assessment* (3rd ed.). New York: Oxford University Press.

Lovell, M. R., & Smith, S. S. (1997). Neuropsychological evaluation of subcortical dementia. In P. D. Nussbaum (Ed.), *Handbook of neuropsychology and aging* (pp. 189–200). New York: Plenum Press.

Malec, J. (1984). Training the brain-injured client in behavioral self-management skills. In

B. A. Edelstein & E. T. Couture (Eds.), *Behavioral assessment and rehabilitation of the traumatically brain-damaged* (pp. 121–150). New York: Plenum Press.

Malec, J. F. (1996). Cognitive rehabilitation. In R. W. Evans (Ed.), *Neurology and trauma* (pp. 231–248). Philadelphia: W. B Saunders.

Malloy, P. F., & Richardson, E. D. (1994). Assessment of frontal lobe functions. *Journal of Neuropsychiatry, 6,* 399–410.

Muir, C. A., & Haffey, W. J. (1990). Psychological and neuropsychological interventions in the mobile mourning process. In B. A. Edelstein & E. T. Couture (Eds.), *Behavioral assessment and rehabilitation of the traumatically brain-damaged* (pp. 247–271). New York: Plenum Press.

Nelson, H. E. (1982). *The National Adult Reading Test (NART): Test manual.* Windsor, UK: NFER-Nelson.

Pennington, B. F. (1997). Dimensions of executive functions in normal and abnormal development. In N. A. Krasnegor, G. R. Lyon, & P. S. Goldman-Rakic (Eds.), *Development of the prefrontal cortex* (pp. 265–281). Baltimore: Paul Brooks.

Raz, N. (1996). Neuroanatomy of the aging brain observed in vivo: a review of structural MRI findings. In E. D. Bigler (Ed.), *Neuroimaging: Vol. 2. Clinical applications* (pp. 153–182). New York: Plenum Press.

Royall, D. R (1994). Precis of executive dyscontrol as a cause of problem behavior in dementia. *Experimental Aging Research, 20,* 73–94.

Royall, D. R., & Mahurin, R. K. (1996). Neuroanatomy, measurement, and clinical significance of the executive cognitive functions. In L. J. Dickstein, J. M. Oldham, & M. B. Riba (Eds.), *Annual review of psychiatry* (Vol. 15, pp. 175–204). Washington, DC: American Psychiatric Press.

Royall, D. R., Mahurin, R. K., & Cornell, J. (1994). Bedside assessment of frontal degeneration: Distinguishing Alzheimer's disease from non-Alzheimer's cortical dementia. *Experimental Aging Research, 20,* 95–103.

Royall, D. R., & Polk, M. P. (1998). Dementias that present with and without posterior cortical features: An important clinical distinction. *Journal of the American Geriatrics Society, 46,* 98–105.

Shallice, T. (1982). Specific impairments of planning. *Philosophical Transactions of the Royal Society of London, 298,* 199–209.

Stuss, D. T., & Benson, D. F. (1986). *The frontal lobes.* New York: Raven Press.

Sufrin, E. M. (1984). The physical rehabilitation of the brain-damaged elderly. In B. A. Edelstein & E. T. Couture (Eds.), *Behavioral assessment and rehabilitation of the traumatically brain-damaged* (pp. 191–226). New York: Plenum Press.

Usman, M. A. (1997). Frontotemporal dementias. In P. D. Nussbaum (Eds.), *Handbook of neuropsychology and aging,* (pp. 159–176). New York: Plenum Press.

10

The Influence of Depression on Cognitive Rehabilitation in Older Adults

NANCY A. PACHANA

BERNICE A. MARCOPULOS

KELLIE A. TAKAGI

Depression is one of the most common mental disorders experienced by older adults (Alexopoulos, Young, Meyers, Abrams, & Shamoian, 1988) and remains a major health concern (National Institute of Health [NIH], 1992). Depressive symptoms have been estimated to occur in 10–25% of community-dwelling older adults aged 65 and over, and in 30% of older adults in residential care settings (Blazer, 1993). Depression and its symptoms are frequently underreported in the elderly (Lyness et al., 1995), and depression remains underdiagnosed and undertreated in this population (NIH, 1992). The distinctions between forms of depression in the elderly (early- vs. late-onset; clinical vs. subclinical manifestations of symptoms) is a focus of ongoing research. What has emerged from the research literature is a profile of depressive symptomatology among older adults that often includes complaints of cognitive dysfunction.

From both an assessment and a rehabilitation standpoint, depressed older adults present a particular challenge. Advancing age and comorbid medical conditions may affect cognitive and emotional presentation in this population. Assessment instruments and corresponding normative data must be chosen with care to ensure adequate reliability and validity for use with the elderly. The differentiation of cognitive decline secondary to depression from such declines resulting from progressive dementing disorders is a common but challenging assessment question. While treatment of depression with medication, psychotherapy, or some combination may have some positive effects on cognitive functioning (e.g., Siegfried, Jansen, & Pahnke, 1984), cognitive impairments may persist despite treatment (Fromm & Schopflocher, 1984). Rehabilitation efforts directed at improving cognitive function in depressed older adults must be designed with the particular complaints as well as the individual's cognitive strengths and weaknesses in mind. Although still a relatively recent area of research, techniques to improve cognitive functioning in older adults in general, and in particular subgroups such as those with mood or dementing disorders, are available.

The nature of depression and its effect on cognition in older adults, as well as issues of assessment and rehabilitation strategies aimed at this group, will be discussed in this chapter.

Types and Etiologies of Depression in Old Age

Prevalence rates of depression in older adults vary in epidemiological studies due to differing methods used to diagnose psychiatric disorders. It has been estimated that the prevalence rate for major depression in older adult community residents is between 1% and 2% (Blazer, Hughes, & George, 1987), and 2% for dysthymia (Blazer, 1989). However, it is not uncommon for older adults to present with a transient recurrence of depressive symptoms that do not meet current diagnostic criteria. "Double depression," in which a major depressive disorder is superimposed on dysthymia or minor depression, has been described in several studies (Keller & Shapiro, 1982; Rounsaville, Sholomskas, & Prusoff, 1980) and may serve to further complicate the diagnostic picture.

Clinicians often distinguish between depressive disorders that develop either before (early-onset) or after (late-onset) the ages of 50–60. Distinguishable differences between late-onset and early-onset depression are in the areas of clinical manifestation and course of the disorder. Late-onset depression is associated with multiple medical disorders (Blazer et al., 1987), lower socioeconomic status, low social integration (Phifer & Murrel, 1986; Turner & Noh, 1988), and structural brain changes (Coffey, Figiel, Djang, & Saunders, 1989; Coffey, Figiel, Djang, & Weiner, 1990) including cerebrovascular disease (Steffens, Hays, George, Krishnan, & Blazer, 1996). Comparisons of early- and late-onset depressive symptomatology indicate that older adults tend to have decreased guilt feelings (Brown, Sweeney, Sweeney, Loutsch, & Kocsis, 1984) along with increases in loss of interest (Post, 1962), psychosis (Myers & Greenberg, 1989) and generalized anxiety (Brown et al., 1984; Myers & Greenberg, 1989). However, differences between early- and late-onset depression are far from clear-cut, with conflicting results reported in the literature (see Caine, Lyness, & King, 1993, for a review).

Both medical disorders and functional disabilities have been found to contribute substantially to the chronicity of depressive symptomatology in older adults (Kennedy, Kelman, & Thomas, 1991). Vulnerability to depression in older adults with a range of illnesses has been reported, including rheumatoid arthritis (Creed & Ash, 1992), stroke, cancer, hypothyroidism, and vitamin deficiencies (Finch, Ramsay, & Katona, 1992). (For an overview of functional impairment, physical disease, and depression in older adults, see Zeiss, Lewinsohn, & Rohde, 1996). However, King, Cox, Lyness, and Caine (1995) found that comorbid medical illness had minimal effect on test performance in same-age depressed and nondepressed elderly. Clearly, while age and medical conditions may impact depressive symptomatology in older adults, this is an area requiring further study.

Difficulties have been encountered in establishing clear boundaries between major depression and dysthymia as diagnostic categories, due to high rates of comorbidity and commonality of symptoms (Clark, Beck, & Beck, 1994; Kocsis & Frances, 1987; Murphy, 1991). Dysthymia is often comorbid with lifetime histories of major depression, anxiety disorders, bipolar disorders, personality disorders (particularly borderline and avoidant personality disorders), or substance abuse. The Epidemiologic Catchment Area (ECA) Study (Weissman, Bruce, Leaf, Florio, & Holzer, 1991) determined that while the onset of major depression and dysthymia was predominantly prior to age 45, a sizable subgroup of dysthymic patients developed the disorder somewhat later in life. Patients with dysthymia frequently lack neurovegetative symptoms but often complain of cognitive and behavioral dysfunction (Keller et al., 1997; Kocsis & Frances, 1987).

Grief reactions may also trigger depression in older adults (Gallagher, Breckenridge, Thompson, & Peterson, 1983); reactions may range from intense emotional symptoms to depression. Generally, while normal grief reactions may include depressive symptoms, feelings of worthlessness, pervasive guilt or hopelessness, and morbid thinking are absent (Gallagher, Breckenridge, Thompson, Dessonville, & Amaral, 1982). Especially after the death of a spouse, older adults are often faced with multiple challenges, including learning new skills. For this group, coping may be hindered by the presence of depressive symptomatology, particularly if cognitive dysfunction is present.

Dementia, "Pseudodementia," and Depression in Older Adults

The relationship between dementia, "pseudodementia," and depression is also multifaceted and continues to challenge clinicians and researchers in the area of evaluation and treatment. An epidemiological link has been found between depression and dementia, leading some clinicians and researchers to propose a possible etiological link. Some researchers have suggested that depression may predispose one to develop dementia and that normality, depression, pseudodementia, and dementia may lie on a progressive continuum, with depression being the first sign of dementia (Cassens, Wolfe, & Zola, 1990). The association between depression and dementia has been viewed from four vantage points: pseudodementia, dementia syndrome of depression, depression as an early symptom of dementia, and coexistence of dementia and depression.

Pseudodementia refers to unrecognized and untreated psychiatric disorders, especially depression, that may cause apparent cognitive deficits (Kiloh, 1961). Caine (1986) reviewed the literature and concluded that pseudodementia is most often associated with depression in elderly patients but can also occur in many other kinds of psychiatric diagnoses in younger patients. The assumption in pseudodementia is that the clinician must differentiate depression from dementia because if the depression is correctly identified and successfully treated, concomitant cognitive deficits may also abate. It is assumed that these two clinical entities are mutually exclusive and that pseudodementia is a reversible dementia.

Early follow-up studies lent support to the concept because in many cases, the diagnosis of "presenile" dementia eventually evolved into depression (Nott & Fleminger, 1975; Ron, Toone, Garralda, & Lishman, 1979). A more recent study found improvement on the Mattis Dementia Rating Scale on Initiation, Perseveration and Memory subtests following electroconvulsive treatment (Stoudemire, Hill, Morris, & Dalton, 1995).

In recent years, the concept of pseudodementia has been criticized, since it implies clinically dichotomous and mutually exclusive diagnostic entities when, in reality, patients can be both demented and depressed. Recent estimates of the prevalence of "reversible" dementias are less than 1% (Walstra, Teunisse, van Gool, & van Crevel, 1997; Weytingh, Bossuyt, & van Crevel, 1995). Patients with low intelligence, low education, physical illness, advanced age, or a history of mental illness are more likely to be diagnosed with pseudodementia, an outcome suggesting some problems with both the diagnostic criteria and the use of cognitive screening measures to aid diagnosis. Several authors have suggested that the term be abandoned (e.g., Bieliauskas, 1993; Lamberty & Bieliauskas, 1993; Marcopulos, 1989; Nussbaum, 1994; Poon, 1992; Reifler, 1982).

In their review, King and Caine (1996) concluded that neuropsychological deficits in depression are not an epiphenomenon but are due to depression-related changes in cerebral functioning, sometimes referred to as the *Dementia syndrome of depression.* Cognitive deficits found in depressed individuals, including inattention and declines in memory recall and spontaneous behavior, are similar to those found in patients with subcortical dementias, so some authors propose that depression be considered a form of subcortical dementia (Caine, 1981; Cummings & Benson, 1984; Folstein & McHugh, 1978; King & Caine, 1990).

Another way to look at this clinical dilemma is that normality, depression, pseudo-dementia, and dementia may lie on a progressive continuum, with depression being the first sign of dementia (Kral & Emery, 1989; Reding, Haycox, & Blass, 1985). Lishman (1987) warned that some cases of pseudodementia might turn out in fact to be a "pseudopseudodementia." Nussbaum, Kaszniak, Allender, and Rapcsak (1991) found that 23% of their depressed patients showed cognitive decline over a 25-month period. These patients had more white-matter MRI, CAT, and EEG abnormalities than those who did not show decline (Reifler, 1982; Reifler, Larson, & Hanley, 1982).

Both retrospective and prospective community studies have found that depressed mood is associated with a moderately increased risk of developing dementia (Buntinx, Kester, Bergers, & Knottnerus, 1996; Devanand et al., 1996; Speck et al., 1995). For example, Alexopoulos, Meyers, Young, Mattis, and Kakuma, (1993) followed a group of patients who had "reversible dementia" for just over 2 years. Reversible dementia was defined as those depressed elderly inpatients who had diagnoses of dementia and depression on admission, but whose dementia and depression improved after treatment; improvement was defined as a Mini-Mental State Exam (MMSE; Folstein, Folstein, & McHugh, 1975) score greater than 24. Alexopoulos et al. found that these patients had a 4.69 times greater risk of developing dementia than patients with a diagnosis of depression only.

It may be that depressed elders who show cognitive impairment may have subtle neurochemical or neurophysiological abnormalities that predispose them to show cognitive impairment in depression or to develop dementia. Zubenko, Henderson, Stiffler, Stabler, Rosen, and Kaplan (1996) found no relationship between depression and the apolipoprotein E (ApoE) and no relationship between MMSE score and ApoE in inpatient elders. However, depressed elders with psychotic features had a higher frequency of the ApoE alleles. Steffens et al. (1997) concluded in their twin study of depression and ApoE that depression may reflect prodromal symptoms rather than increase the risk of developing Alzheimer's disease.

Depressive symptomatology occurs in many forms of dementia; however, there are conflicting reports in the literature on prevalence rates for depression by type of dementia (Ballard, Bannister, Solis, Oyebode, & Wilcock, 1996; Bucht & Adolfsson, 1983; Fischer, Simanyi, & Danielczyk, 1990; Komahashi et al., 1994). In reviews of depression in mixed dementia patients, prevalence rates of coexistence varied between 0% and 87%, with modal rates above 30% (Reifler et al., 1982; Teri & Reifler, 1987; Wragg & Jeste, 1989; for a review, see Teri & Wagner, 1992). In comparisons with nondemented elderly, both AD and vascular dementia patients were more depressed than controls; the two demented groups did not differ in terms of depression (Fischer et al., 1990). Symptoms of depression were reported in the earlier stages of Alzheimer's disease in approximately 10–25% of patients (Rovner, Broadhead, Spencer, Carson, & Folstein, 1989). Clinical features that may signal depression in Alzheimer's patients include increased psychomotor retardation, ideas of worthlessness, recurrent thoughts of death, and early-morning awakening (Greenwald et al., 1989). Depressed Alzheimer's patients also have been found to demonstrate greater severity of cognitive impairment, greater dependency on others for activities of daily living, and higher prevalence of past psychiatric history than to nondepressed Alzheimer's patients (Rovner & Morris, 1989).

In one study (Sulzter, Levin, Mahler, High, & Cummings, 1993), Alzheimer's disease and vascular dementia patients were matched for severity of cognitive impairment, age, and educational background. It was determined that there was no significant relationship between severity of cognitive impairment and noncognitive symptoms such as depression. It was also determined that the vascular dementia patients had more severe behavioral retardation, depression, and anxiety than Alzheimer's disease patients.

In summary, the use of the term and concept of *pseudodementia* has been rejected by most researchers and clinicians. However, the prevalence of cognitive deficits in depressed older persons remains unknown. The dividing line between mild cognitive deficit in depression and mild depression in dementia is far from clear, although several authors have attempted clarification. For example, Emery and Oxman (1997) proposed that depressive dementia may be a "transitional dementia." Much work remains to be done to clarify the relationship in older adults between cognitive deficits and depressive symptoms in both depression and dementia.

The Nature of Cognitive Loss in Depression

With increasing age, many spheres of cognitive functioning change. The impact of depression on cognition must be understood within the context of changes in cognition associated with "normal" or disease-free aging as well as cognitive changes associated with particular disease states, including physiological, neurological, and psychiatric disorders. As the topic of cognitive changes associated with normal aging is covered elsewhere in this book, what follows is a review of changes in cognitive functioning in depressed older adults.

Although there is some neurobiological evidence that depression involves changes in brain structures and substances associated with memory (Bartus, Dean, Beer, & Lippa, 1982; McGaugh, 1983; Nussbaum, 1997), the research evidence as to the prevalence and extent of memory impairment in depressed elderly is equivocal. Many studies suggest various types and degrees of memory impairment in depressed subjects, in terms of learning and short-term memory (Bäckman & Forsell, 1994; Caine, 1986; Gibson, 1981; Raskin, Friedman, & DiMascio, 1982); errors in recall (Henry, Weingartner, & Murphy, 1973; McAllister, 1981; Whitehead, 1973); and less effective coding and memory strategies (Breslow, Kocsis, & Belkin, 1981; Weingartner, Cohen, & Bunney, 1982). Other studies (Derry & Kuiper, 1981; Niederehe & Camp, 1985; Pearlson et al., 1989; Popkin, Gallagher, Thompson, & Moore, 1982) fail to demonstrate impairment in the overall memory performance of depressed subjects. In a study by Williams, Little, Scates, and Blockman (1987), while depressed and nondepressed adults were comparable on memory test performances, the depressed group complained of greater problems in memory than nondepressed adults. Subjective memory complaints are far more common among depressed older adults than among nondepressed controls (cf. Feehan, Knight, & Partridge, 1991); such negative evaluation of memory is congruent with depressed individuals' tendency to negatively evaluate many aspects of their self-worth and capacities.

Other cognitive processes that may impact performance on memory tasks, such as vigilance, attention, and reaction time (Breslow et al., 1981; Frith et al., 1983; Glass, Uhlenhuth, Hartel, Matuzas, & Fischman, 1981) and use of coding and memory strategies (Breslow et al., 1981; Cohen, Weingartner, Smallberg, Pickar, & Murphy, 1982), have also been found to be impaired in depressed patients. Hart, Kwentus, Taylor, and Hamer (1987a) found depressed patients less able than nondepressed elders to benefit from imagery to aid retention of items from a selective reminding task. In their study, Hart et al. (1987a) did find depressed patients able to make good use of cues (reminders).

The degree of cognitive impairment of depressed older adults may vary as a function of demographic variables, levels of care, or the presence of comorbid psychiatric conditions. In a review article, Poon (1992) stated that poor control of variables such as age and education may contribute to conflicting evidence on the impact of depression on cognitive function in late life. Differences in performance on memory tasks has been found between male and female depressed elderly (Cipolli, Neri, Andermarcher, Pinelli, & Lalla, 1990). Cultural differences are also often overlooked in studies of cognition and cognitive remediation, particularly among older adults (Altarriba, 1993; Gilinsky, Ehrlich, & Craik, 1993). Memory impairment has been found to be greater in psychiatric inpatients than in psychiatric outpatients, and greater in mixed unipolar and bipolar depression than in unipolar depression alone (Burt, Zembar, & Niederehe, 1995). King et al. (1995) compared elderly depressed inpatients with community-dwelling elders attending a senior center. They found deficits in attention, word generation, immediate and delayed verbal recall, and constructional praxis in the depressed group. No differences were found on verbal retention or nonverbal learning.

There are several different approaches to the study of memory in depression. Cognitive psychologists study aspects of the *quality* (content and process) of memory, while neuropsychologists often focus on the *quantity* (deficits) of memory functioning in depression and relate it to brain function. From a cognitive processing standpoint, depressed persons recall more negative information than positive, the so-called valence effect of recall (Blaney, 1986; Ingram & Reed, 1986). Hasher and Zacks (1979) proposed that depressed persons have more difficulty with cognitive processes that require effort (i.e., more attentional capacity than automatic processes). The reason may be that depressed persons are using attentional capacity to focus on depression-related thoughts (Hartlage, Alloy, Vazquez, & Dykman, 1993). Burt et al. (1995) found support for the valence effect theory that depressed persons find it easier to remember mood-congruent material (e.g., Blaney, 1986). However, in a study that included older adults, Rohling and Scogin (1993) did not find that depression was associated with effortful memory deficits. (See Hartlage and Clements, 1996, for a review of cognitive processes in depression.)

Although one might assume that the cognitive deficits associated with depression are more prominent in elderly persons, the literature does not support this assumption. Older depressed adults, like younger persons with depression, are able to remember more negative valence material and show mild decrements on memory testing and may demonstrate more problems with "effortful" memory processing. To date, the most comprehensive evaluation of the effect of depression on memory was completed by Burt et al. (1995) via meta-analyses. They found significant and consistent relationships between depression and memory impairment. What was surprising was that they found that this association was stronger in *younger* patients than in older patients. This finding agrees with that of Rohling and Scogin (1993), who found that depressed older adults were not more predisposed to memory loss. Kinderman and Brown (1997) conducted a meta-analysis of 40 studies looking at the effects of depression in older adults. They looked at patient characteristics and memory task factors and compared their results with those of Burt et al. (1995). Mixed unipolar and bipolar patient groups showed larger effect sizes than studies that included only unipolar patients. Also, like Burt et al., Kinderman and Brown found that studies that included younger subjects had larger effect sizes. Consistent with much of the neuropsychological literature, they found larger effect sizes for figural memory tasks than for verbal memory tasks, delayed memory versus immediate memory and recognition versus free recall.

Assessment Strategies for Cognitive Loss in Late-Life Depression

Assessment of older adults brings with it the usual clinical considerations of using appropriate instruments with adequate norms, being aware of patient fatigue or anxiety, possible sensory losses that may influence testing, and the existence of possible comorbid physical, psychiatric, or dementing conditions that may impact testing. Three primary purposes of assessment are diagnostic, descriptive, and longitudinal. It is important to complete a comprehensive enough assessment to determine the causes of cognitive declines while not straining either patient tolerance or clinical common sense. An assessment that provides a good description of the individual patient's strengths and weaknesses will be of enormous value when treatment and rehabilitation plans are devised. Assessments done over time can provide comparisons with baseline measurements in terms of rehabilitative progress or rate and degree of continued decline if dementia is present. Mood as well as cognitive dysfunction needs to be adequately assessed.

Assessment of Mood

A variety of instruments that assess depressed mood have normative data for, or have been developed specifically for use with, older patients (see Pachana, Gallagher, & Thompson, 1992, for a review). Despite its widespread use, the Beck Depression Inventory (BDI; Beck, Ward, Mendelson, Mock, & Erbaugh, 1961) has limitations for use with older adults, although the reliability and validity of the instrument for this population are adequate (see Gallagher, 1986, for a review). The BDI does not sample depressive symptomatology characteristic of the elderly, such as emptiness and helplessness (Weiss, Nagel, & Aronson, 1986). The response format requires choosing from a variety of options the statement that best reflects the respondent's state of mind; cognitively compromised elders may find this task difficult. The number of questions assessing somatic symptoms limits the clinician's ability to distinguish distress due to medical illness from distress secondary to depression (Norris, Gallagher, Wilson, & Winograd, 1987). The Geriatric Depression Scale (GDS; Yesavage, Brink, & Rose, 1983), developed specifically for use with older depressed adults, addresses many of these limitations. Items on the GDS address symptoms commonly presented by older depressed adults and contain virtually no somatic complaints. The simplified yes/no response format of the GDS also reduces cognitive demands on patients. Several studies demonstrate the superiority of the GDS over the BDI and other self-report measures of depression in discriminating depressed and non-depressed elders (Brink et al.,1982; Hyer & Blount, 1984; Kiernan et al., 1986).

The Geriatric Depression Rating Scale (GDRS; Jamison & Scogin, 1992) is an interviewer-based rating scale that uses items from the GDS as topic areas in a structured interview format. Areas assessed include mood, hopefulness, cognitive function, and life satisfaction. This instrument, designed and normed specifically for older adults, includes detailed administration instructions by the authors. Another commonly used interviewer-based rating scale for depression, the Hamilton Rating Scale for Depression (HRSD; Hamilton, 1967) and the more recent refinement of this scale, the Structured Interview Guide for the HRSD (SIGH-D; Williams, 1988) should both be used with caution in an elderly population. Item reliabilities for both instruments are only fair (Pachana et al., 1992); unsophisticated interviewers may fail to record the presence of depressive symptomatology in cognitively compromised frail elders and thus may underestimate depression (Lichtenberg, Marcopulos, Steiner, & Tabscott, 1992). As on the GDS, the fact that many items on the HRSD are somatic may lead to an overestimation of depression in medically compromised elders (Thompson, Futterman, & Gallagher, 1988).

When faced with assessment of depression with comorbid dementia, specialized instruments such as the Cornell Scale for Depression in Dementia (Alexopoulos, Abrams, Young, & Shamoian, 1988) or the Dementia Mood Assessment Scale (Sunderland et al., 1988) may be appropriate. The GDS appears to be a valid measure of depressive symptoms in patients with mild to moderate dementia (Feher, Larrabee, & Crook, 1992); however, in general, the greater the severity of dementia, the more limited the utility of the GDS (Burke, Houston, Boust, & Roccaforte, 1989).

Assessment of Cognition

Neuropsychological tests used for assessment of older populations should have well-constructed age- and education-appropriate norms (e.g., Heaton, Grant, & Matthews, 1991; Ivnik et al., 1992; Spreen & Strauss, 1997). Also important is documentation of predictive and concurrent validity for assessing cognitive impairment in depression and identifying dementia, as well as adequate psychometric properties, including test-retest reliability for assessing change in future assessments (Christensen, Hadzi-Pavlovic, & Jacomb, 1991; LaRue, 1992). Knowledge of how normal cognitive changes differentially affect test scores is crucial. For instance, age effects are greater for memory, cognitive flexibility, and motor speed tasks than purely verbal tests (reviewed in Birren & Schaie, 1990). For this reason, it is better to use neuropsychological tests that have been adequately normed on older adults, rather than using cutoff scores (e.g., the Halstead-Reitan Battery), which tend to overestimate cognitive impairment in older adults (e.g., Moehle & Long, 1989). At a minimum, neuropsychological testing should encompass attention, language, memory, visuospatial skills, cognitive flexibility, and abstract reasoning (Thompson, Gong, Haskins, & Gallagher, 1987). While a discussion of neuropsychological testing of older adults is beyond the scope of this chapter, the reader is referred to several excellent texts and reviews of this subject (Albert, 1981; LaRue, 1992; Woodruff-Pak, 1997).

Assessment of the individual's current problems with cognition and the impact of everyday functioning cannot be overlooked if rehabilitation strategies are to be successfully implemented. As depression may result in the patient's being unable to realistically state current strengths and weaknesses, careful and thorough questioning is essential. Test scores should be used in conjunction with the clinical interview and assessment of prior or current cognitive strategies. A thorough assessment of the patient's developmental history may also be of help when designing rehabilitation strategies (Willis & Schaie, 1988). However, the clinician should be conscious not to tax the patient with too lengthy an assessment in one sitting, as one study (Hayslip, Kennelly, & Maloy, 1989) demonstrated that a lengthy, demanding test battery may exaggerate deficits observed in older depressed adults.

The distinction of dementia from depression on assessment is difficult but is essential for proper treatment recommendations. Behavioral features and qualitative aspects of cognitive performance may assist in such a differentiation (Kaszniak & Christenson, 1994); such features, along with differences on various formal testing measures, are discussed below. However, it is likely that in patients of advanced age, the distinction of the sequelae of depression and dementia may be impossible to make.

Generally, depressed older adults present as acutely aware of any cognitive deficits, which they may describe in great detail and which they report significantly interfere with normal functioning. While cognitive dysfunction is a prominent characteristic of depression in older adults, hopelessness, emptiness, feelings of envy, and a history of depressive feelings (Weiss et al., 1986) are also often present. The progression of these symptoms is often uneven, though their onset is often clear. In terms of test behavior, depressed patients in general display poor motivation and many "I don't know" responses and may display significantly improved performance with prompting and cuing.

In contrast, older mild to moderately demented patients with depression are generally less aware of their degree of impairment and less articulate and forthcoming in their description of symptoms. Particularly in the case of Alzheimer's, the onset of symptoms is insidious, with a relatively steady decline in functioning. On testing, cooperation and motivation may be high, unlike those of depressed patients, but poor performance generally is not helped by prompting or cuing and indeed may be unrecognized as deficient by the patient. While behavior in the demented patient is often congruent with cognitive losses evident on testing, the same is not always true in depression alone (Strub & Black, 1988). However, whereas the social skills of dementia patients are often remarkably well preserved despite cognitive losses, the social skills of depressed elderly patients are often impaired (Mirchandani, 1988). "Sundowning," or the nocturnal worsening of cognitive and behavioral functioning, is often present in dementia patients but generally absent in depression (Mirchandani, 1988).

Depressed persons with and without comorbid dementia may also show differences in cognitive performance. Unlike demented patients, depressed older adults produce few intrusion errors (Marcopulos & Graves, 1990) and usually can benefit from cuing and encoding strategies. Depressed patients have normal serial position curve and normal rates of forgetting, whereas demented patients show rapid loss of information (Hart, Kwentus, Taylor, & Harkins, 1987b; Larrabee, Youngjohn, Sudilovsky, & Crook, 1993; DesRosiers, Hodges, & Berrios, 1995). Because the performance of depressed older adults varies greatly, even within a single testing session, several tests tapping the same cognitive domain may be useful in distinguishing depressed from demented patients, whose performance is much more stable. Naming and simple calculation skills are relatively unimpaired in depressed compared to demented patients (LaRue, 1992).

The following case illustrates an assessment that revealed cognitive impairment associated with depression, but not dementia, which remitted with treatment.

Case I

Referral Question and Background Information: Mr. S, a 67-year-old, right-handed, college-educated, white male, was treated as an outpatient for I year for persistent depressive symptoms. Mr. S had had at least two previous episodes of major depression, which had been successfully treated. This recent episode was precipitated by several significant stressors, including "forced" retirement and marital stress. Testing was requested to further evaluate his recent cognitive decline.

Behavioral Observations and Clinical Interview: Mr. S presented as a well-groomed 67-year-old man, looking his stated age. He reported poor sleep and appetite and complained of anxiety and minor trouble with memory, mostly with remembering names. He had no history of cerebral trauma, although he did have a history of well-controlled non-insulin-dependent diabetes. Mild hearing difficulties and his required glasses for reading were noted. Mr. S showed some difficulty with distractibility and sustained concentration. He was very reluctant to guess at questions, answering many questions with "I don't know." He made numerous self-deprecating comments and had very poor frustration tolerance. He frequently became anxious and overwhelmed by the tests, throwing up his arms and saying, "I can't do this."

Test Results: On intelligence testing, Mr. S received an average IQ score; however, his performance on verbal subtests was significantly better than on performance subtests. He showed a steady decline in subtest performance across time, indicating difficulties with sustained effort. On memory tests, Mr. S achieved above-average scores for both immediate and delayed recall for stories, despite protestations upon hearing instructions for the test that "I can't do that—I'll just fail!" His memory was poorer for learning a list of words, though cued recall was less impaired than free recall. While he showed little impairment on his copy and recall of simple designs, he had great difficulties in correctly drawing a more complex figure, particularly with respect to integrating proportions. A severe deficiency in recalling this figure after 30 minutes resulted in such frustration that testing was discontinued for a short time. Mr. S's naming of common objects was normal. Performance on a test of visual scanning and psychomotor speed was mildly impaired. When this test was made more difficult by requiring Mr. S to keep two concepts in mind simultaneously, his performance was moderately impaired in terms of both accuracy and speed. Motor speed was moderately impaired. Mr. S's score of 27 (out of 30) on the Geriatric Depression Scale indicated a severe level of depression.

Summary and Impression: Mr. S presented as a severely depressed man with neurovegetative symptoms who had mild to moderate cognitive impairment. The test results showed a mild decline in his overall intelligence from high average premorbid estimate to current average/low average. Because his performance declined on his Wechsler Adult Intelligence Scale–Revised (WAIS-R) subtests as the testing progressed, the lowest scores being on those tests administered last, this reduction was probably secondary to fatigue and inability to sustain cognitive effort due to depression rather than a dementia. He became overwhelmed and anxious, especially during performance tasks, and easily gave up his efforts. On concept formation tasks, he performed well. Memory and learning abilities were low average but essentially intact. His ability to learn and remember new material was mildly diminished, compared with that of other persons his age but more consistent with the deleterious effect of a mood disorder than with dementia. The fact that his delayed memory was superior to initial encoding argued against a primary degenerative dementia. He had mildly impaired verbal fluency, but naming was intact. The results were consistent with diminished cognitive efficiency characteristic of moderate to severe depression.

Discussion of Case 1

The typical presentation for a depressed person on neuropsychological testing is depressed mood or pervasive loss of interest coupled with a mild memory deficit (which may be exaggerated by the patient's self-report), a mild to moderate visuospatial impairment, and reduced abstraction and cognitive flexibility. Behavioral observations during testing often reveal considerable self-criticism, underestimations of actual ability, and rejection of positive or encouraging comments made by the examiner. The depressed patient often complains of fatigue or physical distress and complains of poor concentration. This patient's test results represent a classic profile for a depressed person. Memory, especially delayed memory, was intact, including a normal rate of forgetting. Depressed persons typically have a normal rate of forgetting, whereas demented patients show rapid loss (Hart et al., 1987b; Larrabee et al., 1993; DesRosiers et al., 1995). Mr. S's retention of information to be remembered was very good, probably the strongest argument against a diagnosis of primary degenerative dementia (Troster et al., 1993; Welsh, Butters, Hughes, Mohs, & Heyman, 1992). Language, reasoning, and abstraction were intact; these are typically impaired even in persons with mild dementia. Lower scores on Performance compared to Verbal subtests on the WAIS-R were displayed in this patient and are widely reported in depression (LaRue, 1992); dementia patients typically show declines on both Verbal and Performance subtests of the WAIS-R. An interesting observation about this patient's performance is its decline over the duration of testing, so that the tests administered last were the tests with lower scores. This outcome strongly suggests a fatigue or effort component, consistent with depression.

Qualitative aspects of his test performance were appropriate for his age and background; "pathognomonic signs" or other qualitative indicators of dementia such as intrusions, rotations, and confabulations were absent. Tasks that he did perform poorly on (visuospatial and motor speed) are not the most diagnostically significant for dementia and fit more with the most commonly found deficits in depression (Lyness, Eaton, & Schneider, 1994; Veiel, 1997). The onset of functional impairment and memory complaints coincided with the onset of the depressive episode. Although he had mild cognitive deficits that were probably related to his depression, it would be misleading to label his as "pseudodementia" or dementia syndrome of depression (depressive subcortical dementia).

This patient was briefly reassessed 4 months after he had experienced some remission of his depressive symptoms after treatment. Retest data demonstrated no further decline, and in fact, Mr. S showed improvement on nearly all tests readministered. Although one would expect some practice effects, especially on motor and memory tests (e.g., McCaffrey, Ortega, Orsillo, Nelles, & Haase, 1992), the improvements were quite large, and the test-retest interval was too long for the results to be entirely due to simple practice effects. The fact that his test performance improved was evidence that the mild deficits noted on the previous evaluation were related to his depression and not a dementing process.

Rehabilitation Strategies for Cognitive Loss in Late-Life Depression

As the above case illustrates, in older adults treatment of depression often brings about improvement of cognitive complaints. However, as in the course of treatment cognitive awareness and acceptance of improvement often occur after vegetative and mood symptoms remit, it may be necessary to give supportive rehabilitation until the patient's cognitive status improves. Rehabilitation is perhaps most important in depressed elderly patients when cognitive impairments persist despite treatment (Fromm & Schopflocher, 1984).

As the etiology, nature, and degree of cognitive complaints among elders are generally quite variable, an individualized approach to rehabilitation, coupled with a supportive environment, is most likely to achieve successful results (Poon, Fozard, & Treat, 1978). Research on the use of cognitive rehabilitation strategies in a variety of older populations, including depressed, stroke, and dementia patients, is burgeoning and reflects the growing body of research on older populations generally (Gouvier, Webster, & Blanton, 1986).

Research on clinical or practical cognitive training in older adults has identified both inter- and intraindividual variables that may impact the success of such rehabilitation efforts. Several studies (e.g., Schaie & Willis, 1986) have shown differences in cognitive performance after training between young-old and old-old adults, suggesting that more intensive and lengthy training procedures are needed to remediate declines in older cohorts. These group differences may be due in part to differences in arousal levels (Faucheux, Lillie, Baulon, Dupuis, & Bourliere, 1985) and attentional functioning (Kinsbourne, 1980) between young-old and old-old adults. Ability-specific cognitive training approaches are also superior to simple repeated exposure or practice effects, as demonstrated by several extensive studies on test-retest effects in the elderly (Baltes, Dittmann-Kohli, & Kliegl, 1986; Hofland, Willis, & Baltes, 1981). Such approaches appear particularly effective for old-old groups; whereas simple practice was enough to facilitate performance on a wide range of cognitive tasks in young-old cohorts, for older individuals targeted cognitive training was required for remediation (Willis, 1989).

As a consequence of the generally high levels of heterogeneity in the experiences, functioning, and goals of older adults, optimum conditions and strategies for cognitive retraining may need to be highly tailored, so "group approaches" may be less effective in improving performance in specific individuals (Poon, Walsh-Sweeney, & Fozard, 1980; Robertson-Tchabo, 1980; Winograd & Simon, 1980). Barbara Wilson's research on group memory training at Rivermead Hospital has found that group memory training is as yet underresearched, and that both the therapy process itself and the sensitivity of outcome measures require improvement (Wilson & Moffat, 1992). The most useful individualized approaches require a thorough assessment of an individual's cognitive strengths and weaknesses, including preserved abilities that may be recruited to assist those in decline, as well as determination of that individual's responsiveness to aids such as visualization, organizational aids, rehearsal, and retrieval cues. When combined with self-reports of the cognitive problems causing distress in everyday life, such individualized approaches will allow for target abilities to be trained and reasonable individual goals to be achieved (Bäckman, 1989).

For rehabilitation to be most effective, the strategies employed should be easy to use, should address current complaints, and should be taught with an eye to generalization (rather than "teaching the test") and to how learning can be incorporated and used in the patient's daily activities. Ideally, strategies will have feedback mechanisms built in, to increase both motivation and maintenance of gains. Older patients should also be warned that gaining mastery over new strategies to aid cognition may take much time and effort, particularly initially. Such forewarning, coupled with a supportive learning environment, should bolster both compliance and performance.

Available strategies for treatment of specific cognitive complaints in depressed older adults are discussed later, along with interventions for depressed elderly with comorbid dementia.

Attention/Orientation

Intact attentional skills are important for successful completion of most cognitive operations, including learning, encoding, and scanning of information. Older adults may benefit from increased focus on attention, particularly with regard to sustained attention to tasks over time, as some research suggests that older adults may discontinue learning tasks prematurely (Murphy, Sanders, Gabriesheski, & Schmitt, 1981).

In the case of dementia patients, orientation to their environment may be a critical part of any rehabilitation or coping intervention. The use of clocks, calendars, large notes, signs, and the assistance of relatives and staff in orientation for cognitively impaired patients may also increase functioning. Environmental adaptations such as signs on doors not only assist with orientation but also decrease the demands on a patient's cognitive system by reducing the need to remember. Such modifications to the environment, in conjunction with active orientation training, have been shown to be effective both immediately and at follow-up (Gilleard, Mitchell, & Riordan, 1981; Hanley, 1981).

Memory

In order to improve performance of practical, everyday tasks for older depressed adults, techniques should include internal strategies such as organization, visualization, and verbal elaboration, as well as external strategies such as writing notes as reminders, making lists, and using calendars (West, 1989). In a study of strategies used by older and younger adults, Cavanaugh, Grady, and Perlmutter (1983) found that external memory aids are used more frequently than internal aids, and that older adults make use of memory aids more often than younger adults for prospective tasks such as appointments. External strategies such as selected memory places for objects, specific object cues in the environment (such as leaving out in full view an item to be taken to the cleaners), and general reminders such as timers or pill boxes may be successfully used with older adults (West, 1985). Lovelace (1984) reported mental retracing as a common internal aid to remembering used by older adults. Imagery techniques (i.e., pairing objects to be remembered with their location) and the method of loci (pairing items to be recalled with landmarks on a mental "walk") are examples of other internal strategies that have been used successfully with elders (see Treat, Poon, Fozard, & Popkin, 1978, for full descriptions of these and other techniques; see also the chapter by Stigsdotter Neely in this text). Memory strategies may be thought of as being high or low in their familiarity and discriminability (or distinctiveness). More familiar strategies and more distinctive cues and mnemonics have increased success in enhancing older adults' performance (Kotler-Cope & Camp, 1990).

Empirically, whether it is better to utilize familiar, successful strategies or to teach unfamiliar and possibly more powerful memory strategies to older adults remains an open question (West, 1989). A study on older adults' use of the method of loci (Anschutz, Camp, Markley, & Kramer, 1987) suggests that issues of compliance must be addressed if results of training are to be used beyond the rehabilitation setting. Rehabilitation therapists may need to be guided as much by the specific needs, goals, and existing skills and deficits of the depressed older patient as by the extant literature.

However, research with practical memory skills in older adults may suggest fruitful paths for rehabilitation. As older adults often do not spontaneously develop or engage in organizational strategies, techniques promoting their use are a valuable training technique (Craik, 1984). For example, older adults may more easily remember organized than unorganized arrays (Waddell & Rogoff, 1981). Similarly, older adults were as good as younger adults at locating specific items in an unfamiliar supermarket (Kirasic & Allen, 1985). Thus, increasing organization or giving instruction in comparing familiar and unfamiliar organizational plans may increase memory for the location of objects as well as memory for large-scale spaces such as the layout of shops in a street, landmarks, or neighborhood locations (West, 1989). Improving visual scanning and simply encouraging increased interaction with new environments can also be of great assistance.

Organization may also facilitate recall of planned or completed activities, such as hierarchical organization of activities according to goals (Meacham, 1982). While familiar activities are often better recalled than unfamiliar activities (West, 1989), distinctive encoding of tasks, through verbal elaboration or imaginal strategies, for example, may enhance activity memory (Kausler & Hakami, 1983; West, 1985). An improved organizational approach may assist in more fruitful utilization of external memory aids (for example, organizing *where* notes and lists are to be kept).

The use of imagery techniques as mnemonics may have some limitations with elders, as some studies suggest that older adults find it difficult to produce and remember visual images (Poon et al., 1980; Winograd & Simon, 1980). Several studies (Camp, Markley, & Kramer, 1983; Wood & Pratt, 1987) suggest that older adults tend not to use visual imagery and develop verbal strategies more spontaneously. Cermak (1980) suggested that verbal techniques may be more effective than visualization for this population.

Language

A majority of stroke patients, regardless of age, suffer from depression (Robinson, Starr, Kubos, & Price, 1983). Poststroke depression can present a major impediment to rehabilitation and to maximizing quality of life (Hibbard, Grober, Stein, & Gordon, 1992). With elderly stroke patients, age-related physiological changes combined with the presence of depression may seriously impede rehabilitation efforts. A complete discussion of specialized language and cognitive rehabilitation in older stroke patients is beyond the scope of this chapter; the reader is referred to Skilbeck (1996) for an excellent review of the subject.

Executive Abilities

Executive cognitive skills may include problem solving, planning, task initiation and completion, and self-monitoring. Problem-solving abilities have been shown to be amenable to training by researchers using a variety of strategies, including modeling and verbal self-regulation (Denney, Jones, & Krigel, 1979; Meichenbaum, 1974). Training in use of appropriate strategies combined with anxiety reduction training was successful in increasing inductive reasoning performance of older adults (Labouvie-Vief & Gonda, 1976). Practice with prototypical tasks and feedback regarding correctness of responses also appears useful in terms of improved performance (Willis, 1989).

Self-instructional training to improve self-monitoring and metacognition have met with some success in older adults (Adams, Rebok, & King, 1981; Labouvie-Vief & Gonda, 1976). Age-related deficits in metamemory (Cavanaugh, 1989) and failure to initiate newly learned strategies as well as to self-correct strategies if they are not working properly (Poon et al., 1980) suggest that neglect of self-monitoring may inhibit rehabilitation gains. Teaching on-task monitoring of performance may both increase performance and increase utilization and practical application of strategies mastered (West, 1989).

Case 2

Background Information: Mr. W, a 64-year-old, right-handed, high-school-educated, white male, was seen for follow-up testing and possible rehabilitation recommendations following treatment for depression. The patient had suffered a severe corneal injury and diplopia secondary to an eye injury at his place of work 3 years previously. Since the time of the accident, he had had to leave work and had been suffering from symptoms of depression, including apathy, mild dysphoria, poor sleep, and decreased cognitive functioning. After trials on a variety of medications to treat his mood disorder, he had appeared stable on a regime of fluoxetine for the past 6 months. His history was significant for a head injury sustained when he was a teenager; otherwise, he had no prior psychiatric or substance abuse history and had functioned well both occupationally and socially prior to his accident.

Test Results: Mr. W was given a range of neuropsychological tests, the results of which were essentially unchanged from testing 1 year before, despite slight improvement and stabilization of mood. Namely, attention was variable, with poor concentration, especially for more complex tasks, and significant memory impairment was evident for both verbal and nonverbal information. As on previous testing and as noted in the interview, language skills and social behaviors were intact. Mr. W's performance on attentional and memory tasks was very frustrating for him and caused him much distress. He also tended to underestimate his ability to complete tasks and to belittle his performance. Despite its being pointed out to him that his memory was better when he was given cues, he merely repeated that his memory was "not what it used to be, and it used to be perfect."

Rehabilitation Assessment: Mr. W was interviewed at length as to his current difficulties with attention memory. He admitted that his poor memory was having an adverse affect on his relationship with his wife and their friends. For example, in order to keep busy at home, Mr. W had embarked on several small home improvement projects at his wife's urging. These always seemed to turn out badly and resulted in fierce arguments between the pair. Upon further questioning, Mr. W revealed that he never wrote down dimensions or specifications before going to the hardware store to purchase supplies and never measured materials before cutting or joining. Socially, Mr. W enjoyed bowling with friends and was often asked to keep score (his traditional role before his accident). However, he often failed to record scores or made mathematical errors, which irritated his teammates and which had caused several to refuse to play on Mr. W's team.

Summary and Impression: Mr. W continued to complain of mild depressive symptoms, which had improved but not completely resolved with pharmacological treatment. Attention and memory complaints continued to significantly impair his daily functioning and might well inhibit further improvement in mood. Individual therapy as well as the institution of cognitive rehabilitation training was recommended.

Discussion of Case 2

This presentation of cognitive deficits is typical of the cognitive dysfunction accompanying moderate depression. Mr. W's elevated scores on a self-report measure of depressed mood supported this diagnosis, as did his overall presentation and history. The patient's wife concurred that changes in his behavior since the accident had included decreased attention, memory, energy, and self-confidence and increased depression, guilt, and irritability. Short-term (20-session) cognitive behavioral therapy was initiated, along with a program to teach strategies aimed at cognitive rehabilitation.

Internal strategies such as visualization were unappealing to Mr. W, who claimed to have little imagination. External strategies such as use of calendars and extensive note taking were at first rejected on grounds that they would become a "crutch." Slowly, as therapy progressed, strategies for improving memory were combined with homework assignments to bolster therapeutic gains. Strategies such as buying and using a large, simple calculator to assist with scorekeeping, organizing tools and other commonly used materials, and use of a special "home improvement" notebook to record details of ongoing projects helped not only increase memory but also to increase the pleasure derived from participating in these activities. Fostering a supportive environment, particularly in terms of eliciting his wife's support in encouraging active use of memory strategies, was invaluable in increasing both motivation and compliance in this patient.

It should be stressed that not all older adults show improvement in cognition with rehabilitation. In his review of the literature, Poon (1985) stated that memory retraining helps only a portion of elders, and improvements are often not maintained after training. Poon also stated that strategies learned in training are often not applied in daily life, and that issues of motivation and generalization need to be addressed when implementing rehabilitation. In the case of Mr. W, learning to monitor his own cognitions, and to implement appropriate strategies when information needed to be encoded or recalled, was an immense help in reinforcing the use of strategies learned in rehabilitation.

The effect of improvement in mood on cognitive performance, regardless of intervention, may be significant. Zarit, Gallagher, and Kramer (1981) found that subjects receiving memory training and subjects participating in "growth" sessions such as relaxation or social skills training showed increased memory performance and decreased subjective memory complaints. Decreases in depressive mood, rather than improved memory performance, were related to decreases in memory complaints. The current level of depressive symptomatology experienced by the patient is an important and potentially fluctuating variable to be conscious of throughout the course of assessment and rehabilitation.

While the ability to learn new information may be denied by the depressed patient, the potential for learning is often overlooked by professionals when dealing with older adults with a dementing disorder. Although learning in dementia patients is unquestionably impaired, some limited and potentially valuable learning opportunities may be fruitfully identified and used by clinicians (see Miller & Morris, 1993, pp. 113–115). Many studies suggest that demented elderly are less able to benefit from manipulations on the processing of information, such as deep processing (Corkin, 1982; Wilson, Kazniak, Bacon, Fox, & Kelly, 1982), organizational instructions (Diesfeldt, 1984; Weingartner et al., 1982), or copy cues (Miller, 1975). Thus, for depressed patients with comorbid dementia, the key is to focus on select targets of high utility, to have realistic expectations of what may be gained, and to elicit the aid of family and staff wherever practical. External supports to cognitive functioning, such as message boards, large signs, name tags, printed directional arrows, and warning signs may be immediately useful for the patient. Such an approach also redirects the patient's family and other caregivers away from attempts to "restore" prior ability levels and instead focuses energy on working with the person's own cognitive strengths and weaknesses to maximize current functioning.

Case 3

Background Information: Mrs. L, an 80-year old, right-handed, widowed, Caucasian female with 16 years of education, was seen for neuropsychological testing to diagnose possible dementia. She reported insidious onset and progressive memory impairment over the last 4 years, which were followed by social isolation, fatigue, irritability, and feelings of sadness.

Interviews with family members confirmed the presence of significant and progressive memory impairments, which had resulted in the hiring of a full-time professional caretaker to assist Mrs. L with activities of daily living. MRI and PET scan results showed some diffuse atrophy with mild bilateral frontal hypometabolism; other laboratory results were normal. No psychiatric history, chronic medical problems, personal or family history of suicide, or history of substance abuse was reported. The patient's three children lived at some distance but had traveled to the clinic to participate in the clinical evaluation. Significant losses in the patient's recent history included the death of a much-loved family pet and her youngest daughter's recent move out of the state.

Behavioral Observations: Upon her arrival at the clinic, Mrs. L appeared somewhat disheveled and was vague when asked the purpose of her evaluation. She was generally cooperative during the testing until the examiner asked her to draw the same figure a second time without the benefit of the model. She quickly drew the figure, then erased it, and finally threw both pencil and paper at the examiner in frustration. Mood ranged from anxious to depressed, and affect was restricted. Her speech was loud, rapid, and generally content-appropriate, although occasionally perseverative. She tended to sacrifice accuracy in tasks due to her carelessness. There was no evidence of hallucinations, but there was evidence of delusions, such as other people moving her furniture without her consent.

Test Results: Mrs. L scored 19/30 on the MMSE, a score suggesting impaired cognitive functioning. While her performance on tests of simple attention was within normal limits, sustained concentration was poor. Mrs. L had no difficulty rapidly counting backward and reciting the alphabet but demonstrated difficulty counting by 3s. On a test of concentration, visual scanning, psychomotor speed, and sequencing abilities (Trials A), she was within the low average range. During Trials B, a more demanding task, she utilized verbal mediation in order to complete the task but still scored in the impaired range. Naming was poor, with phonemic cues of only limited value in eliciting additional responses. Verbal fluency was also in the borderline range. The Fuld Object Memory Evaluation, a test of verbal learning and retrieval by categories, was used to assess memory functioning. In the categories of female names, Mrs. L scored in the low average range; with the categories of food and vegetables, she was in the severely impaired range. She did not show a learning curve, and recognition memory was borderline impaired. Both immediate and delayed recall of short stories, word pairs, and drawings from the Wechsler Memory Scale-Revised (WMS-R) were impaired. Performance on a complex figure was discontinued due to increasing patient agitation. Psychomotor speed was in the low average range across several tasks. The patient demonstrated a tendency toward concrete thinking, impaired judgment, and perseveration. Other evidence of frontal impairment came from impulsivity and carelessness shown on many tests. Mrs. L endorsed 12 of 30 items on the Geriatric Depression Scale. She stated that she felt sad and depressed but that she had not experienced a change in sleep, appetite, or weight. Suicidal ideation was denied.

Summary and Impression: The major finding of this assessment was of impairments in short-term memory, visual and verbal learning, judgment and reasoning, and complex attention. Neuroimaging studies, psychiatric findings such as paranoid ideations, and impaired cognitive functioning pointed to the probable presence of a primary degenerative dementia syndrome. Mrs. L had several areas of relatively intact cognitive functioning, including intact simple attention and good motivation despite moderate dysphoria. It is important to note that her performance on tests and current deficits were compounded by her rapid performance on all tasks, her lack of care on tasks, and her lack of questions for clarification regarding instructions.

Discussion of Case 3

This patient had experienced profound losses that all agreed had accelerated her cognitive declines, particularly her lack of care with regard to herself or any tasks she undertook. The patient was started on a low dose of Zoloft, with the aim of decreasing dysphoria and agitation. Cognitive rehabilitation was aimed at establishing routines and behavioural patterns that would increase Mrs. L's level of functioning. A number of external cognitive aids, such as large calendars, prominent wall clocks, and a wristwatch with a beeper to remind her to take her medication, were successfully introduced. The combination of increased daily structure, external memory aids to decrease cognitive load, and pharmacotherapy combined to allow for a decrease in caregiving required while increasing quality of life for this patient.

Studies examining the maintenance of training effects unfortunately often only look at gains maintained over relatively short periods, although a few studies (e.g., Anschutz et al., 1987; Baltes & Willis, 1982; Sheikh, Hill, & Yesavage, 1986) have examined gains after 6 months or more. Since retest studies have shown that repeated testing often results in a significant increase in items attempted, which thus can increase number of correct responses over time, error analyses should be conducted to examine more closely what behaviors have been affected and what gains have accrued from training (Willis, 1989). Unfortunately, a variety of studies have shown that continued use of cognitive strategies after completion of formal rehabilitation is low in older adults (Kotler-Cope & Camp, 1990). Older adults have a sizable developmental reserve capacity, which current rehabilitation strategies may not yet be fully utilizing (Kliegl, Smith, & Baltes, 1989). Kotler-Cope and Camp (1990) suggested that particularly with older depressed adults, use of creative and research-grounded cognitive interventions be linked with strategies aimed at increasing confidence and decreasing anxiety concerns about levels of functioning.

Finally, and perhaps most significantly, research on lifestyle antecedents of cognitive change indicates that in the natural environment, active lifestyles involving high levels of stimulation are associated with maintenance of previous performance levels in older adults, whereas a restrictive lifestyle, associated with low activity levels and loss of family supports, is associated with decline of performance (Gribbin, Schaie, & Parham, 1980; Stone, 1980). Thus, the environment to which an individual returns will have an important effect on the maintenance of rehabilitation gains (Willis, 1989).

Conclusion

In order both to study the true efficacy of cognitive rehabilitation strategies and to be able to effectively provide such treatment to older adults with depression, many issues must be considered. A good understanding of the biological and psychosocial factors influencing normal and abnormal cognition and psychiatric function in older adults is critical. Careful diagnostic workup of patients, especially those with pronounced cognitive deficits or suspicion of dementia, will guide all phases of assessment and treatment. A clear delineation of individuals' strengths and weaknesses, as well as their particular goals in rehabilitation, will maximize therapeutic gains.

Cognitive rehabilitation of older adults with a diagnosis of depression is an area of growing research interest. Problems with cognitive functioning can significantly impair daily functioning and quality of life for these patients. Despite adequate diagnostic workup and treatment for depression, residual cognitive effects may remain; this is especially true for those who may suffer from depression with comorbid dementia. The implementation of rehabilitation strategies to improve functioning, enhance quality of life, and preserve independence is possible with careful consideration of an individual's unique presentation, a good working knowledge of rehabilitation strategies, and an understanding of the cognitive and psychiatric considerations involved in working with older adults.

References

Adams, C. C., Rebok, G. W., & King, M. H. (1981, November). *Facilitating intellectual functioning in older adults: A metacognitive approach.* Paper presented at a meeting of the Gerontological Society of America, Toronto.

Albert, M. S. (1981). Geriatric neuropsychology. *Journal of Consulting and Clinical Psychology, 49,* 835–850.

Alexopoulos, G. S., Abrams, R. C., Young, R. C., & Shamoian, C. A. (1988). Cornell scale for depression in dementia. *Biological Psychiatry, 23,* 271–284.

Alexopoulos, G. S., Meyers, B. S., Young, R. C., Mattis, S., & Kakuma, T. (1993). The course of depression with "reversible dementia": A controlled study. *American Journal of Psychiatry, 150,* 1693–1699.

Alexopoulos, G., Young, R. C., Meyers, B. S., Abrams, R. C., & Shamoian, G. A. (1988). Late-onset depression. *Psychiatric Clinics of North America, 11,* 101–115.

Altarriba, J. (1993). Cognition and culture: A cross-cultural approach to cognitive psychology. *Advances in Psychology* (Vol. 103). Amsterdam: North-Holland/Elsevier.

Anschutz, L., Camp, C. J., Markley, R. P., & Kramer, J. J. (1987). Remembering mnemonics: A 3-year follow-up on the effects of mnemonics training in elderly adults. *Experimental Aging Research, 13,* 141–143.

Bäckman, L. (1989). Memory compensation and aging. In L. W. Poon, D. C. Rubin, & B. A. Wilson (Eds.), *Everyday cognition in adulthood and late life* (pp. 509–544). Cambridge: Cambridge University Press.

Bäckman, L., & Forsell, Y. (1994). Episodic memory functioning in a community-based sample of old adults with major depression: Utilization of cognitive support. *Journal of Abnormal Psychology, 103,* 361–370.

Ballard, C., Bannister, C., Solis, M., Oyebode, F., & Wilcock, G. (1996). The prevalence, associations, and symptoms of depression amongst dementia sufferers. *Journal of Affective Disorders, 36,* 135–144.

Baltes, P. B., Dittman-Kohli, F., & Kliegl, R. (1986). Reserve capacity of the elderly in aging-sensitive tests of fluid intelligence: Replication and extension. *Psychology and Aging, 1,* 172–177.

Baltes, P. B., & Willis, S. L. (1982). Enhancement (plasticity) of intellectual functioning in old age: Penn State's Adult Development and Enrichment Project (ADEPT). In F. I. M. Craik & S. E. Trehub (Eds.), *Aging and cognitive processes* (pp. 353–389). New York: Plenum Press.

Bartus, R. T., Dean, R. L., Beer, B., & Lippa, A. S. (1982). The cholinergic hypothesis of geriatric memory dysfunction. *Science, 217,* 408–417.

Beck, A. T., Ward, C. H., Mendelson, M., Mock, J., & Erbaugh, J. (1961). An inventory for measuring depression. *Archives of General Psychiatry, 4,* 561–571.

Bieliauskas, L. A. (1993). Depressed or not depressed? *Journal of Clinical and Experimental Neuropsychology, 15,* 119–134.

Birren, J. E., & Schaie, K. W. (Eds.). (1990). *Handbook of the psychology of aging* (3rd ed.). San Diego: Academic Press.

Blaney, P. H. (1986). Affect and memory: A review. *Psychological Bulletin, 99,* 229–246.

Blazer, D. (1989). Current concepts: Depression in the elderly. *New England Journal of Medicine, 320,* 164–166.

Blazer, D. (1993). *Depression in late-life* (2nd ed.). St. Louis: Mosby.

Blazer, D., Hughes, D. C., & George, L. K. (1987). The epidemiology of depression in an elderly community population. *Gerontologist, 27,* 281–287.

Breslow, R., Kocsis, J., & Belkin, B. (1981). The contribution of the depressive perspective to memory function in depression. *American Journal of Psychiatry, 138,* 227–230.

Brink, T. L., Yesavage, J. A., Lunn, O., Hersema, P. H., Adey, M., & Rose, T. L. (1982). Screening tests for geriatric depression. *Clinical Gerontologist, 1,* 37–43.

Brown, R. P., Sweeney, J., Sweeney, J., Loutsch, E., & Kocsis, J. (1984). Involutional melancholia revisited. *American Journal of Psychiatry, 141,* 24–28.

Bucht, G., & Adolfsson, R. (1983). The Comprehensive Psychopathological Rating Scale in patients with dementia of the Alzheimer's type and multi-infarct dementia. *Acta Psychiatrica Scandinavica, 64,* 263–270.

Buntinx, F., Kester, A., Bergers, J., & Knottnerus, J. A. (1996). Is depression in elderly people followed by dementia? A retrospective cohort study based in general practice. *Age and Ageing, 25,* 231–233.

Burke, W. J., Houston, M. J., Boust, S. J., & Roccaforte, W. H. (1989). Use of the Geriatric Depression Scale in dementia of the Alzheimer's type. *Journal of the American Geriatrics Society, 37,* 856–860.

Burt, D. B., Zembar, M. J., & Niederehe, G. (1995). Depression and memory impairment: A meta-analysis of the association, its pattern and specificity. *Psychological Bulletin, 117,* 285–305.

Caine, E. D. (1981). Pseudodementia: Current concepts and future directions. *Archives of General Psychiatry, 38,* 1359–1364.

Caine, E. D. (1986). The neuropsychology of depression: The pseudodementia syndrome. In I. Grant & K. M. Adams (Eds.), *Neuropsychological assessment of neuropsychiatric disorders* (pp. 221–243). New York: Oxford University Press.

Caine, E. D., Lyness, J. M., & King, D. A. (1993). Reconsidering depression in the elderly. *American Journal of Geriatric Psychiatry, 1,* 4–20.

Camp, C. J., Markley, R. P., & Kramer, J. J. (1983). Spontaneous use of mnemonics by elderly individuals. *Educational Gerontology, 9,* 57–71.

Cassens, G., Wolfe, L., & Zola, M. (1990). The neuropsychology of depressions. *Journal of Neuropsychiatry and Clinical Neurosciences, 2,* 202–213.

Cavanaugh, J. C. (1989). The importance of awareness in memory aging. In L. W. Poon, D. C. Rubin, & B. A. Wilson (Eds.), *Everyday cognition in adulthood and late life* (pp. 416–436). Cambridge: Cambridge University Press.

Cavanaugh, J. C., Grady, J. G., & Perlmutter, M. (1983). Forgetting and use of memory aids in 20-to 70-year-old's everyday life. *International Journal of Aging and Human Development, 17,* 113–122.

Cermak, L. S. (1980). Comments on imagery as a therapeutic mnemonic. In L. W. Poon, J. L. Fozard, L. S. Cermak, D. Arenberg, & L. W. Thompson (Eds.), *New directions in memory and aging: Proceedings of the George A. Talland memorial conference* (pp. 507–510). Hillsdale, NJ: Erlbaum.

Christensen, H., Hadzi-Pavlovic, D., & Jacomb, P. (1991). The psychometric differentiation of dementia from normal aging: A meta-analysis. *Psychological Assessment, 3,* 147–155.

Cipolli, C., Neri, M., Andermarcher, E., Pinelli, M., & Lalla, M. (1990). Self-rating and objective memory testing of normal and depressed elderly. *Aging, 2*, 39–48.

Clark, D. A., Beck, A. T., & Beck, J. S. (1994). Symptom differences in major depression, dysthymia, panic disorder, and generalized anxiety disorder. *American Journal of Psychiatry, 151*, 205–209.

Coffey, C. E., Figiel, G. S., Djang, W. T., & Saunders, W. B. (1989). White matter hyperintensity on magnetic resonance imaging: Clinical and neuroanatomical correlates in the depressed elderly. *Journal of Neuropsychiatry and Clinical Neurosciences, 1*, 135–144.

Coffey, C. E., Figiel, G. S., Djang, W. T., & Weiner, R. D. (1990). Subcortical hyperintensity on magnetic resonance imaging: A comparison of normal and depressed elderly subjects. *American Journal of Psychiatry, 147*, 187–189.

Cohen, R. M., Weingartner, H., Smallberg, S. A., Pickar, D., & Murphy, D. (1982). Effort and cognition depression. *Archives of General Psychiatry, 39*, 593–597.

Corkin, S. (1982). Some relationships between global amnesias and the impairments in Alzheimer's disease. In S. Corkin, K. L. Davis, J. H. Growden, E. Usdin, & R. J. Wurtman (Eds.), *Alzheimer's disease: A report of progress in research*. New York: Raven Press.

Craik, F. I. M. (1984). Age differences in remembering. In L. R. Suire & N. Butters (Eds.), *Neuropsychology of memory* (pp. 3–12). New York: Guilford Press.

Creed, F., & Ash, G. (1992). Depression in rheumatoid arthritis: Aetiology and treatment. *International Review of Psychiatry, 4*, 23–34.

Cummings, J. L., & Benson, D. F. (1984). Subcortical dementia: Review of an emerging concept. *Archives of Neurology, 41*, 874–879.

Cummings, J. L., & Benson, D. F. (1992). *Dementia: A clinical approach* (2nd ed.). Boston: Butterworth-Heinemann.

Denney, N. W., Jones, F., & Krigel, S. (1979). Modifying the questioning strategies of young children and elderly adults. *Human Development, 22*, 23–36.

Derry, P. A., & Kuiper, N. A. (1981). Schematic processing and self-reference in clinical depression. *Journal of Abnormal Psychology, 90*, 286–297.

DesRosiers, G., Hodges, J. R., & Berrios, G. (1995). The neuropsychological differentiation of patients with very mild Alzheimer's disease and/or major depression. *Journal of the American Geriatrics Society, 43*, 1256–1263.

Devanand, D. P., Sano, M., Tang, M. X., Taylor, S., Gurland, B. J., Wilder, D., Stern, Y., & Mayeux, R. (1996). Depressed mood and the incidence of Alzheimer's disease in the elderly living in the community. *Archives of General Psychiatry, 53*, 175–182.

Diesfeldt, H. F. A. (1984). The importance of encoding instructions and retrieval cues in the assessment of memory in senile dementia. *Archives of Gerontology and Geriatrics, 3*, 51–57.

Emery, V. O. B., & Oxman, T. E. (1997). Depressive dementia: A "transitional dementia"? *Clinical Neuroscience, 4*, 23–30.

Faucheux, B. A., Lillie, F., Baulon, A., Dupuis, C., & Bourliere, F. (1985). Adjustment to the stress induced by mental tasks, in middle-aged and elderly men [Abstract]. *Proceedings of the 13th International Congress of Gerontology* (p. 132).

Feehan, M., Knight, R. G., & Partridge, F. M. (1991). Cognitive complaint and test performance in elderly patients suffering depression and dementia. *International Journal of Geriatric Psychiatry, 6*, 287–293.

Feher, E. P., Larrabee, G. J., & Crook, T. H. (1992). Factors attenuating the validity of the geriatric depression scale in a dementia population. *Journal of the American Geriatrics Society, 40*, 906–909.

Finch, E. J. L., Ramsay, R., & Katona, C. L. E. (1992). Depression and physical illness in the elderly. *Clinics in Geriatric Medicine, 8*, 275–287.

Fischer, P., Simanyi, M., & Danielczyk, W. (1990). Depression in dementia of the Alzheimer's type and in multi-infarct dementia. *American Journal of Psychiatry, 147,* 1484–1487.

Folstein, M. F., Folstein, S. E., & McHugh, P. R. (1975). "Mini-mental state": A practical method for grading the mental state of patients for the clinician. *Journal of Psychiatric Research, 12,* 189–198.

Folstein, M. F., & McHugh, P. R. (1978). Dementia syndrome of depression. In R. Katzman, R. D. Terry, & K. L. Bick (Eds.), *Alzheimer's disease, senile dementia and related disorders* (pp. 281–289). New York: Raven Press.

Frith, C. D., Stevens, M., Johnstone, E. C., Deakin, J. F. W., Lawler, P., & Crow, T. J. (1983). Effects of ECT and depression on various aspects of memory. *British Journal of Psychiatry, 142,* 610–617.

Fromm, D., & Schopflocher, D. (1984). Neuropsychological test performance in depressed patients before and after drug therapy. *Biological Psychiatry, 19,* 55–72.

Gallagher, D. (1986). The Beck Depression Inventory and older adults: Review of its development and utility. *Clinical Gerontologist, 5,* 149–163.

Gallagher, D. E., Breckenridge, J. N., Thompson, L. W., Dessonville, C., & Amaral, P. (1982). Similarities and differences between normal grief and depression in older adults. *Essence, 5,* 127–140.

Gallagher, D. E., Breckenridge, J. N., Thompson, L. W., & Peterson, J. A. (1983). Effects of bereavement on indicators of mental health in elderly widows and widowers. *Journal of Gerontology, 38,* 565–571.

Gibson, A. (1981). A further analysis of memory loss in dementia and depression in the elderly. *British Journal of Clinical Psychology, 20,* 1048–1051.

Gilinsky, A. S., Ehrlich, M.-F., & Craik, F. I. M. (1993). Aging and cognitive function: Cross-cultural studies. In C. Izawa (Ed.), *Cognitive psychology applied* (pp. 225–237). Hillsdale, NJ: Erlbaum.

Gilleard, C., Mitchell, R. G., & Riordan, J. (1981). Ward orientation training with psychogeriatric patients. *Journal of Advanced Nursing, 6,* 96–98.

Glass, R. M., Uhlenhuth, E. H., Hartel, F. W., Matuzas, W., & Fischman, M. W. (1981). Cognitive function and imipramine in outpatient depressives. *Archives of General Psychiatry, 38,* 1048–1051.

Gouvier, W. D., Webster, J. S., & Blanton, P. D. (1986). Cognitive retraining with brain-damaged patients. In D. Weddington, A. M. Horton, & J. Webster (Eds.), *The neuropsychology handbook: Behavioral and clinical perspectives* (pp. 278–324). New York: Springer.

Greenwald, B. S., Kramer-Ginsburg, E., Marin, D. B., Laitman, L. B., Hermann, C. K., Mohls, R. C., & Davis, K. L. (1989). Dementia with co-existent major depression. *American Journal of Psychiatry, 146,* 1472–1478.

Gribbin, K., Schaie, K. .W, & Parham, I. (1980). Complexity of lifestyle and maintenance of intellectual abilities. *Journal of Social Issues, 21,* 47–61.

Hamilton, M. (1967). Development of a rating scale for primary depressive illness. *British Journal of Social and Clinical Psychology, 6,* 278–296.

Hanley, I. G. (1981). The use of signposts and active training to modify ward disorientation in elderly patients. *Journal of Behavoir Therapy and Experimental Psychiatry, 12,* 241–247.

Hart, R. P., Kwentus, J. A., Taylor, J. R., & Hamer, R. M. (1987a). Selective reminding procedure in depression and dementia. *Psychology and Aging, 2,* 111–115.

Hart, R. P., Kwentus, J. A., Taylor, J. R., & Harkins, S. W. (1987b). Rate of forgetting in dementia and depression. *Journal of Consulting and Clinical Psychology, 55,* 101–105.

Hartlage, S., Alloy, L. B., Vazquez, C., & Dykmen, B. (1993). Automatic and effortful processing in depression. *Psychological Bulletin, 13,* 247–278.

Hartlage, S., & Clements, C. (1996). Cognitive deficits in depression. In P. W. Corrigan &

S. C. Yudofsky (Eds.), *Cognitive rehabilitation for neuropsychiatric disorders* (pp. 101–127). Washington, DC: American Psychiatric Press.

Hasher, L., & Zacks, R. T. (1979). Automatic and effortful processes in memory. *Journal of Experimental Psychology: General, 108,* 356–388.

Hayslip, B., Kennelly, K., & Maloy, R. (1989, November). *Fatigue, depression, and cognitive performance among aged persons.* Paper presented at a meeting of the Gerontological Society of America Meeting, Minneapolis.

Heaton, R. K., Grant, I., & Matthews, C. G. (1991). *Comprehensive norms for an extended Halstead-Reitan Battery.* Odessa, FL: Psychological Assessment Resources.

Henry, G. M., Weingartner, H., & Murphy, D. L. (1973). Influence of affective states and psychoactive drugs on verbal learning and memory. *American Journal of Psychiatry, 130,* 966–971.

Hibbard, M. R., Grober, S. E., Stein, P. N., & Gordon, W. A. (1992). Poststroke depression. In A. Freeman & F. M. Dattilio (Eds.), *Comprehensive casebook of cognitive therapy* (pp. 303–312). New York: Plenum Press.

Hofland, B. F., Willis, S. L., & Baltes, P. B. (1981). Fluid intelligence performance in the elderly: Intraindividual variability and conditions of assessment. *Journal of Educational Psychology, 73,* 573–586.

Hyer, L., & Blount, J. (1984). Concurrent and discriminative validities of the Geriatric Depression Scale with older psychiatric inpatients. *Psychological Reports, 54,* 611–616.

Ingram, R. E., & Reed, M. R. (1986). Information encoding and retrieval processes in depression: Findings, issues and future direction. In R. E. Ingram (Ed.), *Information processing approaches to clinical psychology* (pp. 3–21). San Diego: Academic Press.

Ivnik, R. J., Malec, J. F., Smith, G. E., Tangalos, E. G., Petersen, R. C., Kokmen, E., & Kurland, L. T. (1992). Mayo's older Americans normative studies: WAIS-R, WMS-R, and AVLT norms for ages 56 to 97. *Clinical Neuropsychologist, 6*(Suppl), 1–104.

Jamison, C., & Scogin, F. (1992). Development of an interview-based geriatric depression rating scale. *International Journal of Aging and Human Development, 35,* 193–204.

Kaszniak, A. W. & Christenson, G. D. (1994). Differential diagnosis of dementia and depression. In M. Storandt & G. R. Vanden Bos (Eds.), *Neuropsychological assessment of dementia and depression in older adults: A clinician's guide* (pp. 81–117). Washington, DC: American Psychological Association.

Kausler, D. H., & Hakami, M. K. (1983). Memory for activities: Adult age differences and intentionality. *Developmental Psychology, 19,* 889–894.

Keller, M. B., Klein, D. N., Hirshfeld, R. M. A., Kocsis, J. H., McCullough, J. P., Miller, I., First, M. B., Holzer, C. P., Keiter, G. I., Marin, D. B., & Shea, T. (1997). Results of the DSM-IV mood disorders field trial. *American Journal of Psychiatry, 152,* 843–849.

Keller, M. B., & Shapiro, R. W. (1982). "Double depression": Superimposition of acute depressive episodes on chronic depressive disorders. *American Journal of Psychiatry, 139,* 438–442.

Kennedy, G. J., Kelman, H. R., & Thomas, C. (1991). Persistence and remission of depressive symptoms in late life. *American Journal of Psychiatry, 148,* 174–178.

Kiernan, B. U., Wilson, D., Suter, N., Naqvi, A., Moltzen, J., & Silver, G. (1986). Comparison of the Geriatric Depression Scale and Beck Depression Inventory in a nursing home setting. *Clinical Gerontologist, 6,* 54–56.

Kiloh, L. G. (1961). Pseudo-dementia. *Acta Psychiatrica Scandinavica, 37,* 336–361.

Kinderman, S. S., & Brown, G. G. (1997). Depression and memory in the elderly: A meta-analysis. *Journal of Clinical and Experimental Neuropsychology, 19,* 625–642.

King, D. A., & Caine, E. D. (1990). Depression. In J. L. Cummings (Ed.), *Subcortical dementia* (pp. 218–230). New York: Oxford University Press.

King, D. A., & Caine, E. D. (1996). Cognitive impairment and major depression: Beyond the pseudodementia syndrome. In I. Grant & K. M. Adams (Eds.), *Neuropsychological assessment of neuropsychiatric disorders* (2nd ed., pp. 200–217). New York: Oxford University Press.

King, D. A., Caine, E. D., & Cox, C. (1993). Influence of depression and age on selected cognitive functions. *The Clinical Neuropsychologist, 7,* 443–453.

King, D. A., Cox, C., Lyness, J. M., & Caine, E. D. (1995). Neuropsychological effects of depression and age in an elderly sample: A confirmatory study. *Neuropsychology, 9,* 399–408.

Kinsbourne, M. (1980). Attentional deficits and the elderly: Theoretical models and research perspectives. In L. W. Poon, J. L. Fozard, L. S. Cermak, D. Arenberg, & L. W. Thompson (Eds.), *New directions in memory and aging* (pp. 113–130). Hillsdale, NJ: Erlbaum.

Kirasic, K. C., & Allen, G. L. (1985). Aging, spatial performance, and spatial competence. In N. Charness (Ed.), *Aging and human performance* (pp. 191–223). Chichester, UK: Wiley.

Kliegl, R., Smith, J., & Baltes, P. B. (1989). Testing the limits and the study of adult age differences in cognitive plasticity of a mnemonic skill. *Developmental Psychology, 25,* 247–256.

Kocsis, J. H., & Frances, A. J. (1987). A critical discussion of DSM-III dysthymic disorder. *American Journal of Psychiatry, 144,* 1534–1542.

Komahashi, T., Ohmori, K., Nakano, T., Fujinuma, H., Higashimoto, T., Nakaya, M., Kuroda, J., Asahi, H., Yoshikawa, J., Matsumura, S., et al. (1994). Epidemiological survey of dementia and depression among the aged living in the community in Japan. *Japanese Journal of Psychiatry and Neurology, 48,* 517–526.

Kotler-Cope, S., & Camp, C. J. (1990). Memory interventions. In E. A. Lovelace (Ed.), *Aging and cognition: Mental processes, self-awareness and interventions.* Amsterdam: North-Holland.

Kral, V. A., & Emery, O. B. (1989). Long-term follow-up of depressive-pseudodementia of the aged. *Canadian Journal of Psychiatry, 34,* 445–446.

Labouvie-Vief, G., & Gonda, J. N. (1976). Cognitive strategy training and intellectual performance in the elderly. *Journal of Gerontology, 31,* 327–332.

Lamberty, G. J., & Bieliauskas, L. A., (1993). Distinguishing between depression and dementia in the elderly: A review of neuropsychological findings. *Archives of Clinical Neuropsychology, 8,* 149–170.

Larrabee, G. J., Youngjohn, J. R., Sudilovsky, A., & Crook, T. H. (1993). Accelerated forgetting in Alzheimer-type dementia. *Journal of Clinical and Experimental Neuropsychology, 15,* 713–712.

LaRue, A. (1992). *Aging and neuropsychological assessment.* New York: Plenum Press.

Lichtenberg, P.A., Marcopulos, B. A., Steiner, D. A., & Tabscott, J. A. (1992). Comparison of the Hamilton Depression Rating Scale and the Geriatric Depression Scale: Detection of depression in dementia patients. *Psychological Reports, 70,* 515–521.

Lishman, W. A. (1987). *Organic psychiatry* (2nd ed.). Oxford: Blackwell Scientific.

Lovelace, E. A. (1984, August). *Reported mnemonics and perceived memory changes with aging.* Paper presented at a meeting of the American Psychological Association, Toronto.

Lyness, J. M., Cox, C., Curry, J., Conwell, Y., King, D. A., & Caine, E. D. (1995). Older age and the underreporting of depressive symptoms. *Journal of the American Geriatrics Society, 43,* 216–221.

Lyness, S. A., Eaton, E. E., & Schneider, L. S. (1994). Cognitive performance in older and middle-aged depressed outpatients and controls. *Journal of Gerontology: Psychological Sciences, 49,* 129–136.

Marcopulos, B. A. (1989). Pseudodementia, dementia, and depression: Test differentiation. In T. Hunt & C. J. Lindley (Eds.), *Testing older adults* (pp. 70–91). Austin, TX: Pro-Ed.

Marcopulos, B. A., & Graves, R. E. (1990). Antidepressant effect on memory in depressed older persons. *Journal of Clinical and Experimental Neuropsychology, 12*, 655–663.

McAllister, T. W. (1981). Cognitive functions in the affective disorders. *Comprehensive Psychiatry, 22*, 572–586.

McCaffrey, R. J., Ortega, A., Orsillo, S. M., Nelles, W. B., & Haase, R. F. (1992). Practice effects in repeated neuropsychological assessments. *Clinical Neuropsychologist, 6*, 32.42.

McGaugh, J. L. (1983). Preserving the presence of the past: Hormonal influences on memory storage. *American Psychologist, 38*, 161–174.

Meacham, J. A. (1982). A note on remembering to execute planned actions. *Journal of Applied Developmental Psychology, 3*, 121–133.

Meichenbaum, D. (1974). Self-instruction strategy training: A cognitive prosthesis for the aged. *Human Development, 17*, 273–280.

Miller, E. (1975). Impaired recall and the memory disturbance in presenile dementia. *British Journal of Social and Clinical Psychology, 14*, 73–79.

Miller, E., & Morris, R. (1993). *The psychology of dementia*. Chichester, UK: Wiley.

Mirchandani, I. C. (1988). Depression in the elderly. *Resident and Staff Physician, 34*, 31–42.

Moehle, K. A., & Long, C. J. (1989). Models of aging and neuropsychological test performance decline with aging. *Journal of Gerontology: Psychological Sciences, 44*, 176–177.

Murphy, D. G. (1991). The classification and treatment of dysthymia. *British Journal of Psychiatry, 158*, 106–109.

Murphy, M. D., Sanders, R. E., Gabriesheski, O. O., & Schmitt, F. A. (1981). Metamemory in the aged. *Journal of Gerontology, 36*, 185–193.

Myers, B. S., & Greenberg, R. (1989). Late-life delusional depression. *Journal of Affective Disorders, 11*, 133–137.

National Institutes of Health. (1992). Diagnosis and treatment of depression in late life: NIH Consensus Development Panel on Depression in late life. *Journal of the American Medical Association, 268*, 1018–1024.

Niederehe, G., & Camp, C. J. (1985). Signal detection analysis of recognition memory in depressed elderly. *Experimental Aging research, 11*, 207–213.

Norris, J. T., Gallagher, D., Wilson, A., & Winograd, C. H. (1987). Assessment of depression in geriatric medical outpatients: The validity of two screening measures. *Journal of the American Geriatrics Society, 35*, 989–995.

Nott, P. N., & Fleminger, J. J. (1975). Pre-senile dementia: The difficulty of early diagnosis. *Acta Psychiatrica Scandinavica, 41*, 210–217.

Nussbaum, P. D. (1994). Pseudodementia: A slow death. *Neuropsychology Review, 4*, 71–90.

Nussbaum, P. D. (1997). Late life depression: A neuropsychological perspective. In P. D. Nussbaum (Ed.), *Handbook of neuropsychology and aging: Critical issues in neuropsychology*. New York: Plenum Press.

Nussbaum, P. D., Kaszniak, A. W., Allender, J., & Rapcsak, S. Z. (1991). Depression and cognitive deterioration in the elderly: A follow-up study [Abstract]. *Journal of Clinical and Experimental Neuropsychology, 13*, 100–101.

Pachana, N. A., Gallagher, D., & Thompson, L. W. (1992). Assessment of depression. In M. P. Lawton & J. A. Teresi (Vol. Eds.), *Annual review of gerontology and geriatrics: Vol. 14. Focus on assessment techniques* (pp. 234–256). New York: Springer.

Pearlson, G. D., Rabins, P. V., Kim, V. S., Speedie, L. J., Moberg, P. J., Burns, A., & Bascom, M. J. (1989). Structural brain CT changes and cognitive deficits in elderly depressives with and without reversible dementia ("pseudodementia"). *Psychological Medicine, 19*, 573–584.

Phifer, J. F., & Murrell, S. A. (1986). Etiological factors in the onset of depressive symptoms in older adults. *Journal of Abnormal Psychology, 95*, 282–291.

Poon, L. W. (1985). Differences in human memory and aging: Nature of causes and clinical implications. In J. E. Birren & K. W. Schaie (Eds.), *Handbook of the psychology of aging* (2nd ed., pp. 427–462). New York: Van Nostrand Reinhold.

Poon, L. W. (1992). Toward an understanding of cognitive functioning in geriatric depression. *International Psychogeriatrics, 4*(Suppl. 2), 41–66.

Poon, L. W., Fozard, J. L., & Treat, N. J. (1978). From clinical and research findings on memory to intervention programs. *Experimental Aging Research, 4,* 235–253.

Poon, L. W., Walsh-Sweeney, L., & Fozard, J. L. (1980). Memory skill training for the elderly: Salient issues on the use of imagery mnemonics. In L. W. Poon, J. L. Fozard, L. S. Cermak, D. Arenberg, & L. W. Thompson (Eds.), *New directions in memory and aging* (pp. 461–484). Hillsdale, NJ: Erlbaum.

Popkin, S. J., Gallagher, D., Thompson, L. W., & Moore, M. (1982). Memory complaint and performance in normal and depressed older adults. *Experimental Aging Research, 8,* 141–145.

Post, F. (1962). *The significance of affective symptoms in old age.* London: Oxford University Press.

Raskin, A., Friedman, A. S., & DiMascio, A. (1982). Cognitive and performance deficits in depression. *Psychopharmacology Bulletin, 18,* 196–202.

Reding, M., Haycox, J., & Blass, J. (1985). Depression in patients referred to a dementia clinic. *Archives of Neurology, 42,* 894–896.

Reifler, B. V. (1982). Arguments for abandoning the term pseudodementia. *Journal of the American Geriatrics Society, 30,* 665–668.

Reifler, B. V., Larson, E., & Hanley, R. (1982). Coexistence of cognitive impairment and depression in geriatric outpatients. *American Journal of Psychiatry, 139,* 623–629.

Robertson-Tchabo, E. A. (1980). Cognitive-skill training for the elderly: Why should "old dogs" acquire new tricks? In L. W. Poon, J. L. Fozard, L. S. Cermak, D. Arenberg, & L. W. Thompson (Eds.), *New directions in memory and aging. Hillsdale* (pp. 511–518). Hillsdale, NJ: Erlbaum.

Robinson, R. G., Starr, L. B., Kubos, K. L., & Price, T. R. (1983). A two-year longitudinal study of post-stroke mood disorders: Findings during the initial evaluation. *Stroke, 14,* 736–741.

Rohling, M. L., & Scogin, F. (1993). Automatic and effortful memory processes in depressed persons. *Journal of Gerontology, 48,* P87-P95.

Ron, M. A., Toone, B. K., Garralda, M. E., & Lishman, W. E. A. (1979). Diagnostic accuracy in presenile dementia. *British Journal of Psychiatry, 134,* 161–168.

Rounsaville, B. J., Sholomskas, D., & Prusoff, B. A. (1980). Chronic mood disorders in depressed outpatients. *Journal of Affective Disorders, 2,* 73–88.

Rovner, B. W., Broadhead, J., Spencer, C., Carson, K., & Folstein, M. F. (1989). Depression and Alzheimer's Disease. *American Journal of Psychiatry, 146,* 350–353.

Rovner, B. W., & Morris, R. K. (1989). Depression in Alzheimer's Disease. In R. Robinson & R. Rabins (Eds.). *Depression and co-existing disease* (pp. 201–212). New York: Lgaku-Shoin.

Schaie, K.W., & Willis, S. L. (1986). Can decline in adult intellectual functioning be reversed? *Developmental Psychology, 22,* 223–232.

Scogin, F., & Bienias, J. L. (1988). A three-year follow-up of older adult participants in a memory-skills training program. *Psychology and Aging, 3,* 334–337.

Sheikh, J. I., Hill, R. D., & Yesavage, J. A. (1986). Long term efficacy of cognitive training for age-associated memory impairment: Six month follow-up study. *Developmental Neuropsychology, 2,* 413–421.

Siegfried, K. R., Jansen, W., & Pahnke, K. (1984). Cognitive dysfunction in depression: Difference between depressed and nondepressed patients and differential cognitive effects of Nomifensine. *Drug Development Research, 4,* 533–553.

Skilbeck, C. (1996). Psychological aspects of stroke. In R.T. Woods (Ed.), *Handbook of the clinical psychology of aging* (pp. 283–301). Chichester, UK: Wiley.

Speck, C. E., Kukull, W. A., Brenner, D. E., Bowen, J. D., McCormick, W. C., Teri, L., Pfanschmidt, M. L., Thompson. J. D., & Larson, E. B. (1995). History of depression as risk factor for Alzheimer's disease. *Epidemiology, 6,* 333–339.

Spreen, O., & Strauss, E. (1997). *A compendium of neuropsychological tests: Administration, norms, and commentary* (2nd ed.). New York: Oxford University Press.

Squire, L. R. (1974). Remote memory as affected by aging. *Neuropsychologia, 12,* 429–435.

Steffens, D. C., Hays, J., George, L. K., Krishnan, K. R. R., & Blazer, D. G. (1996). Socio-demographic and clinical correlates of number of previous depressive episodes in the depressed elderly. *Journal of Affective Disorders, 39,* 99–106.

Steffens, D. C., Plassman, B. L., Helms, M. J., Welsh-Bohmer, K. A., Saunders, A. M., & Breitner, J. C. S. (1997). A twin study of late-onset depression and apolipoprotein E e4 as risk factors for Alzheimer's disease. *Biological Psychiatry, 41,* 851–856.

Stone, V. (1980). *Structural modeling of the relations among environmental variables, health status and intelligence in adulthood.* Unpublished doctoral dissertation, University of Southern California, Los Angeles.

Stoudemire, A., Hill, C. D., Morris, R., & Dalton, S. T. (1995). Improvement in depression-related cognitive dysfunction following ECT. *Journal of Neuropsychiatry and Clinical Neurosciences, 7,* 31–34.

Strub, R. L., & Black, F. W. (1988). *Neurobehavioral disorders: A clinical approach.* Philadelphia: F. A. Davis.

Sultzer, D. L., Levin, H. S., Mahler, M. E., High, W. M., & Cummings, J. L. (1993). A comparison of psychiatric symptoms in vascular dementia and Alzheimer's disease. *American Journal of Psychiatry, 150,* 1806–1812.

Sunderland, T., Alterman, I. S., Yount, D., Hill, J. L., Tariot, P. N., Newhouse, P. A., Mueller, E. A., Mellow, A. M., & Cohen, R. M. (1988). A new scale for the assessment of depressed mood in dementia patients. *American Journal of Psychiatry, 145,* 955–959.

Teri, L., & Reifler, B. V. (1987). Depression and dementia. In L. Carstensen & B. Edelstein (Eds.), *Handbook of clinical gerontology* (pp. 112–119). New York: Pergamon Press.

Teri, L., & Wagner, A. (1992). Alzheimer's disease and depression. *Journal of Consulting and Clinical Psychology, 60,* 379–391.

Thompson, L. W., Futterman, A., & Gallagher, D. (1988). Assessment of late-life depression. *Psychopharmacological Bulletin, 24,* 577–586.

Thompson, L. W., Gong, V., Haskins, E., & Gallagher, D. (1987). Assessment of depression and dementia in later years. In K. W. Schaie (Ed.), *Annual review of gerontology and geriatrics: Vol. 7. Experimental and applied psychology* (pp. 295–324). New York: Springer.

Treat, N. J., Poon, L. W., Fozard, J. L., & Popkins, S. J. (1978). Toward applying cognitive skill training to memory problems. *Experimental Aging Research, 4,* 305–319.

Troster, A. I., Butters, N., Salmon, D. P., Cullum, D. P., Jacobs, D., Brandt, J., & White, R. (1993). The diagnostic utility of savings scores: Differentiating Alzheimer's and Huntington's disease with the Logical Memory and Visual Reproduction Tests. *Journal of Clinical and Experimental Neuropsychology, 15,* 773–788.

Turner, R. J., & Noh, S. (1988). Physical disability and depression: A longitudinal analysis. *Journal of Health and Social Behavior, 29,* 23–37.

Veiel, H. O. F. (1997). A preliminary profile of neuropsychological deficits associated with major depression. *Journal of Clinical and Experimental Neuropsychology, 19,* 587–603.

Waddell, K. J., & Rogoff, B. (1981). Effect of contextual organization on spatial memory of middle-aged and older women. *Developmental Psychology, 17,* 878–885.

Walstra, G. J. M., Teunisse, S., van Gool, W. A., & van Crevel, H. (1997). Symptomatic treatment of elderly patients with early Alzheimer's disease at a memory clinic. *Journal of Geriatric Psychiatry and Neurology, 10,* 33–38.

Weingartner, H., Cohen, R. M., & Bunney, W. E. (1982). Memory-learning impairments in progressive dementia and depression. *American Journal of Psychiatry, 139,* 135–136.

Weingartner, H., Kaye, W., Smallberg, S., Cohen, R., Ebert, M. H., Gillin, J. C., & Gold, P. (1982). Determinants of memory failures in dementia. In S. Corkin, K. L. Davis, J. H. Growdon, E. Usdin, & R. J. Wurtman (Eds.), *Alzheimer's disease: A report of progress in research.* New York: Raven Press.

Weiss, I. K., Nagel, C. L., & Aronson, M. K. (1986). Applicability of depression scales to the old old person. *Journal of the American Geriatrics Society, 34,* 215–218.

Weissman, M. M., Bruce, M. L., Leaf, P. J., Florio, L. P., & Holzer, C. (1991). Affective disorders. In L. N. Robins, & D. A. Regier (Eds.), *Psychiatric disorders in America: The epidemiologic catchment area study* (pp. 53–80). New York: Free Press.

West, R. L. (1985). *Memory fitness over 40.* Gainesville, FL: Triad.

West, R. L. (1989). Planning practical memory training for the aged. In L. W. Poon, D. C. Rubin, & B. A. Wilson (Eds.), *Everyday cognition in adulthood and late life* (pp. 573–597). Cambridge: Cambridge University Press.

Weytingh, M. D., Bossuyt, P. M. M., & van Crevel, H. (1995). Reversible dementia: more than 10% or less than 1%? *Journal of Neurology, 242,* 466–471.

Whitehead, A. (1973). Verbal learning and memory in elderly depressives. *British Journal of Psychiatry, 136,* 895–900.

Williams, J. B.W. (1988). A structured interview guide for the Hamilton Depression Rating Scale. *Archives of General Psychiatry, 45,* 742–747.

Williams, J. M., Little, M. M., Scates, S., & Blockman, N. (1987). Memory complaints and abilities among depressed older adults. *Journal of Consulting and Clinical Psychology, 55,* 595–598.

Willis, S. L. (1989). Cognitive training: Which old dogs learn what tricks? In L. W. Poon, D. C. Rubin, & B. A. Wilson (Eds.), *Everyday cognition in adulthood and late life* (pp. 545–569). Cambridge: Cambridge University Press.

Willis, S. L., & Schaie, K. W. (1988). Gender differences in spatial ability in old age: Longitudinal and intervention findings. *Sex Roles, 18,* 189–203.

Wilson, B., & Moffat, N. (1992). The development of group memory therapy. In B. A. Wilson & N. Moffat (Eds.), *Clinical management of memory problems* (pp. 240–270). London: Chapman & Hall.

Wilson, R. S., Kazniak, A. W., Bacon, L. D., Fox, J. H., & Kelly, H. P. (1982). Facial recognition in dementia. *Cortex, 18,* 329–336.

Winograd, E. & Simon, E. W. (1980). Visual memory and imagery in the aged. In L. W. Poon, J. L. Fozard, L. S. Cermak, D. Arenberg, & L. W. Thompson (Eds.), *New directions in memory and aging* (pp. 485–506). Hillsdale, NJ: Lawrence Erlbaum.

Wood, L. E., & Pratt, J. D. (1987). Pegword mnemonic as an aid to memory in the elderly: A comparison of 4 age groups. *Educational Gerontology, 13,* 325–339.

Woodruff-Pak, D. S. (1997). *The neuropsychology of aging.* Malden, MA: Blackwell.

Wragg, R. E., & Jeste, D. V. (1989). Overview of depression and psychosis in Alzheimer's disease. *American Journal of Psychiatry, 146,* 577–587.

Yesavage, J. A., Brink, T. L., & Rose, T. L. (1983). Development and validation of a geriatric depression scale: A preliminary report. *Journal of Psychiatric Residents, 17,* 37–49.

Zarit, S. H., Gallagher, D., & Kramer, N. (1981). Memory training in the community aged: Effects on depression, memory complaint, and memory performance. *Educational Gerontology, 6,* 11–27.

Zeiss, A. M., Lewinsohn, P. M., & Rohde, P. (1996). Functional impairment, physical disease, and depression in older adults. In P. M. Kato & T. Mann (Eds.), *Handbook of diversity issues in health psychology* (pp. 161–184). New York: Plenum.

Zepelin, H., Wolfe, C. S., & Kleinplatz, F. (1981). Evaluation of a year-long reality orientation program. *Journal of Gerontology, 36,* 70–77.

Zubenko, G. S., Henderson, R., Stiffler, J. S., Stabler, S., Rosen, J., & Kaplan, B. B. (1996). Association of the APOE e4 allele with clinical subtypes of late life depression. *Biological Psychiatry, 40,* 1008–1016.

PART IV

REHABILITATION STRATEGIES FOR COGNITIVE LOSS IN AGE-RELATED DISEASE

II

Issues in the Clinical Evaluation of Suspected Dementia

Implications for Intervention

THOMAS SCHENKENBERG

PATRICK J. MILLER

Part IV of this volume addresses rehabilitation strategies for dealing with cognitive loss in age-related disease. In keeping with the long-held tradition of diagnosing before proceeding with treatment, this chapter will focus on the clinical issues involved in the assessment of possible cognitive decline in the elderly patient.

For the practicing clinician, the assessment questions are straightforward:

1. Is *this* patient experiencing a clinically significant impairment in cognitive functioning?
2. If so, what is causing this impairment?
3. What can be done about the cause?

While these clinical questions can be posed in this rather straightforward manner, the process for answering these questions is complicated at every turn. For example, a 75-year-old man who has become somewhat forgetful over the preceding year might be experiencing only a mild decline in memory function that is within expected limits for a person his age. Conversely, his forgetfulness might reflect the presence of a clinical entity such as a meningioma that has a potential for curative surgical intervention or a dementing disorder such as Dementia of the Alzheimer's Type (DAT), which is inevitably progressive despite new medications that have become available in recent years. The practicing clinician must address the range of possibilities in each older adult who presents with possible cognitive decline.

Is *This* Patient Experiencing a Clinically Significant Cognitive Impairment?

One of the most common issues confronting the clinician is whether the performance seen on examination represents a level of performance that is to be expected for *this* patient at *this* age. Thus, the clinician must understand the individual patient's cognitive background, the expected changes with increasing age, and the way those changes would present in this patient. It is only by "subtracting out" the expected changes that occur with increasing age that one can interpret the clinical significance of the examination findings.

Normal Aging and Cognitive Functioning

Older adults are at increased risk of central nervous system (CNS) dysfunction and frequently present in clinical settings with cognitive complaints. Additionally, chronic medical illness and the extensive medication regimens of elderly individuals can compromise their mental status. Since normal age-associated cognitive declines must often be distinguished from changes resulting from pathological causes, an understanding of the changes that can be expected in the brain and in cognitive functioning with advancing age is essential.

Physiological Changes in Brain Structure and Function

With increasing age, deterioration occurs across the various organ systems, including the central nervous system. Neurobiological findings in normal aging clearly indicate anatomical, neurochemical, and electrical changes in the brain and other nervous system structures. Brain weight declines with age in both men and women, averaging losses in peak weight of 7–8% (Kemper, 1984). Cortical atrophy is a frequent finding and tends to be maximal in frontal and temporal association cortex. Specific subcortical areas also show reduction in volume on MRI scans (Scheibel, 1992). This shrinkage in size and weight appears to be due primarily to reduction in neuronal size, rather than to significant decrease in the number of neurons (Terry, DeTeresa, & Hansen, 1987). Decreased interconnections within the older brain are reflected in the reduction of dendritic branching and declines in the neurotransmitter substances acetylcholine, dopamine, and norepinephrine (Scheibel, 1992). Mild decline in brain metabolism is suggested by evidence of reduced regional cerebral blood flow and slowed glucose metabolism in older adults as compared to younger controls (Metter, 1988). Age-related changes in brain wave frequencies and amplitudes have also been consistently reported (Dustman, Shearer, & Emmerson, 1991).

Cognitive Changes Associated with Normal Aging

Given the occurrence of neurobiological changes in the central nervous system with aging, it is not surprising that cognitive changes are frequently observed in neuropsychological studies of normal older adults. The research in this area suggests that there is increase in both interindividual and intraindividual variability with age (Albert, 1994). The intraindividual variability is a reflection of the fact that within a single individual, some functions may change, while others do not. Perhaps more striking is the interindividual variability observed among people as they age. Gerontological research has consistently demonstrated that some older persons show little cognitive, physiological, or functional loss when compared with their younger counterparts, even though the mean level of performance for their age group may have declined. It has also been reported that lifestyle factors (e.g., nutrition and exercise) may exaggerate or ameliorate so-called age-related changes (Rosenberg & Miller, 1992; Dustman, Emmerson, & Shearer, 1990). The terms "*successful*" and "*usual*" aging have been suggested (Rowe & Kahn, 1987) to differentiate persons who demonstrate little or no loss in function ("*successful aging*") from those with clinically manifest age-related changes ("*usual aging*").

The study of effects of aging on cognitive abilities is further complicated by methodological difficulties, one of the most important of which concerns subject sampling and generational differences (Albert, 1994). Cross-sectional testing tends to maximize differences between age groups because of factors that confound comparisons of older and younger age groups, such as improved nutrition or increased level of education over successive generations. On the other hand, longitudinal studies may minimize differences due to the loss of at-risk individuals over time. Decreased survival of persons with poor cognitive performance (due to other factors that are correlated with both level of cognitive abilities and longevity) may skew the study toward the remaining subjects, who were "supernormal" at entry (Morris & McManus, 1991). Yet another potential confound in aging research is the possibility that "normal" control groups of apparently healthy and intact elderly persons include at least a few subjects who have undetected early or subtle brain disease.

Despite these difficulties, which complicate the interpretation of cognitive test results for the individual elderly person, it is clear from a growing body of research that normal aging is associated with somewhat predictable declines in cognitive function and test performance and that various abilities differ in their stability or rate of decline (Benton & Sivan, 1984).The nature of this aging pattern remains a cause of considerable debate. Some researchers have invoked the concepts of "*crystallized*" and "*fluid*" *intelligence* (Horn & Cattell, 1967) to account for the fact that some abilities (primarily verbal skills) hold up with advancing age, while others do not.According to this model, overlearned, well-practiced, and familiar skills, abilities, and knowledge (i.e., "*crystallized*") are affected little by advancing age. Conversely, activities requiring "fluid" intelligence (reasoning and problem solving for which familiar solutions are not available) follow a typical pattern of relatively slow decline until the late 50s or early 60s, after which decline proceeds at an increasingly rapid pace. This explanation has been posited by some (e.g., Kaufman, Reynolds, & McLean, 1989) for the finding of greater declines in Performance IQ than Verbal IQ across the life span on the Wechsler Adult Intelligence Scales. Critics of the model have suggested that Verbal-Performance differences are artifactual, reflecting practice effects of different skills or psychomotor slowing rather than neuropsychological declines (Mittenberg, Seidenberg, O'Leary, & DiGiulio, 1989; Storandt, 1990).

Research regarding changes in cognitive abilities with normal aging has produced some general conclusions (American Psychological Association [APA], 1997). There appear to be age-related declines in information-processing speed, several aspects of attention (e.g., vigilance or sustained attention, divided attention, selective attention, ability to switch attention rapidly among stimuli), some aspects of language (especially word finding/naming and rapid generation of word lists), visuospatial abilities, abstraction, and mental flexibility. Memory problems constitute one of the most common complaints of elderly persons (Bolla, Lindgren, Bonaccorsy, & Bleecker, 1991). As in other areas of cognitive activity, different aspects of memory and learning differ in how they hold up with advancing age (Cullum & Rosenberg, 1998). Remote memory tends to be stable, as does short-term memory for small amounts of information that are passively retained and reproduced in an untransformed fashion. Similarly, "gist" memory, or ability to recall the general idea, is relatively unaffected by aging. On the other hand, working memory, which involves simultaneous processing and storing of information, shows steady decline beginning at about age 50 (Albert, 1994). Long-term memory also shows substantial age changes, although the decline is greater for recall than for recognition, and performance generally benefits from cuing.

It is important to note that in general, the cognitive decline associated with normal aging is modest, and changes in mental ability are not invariably present in all older persons across all domains of function. Some elderly individuals may, in fact, perform as well on some measures as individuals several decades younger. For those functions that do decline, the change is generally not severe enough to cause significant impairment in daily occupational or social functioning, as occurs with dementing disorders.

Assessment of Suspected Pathological Cognitive Decline

It is clear from the preceding discussion that results from examinations of intellectual, memory, and other abilities must be interpreted in light of characteristic changes with normal aging, in order to decide whether performance represents the effects of a pathological process. Several additional considerations are also of importance in the clinical evaluation of suspected disease-related decline: (a) determining whether current performance represents a significant change for the individual patient, compared to some previous level of functioning; (b) choosing the most useful and appropriate measures for assessment of current performance and having an awareness of the patient's strengths and weaknesses; and (c) deciding whether current findings are indicative of clinically significant decline.

Estimating Premorbid Functioning

An estimation of expected or premorbid level of functioning is essential in determining whether performance on current measures for an individual represents a decrement or impairment. For example, a finding of a WAIS-R Full Scale IQ of 100 may suggest differing conclusions in regard to the possibility of acquired brain impairment, depending on whether the patient in question was previously intellectually gifted or average. Various methods for estimating premorbid level have been proposed: (a) historical achievement-based estimates (previous standardized testing, educational/vocational achievement, military service rank, occupation, etc.); (b) estimates based on current ability, as reflected in performance on so-called hold tests, typically tasks involving verbal skills (Blair & Spreen, 1989; McFie, 1975); (c) regression formulas based on demographics (e.g., Barona, Reynolds, & Chastain, 1984) or on combinations of demographic and current performance data (Vanderploeg & Schinka, 1995); and (d) estimates based on "best performance" or highest level of functioning, whether derived from test scores, other observations, or historical achievement (Lezak, 1995).

There are inherent limitations in each approach. Past indications of level of ability would provide the best and most reliable estimate of premorbid functioning. Unfortunately, in the clinical situation, these data (e.g., previously administered standardized tests, placement or aptitude tests, grade point average, relative class placement) are not always readily available, if they exist at all. Even educational and vocational attainment may provide spuriously low premorbid ability estimates, especially among older adults, whose educational and career opportunities may have been limited due to social, financial, or historical factors.

Current ability approaches depend on a measure or measures of cognitive ability that are thought to be relatively resistant to the effects of increasing age and therefore may provide a more valid estimate of previous level of cognitive functioning. Traditionally, these measures have involved vocabulary or other verbal skills and more recently the use of measures, such as the North American Adult Reading Test (Blair & Spreen, 1989), that assess a person's ability to pronounce phonetically "irregular" words, a skill that implies previous familiarity with the words. These approaches have been criticized as underestimating the premorbid ability of many patients, including those with some types of brain dysfunction, including dementing illnesses (Larrabee, Largen, & Levin, 1985; Stebbins, Wilson, Gilley, Bernard, & Fox, 1990).

Demographic regression approaches involve the use of differentially weighted variables (such as age, sex, race, education, occupation, and geographic region) in estimation formulas. This type of approach has been found to suffer from significant prediction errors, performing essentially at chance levels, due to a tendency to predict scores toward the population mean (Sweet, Moberg, & Tovian, 1990). Approaches that combine demographic data with current ability measures (e.g., Vanderploeg & Schinka, 1995) perform much better.

The "best performance" approach suffers from a tendency to overestimate premorbid abilities and therefore to overestimate decline, due to its underlying assumption that premorbid performance across multiple premorbid measures is comparable to the best performance on any one current measure (Mortensen, Gade, & Reinisch, 1991). The value of this method also depends on the appropriateness of the data on which estimates of premorbid ability are based and on the skill of the examiner at making what often must be subjective judgments regarding the relative weighting of different pieces of data.

Once the examiner has chosen a comparison standard, the presence or absence of deficit may be assessed by comparing the level of the patient's present cognitive performances with the expected level. A significant discrepancy between expected and observed performance levels suggests a true cognitive deficit. Obtaining significant discrepancies for multiple performance measures may reveal a pattern of deficits.

Measurement of Suspected Clinically Signficant Cognitive Decline

A number of measures are available for the clinical evaluation of suspected cognitive decline. Generally, these can be divided into two assessment domains: neuropsychological measures and measures of functional ability (Kaszniak, 1990). Both provide unique contributions to the evaluation of the older adult. A comprehensive review of the numerous instruments available to the clinician is beyond the scope of this chapter (see Lezak, 1995). Rather, the following section offers a brief description of (a) neuropsychological assessment, (b) assessment of functional abilities, and (c) issues in the assessment of older adults.

NEUROPSYCHOLOGICAL ASSESSMENT Neuropsychological assessment is frequently employed in clinical settings with older adults for a variety of purposes, including differentiating between age-associated cognitive declines and those related to degenerative neurological disorders, distinguishing between neurological and psychiatric disorders (e.g., dementia vs. depression), and addressing questions about legal or financial competency or ability to live independently.

Approaches to neuropsychological assessment have been divided into two major traditions, one of which relies upon a fixed battery of standard tests and the other of which employs a more flexible, individualized approach. The most popular of the neuropsychological test batteries is the Halstead-Reitan Neuropsychological Battery (HRNB; Reitan & Wolfson, 1985). The HRNB is composed of numerous tests of ability and problem solving that measure psychomotor, visuospatial, and abstract reasoning abilities. Also included in the battery are brief tests of language, motor, and sensory functions. Additionally, the Wechsler Adult Intelligence Scale and the Minnesota Multiphasic Personality Inventory are often included to assess intellectual and personality factors. Five of the tests in the battery (the Category Test, Tactual Performance, Rhythm, Speech Sounds Perception, and Finger Tapping), thought to be most sensitive to central nervous system dysfunction, yield scores that can be compared to cutoff scores to calculate an impairment index that is thought to reflect the severity of brain dysfunction.

Numerous studies have shown strong age effects on tests in the HRNB, with large percentages of normal older adults being classified as brain-damaged (Heaton, Grant, & Matthews, 1986; Schear, 1988). Refined normative data are available for interpreting results for older adults (Heaton, Grant, & Matthews, 1991). A significant practical drawback of the HRNB is that the length of administration (typically 5 hours) and the difficulty level of some of the subtests may make it inappropriate for older adults (Kaszniak, 1990).

Within flexible, individualized approaches to neuropsychological assessment, the choice of particular tests is dependent upon the nature of the assessment questions to be answered, as well as patient factors such as age and physical status (Bigler, 1988; Lezak, 1995). A basic or core battery that assesses the major functions of the individual is administered initially, and decisions regarding further testing are based on these results. Bigler (1988) proposed that, at a minimum, a core battery should include measures of intelligence, motor function, language, visuospatial skills, memory, and sensory abilities. Obviously, a thorough knowledge of neuropsychological assessment devices, relevant research literature, and test result patterns associated with different diagnoses is essential when utilizing a flexible battery. Nevertheless, the flexible approach may be quite suited to the assessment of older adults because of its emphasis on adaptation to the needs of the individual patient.

ASSESSMENT OF FUNCTIONAL ABILITIES Optimal functioning from day to day requires a host of skills or behaviors of varying complexity. Older persons are at risk for functional impairment and associated dependency in activities of daily living (ADLs) and instrumental activities of daily living (IADLs). ADLs include such basic self-care abilities as grooming, dressing, toileting, feeding, and transferring (i.e., moving in and out of bed). IADLs involve activities beyond simple self-care, such as using the telephone, shopping, preparing meals, using transportation, and managing personal finances. Impairment in functional abilities frequently results in inability to live independently in the community and in a lower quality of life for older persons and their caregivers.

Many instruments and approaches are available for assessing functional abilities. This process is an essential part of the evaluation of suspected decline in an elderly person. While functional ability level is correlated with cognitive status, extrapolation from findings on cognitive tests to disturbances in activities of daily living should be done with caution. Methods for assessing functional abilities include self-report measures, observational measures, and questionnaires designed to be administered to a caregiver of the patient. Some instruments assess a single area of functional ability (e.g., the Katz ADL Scale; Katz, Ford, & Moskowitz, 1963), while others (e.g., the Multidimensional Functional Assessment Questionnaire; Pfeifer, 1975) assess functional status across a number of categories, such as physical health, mental health, ADLs and IADLs, social functioning, and economic/financial status.

While, for the most part, no one instrument has been shown to be better than others that assess the same domain, there are potential methodological problems associated with the various approaches. For example, accuracy of self-reported estimates of functional ability has been questioned by some researchers. It has been noted that geriatric patients in a medical setting often overestimate their functional ability (Rubenstein, Schairer, Wieland, & Kane, 1984), while affectively impaired older adults may underestimate their own abilities (Kuriansky, Gurland, & Fleiss, 1976). Other research indicates that individual older adults may both under- and overestimate their ability to complete activities of daily living compared to performance-based measures (Sager et al., 1992). Cognitively impaired elderly pose a special challenge to clinicians, since it appears that as levels of cognitive impairment increase, validity of self-report decreases (Sager et al., 1992).

The report-by-other methodology is typically used to supplement and/or verify information obtained via self-report. External validation with other sources of information can be particularly important in the case of cognitively impaired elderly. However, when multiple reports are involved, there is always the issue of whose report is the most accurate. Rubenstein et al. (1984), for example, found that the discrepancy between the functional status of the subject and the rater's report was greater when a spouse responded rather than a child, another relative, or a friend. They also found that nurses and community proxies tended to rate patients as more dysfunctional than more objective indices suggested.

Direct observation of specific behaviors and activities of daily living frequently provides data that are more reliable and valid than those obtained from self-report or other-report approaches. Older adults may be observed in natural settings or in similar, contrived situations. While there are obvious advantages of using direct observations, there are also limitations. Direct observations of ADLs such as bathing and toileting may be intrusive and aversive for many older adults. Furthermore, functional assessment of a patient in an acute state (e.g., a patient transferred from a natural environment to the alien world of the hospital) is often invalid. It is also critical to be aware of which functions are actually required of the patient in daily life. For example, deficits in ability to manage one's finances take on a different meaning depending upon whether the person is in an assisted-living situation or attempting to live independently in the community.

ISSUES IN THE ASSESSMENT OF OLDER ADULTS   Assessment devices designed specifically for older adults are limited, so it is often difficult to find age-appropriate measures for the variables of interest. The literature suggests, however, that the differences between older adults and other age groups are significant enough to require the use of instruments that have been normed or validated with older persons. Issues involving reliability and validity of assessment results obtained with older adults have been thoroughly discussed elsewhere (e.g., Edelstein, Staats, Kalish, & Northrop, 1996; Kaszniak, 1990). It is well known, across all age groups, that failure to consider the psychometric properties of assessment instruments and methods can lead to inaccurate assessment results. Thus, when tests are used with older adult patients that have not been studied in terms of reliability, validity, and normative data for older subjects, the possibility of measurement errors and interpretation errors should be mentioned in reports on results of these tests.

Often the most important factor in examining older persons is their cooperation. Older adults, especially those with limited formal education, are often less familiar with testing than younger adults and may be more cautious in responding or may view testing as a nuisance or invasion of privacy. The testing situation may be particularly aversive to a patient who is not feeling well or is already concerned about diminishing cognitive ability. Familiarizing the older adult with the purpose and procedures of testing is essential to obtaining optimal performance and may require more time than with younger people. Since older adults fatigue more easily, it may be necessary to adjust testing time with frequent breaks and/or multiple testing sessions. In the case of a patient who is ill or convalescing, the examiner needs to be especially alert to signs of fatigue and sensitive to effects of pain, discomfort, or current medications on performance.

Determining Clinical Significance of Decline

After the clinician has selected measures appropriate to the assessment question, determined a reasonable comparison standard, and obtained performance results suggestive of deficit(s), the question of whether the findings are clinically meaningful in regard to this individual must be considered. This question is complicated by evidence of a significant rate of "false positive" neuropsychological results among even healthy, well-screened older adults when cutoff scores are used to identify a performance as "impaired." Palmer, Boone, Lesser, and Wohl (1998), for example, administering a "flexible" battery of tests to a group of neurologically healthy older subjects, found that 37% earned at least one impaired-range score (at least 2.0 standard deviations below the mean) and 20% earned at least two impaired-range scores on separate tests. Such findings illustrate the problems in interpreting isolated "abnormal" scores and underline the importance of gathering additional data regarding an individual's level of functioning.

Even clear evidence of decrease in cognitive function may not be indicative of functional impairment. In a study of a large, community-based, representative sample of nondemented elderly (Corey-Bloom et al., 1996), subjects 85 years of age and older were compared with others aged 65–84 on measures of cognitive and functional status. The individuals older than 84 performed significantly worse on 13 of 27 cognitive measures than the subjects 84 and younger. Poorer performance of the oldest of the older subjects was observed predominantly on verbal and nonverbal memory, psychomotor/executive tasks, and category verbal fluency. However, while cognitive decline appeared to be associated with advancing age, there were no differences in functional ability between the two groups.

Clearly, the judgment regarding the presence of significant decline in the individual elderly patient can be a complicated one for the clinician. Growing numbers of patients who have cognitive changes but who are not demented are presenting for clinical evaluation (Devanand, Folz, Gorlyn, Moeller, & Stern, 1997; Graham et al., 1997). In this context, it has become increasingly apparent that the thorough assessment of the older adult requires consideration of the intimate interplay of physical, psychological, and environmental variables.

If This Patient Is Displaying a Clinically Significant Cognitive Impairment, What Is Causing This Impairment?

As noted above, many factors can contribute to impaired efficiency in cognitive tasks both in day-to-day life and in terms of formal test performance. It is the clinician's responsibility to sort through these possibilities in a systematic fashion with the initial, primary objective being to identify, if possible, the underlying cause or causes of this inefficiency.

The standard definitions of dementia according to such formulations as the *International Classification of Disease* (World Health Organization, 1992) and the *Diagnostic and Statistical Manual (DSM)* (APA, 1994) reinforce the necessity of pursuing various possible causes of the cognitive impairment. The process is one of systematically ruling in or ruling out various possibilities on the basis of the history, the nature, and the progression of the impairment and the results of various examinations and special diagnostic procedures. Several authors have provided algorithms reflecting the logical process by which the clinician sorts through the differential possibilities (Corey-Bloom et al., 1995; Geldmacher & Whitehouse, 1996; U.S. Department of Veterans Affairs [VA], 1997).

The underlying clinical purpose of this differential diagnostic process is, when possible, to isolate an etiology that would lead to a specific treatment regimen. While some individuals seem to assume that the underlying causes of cognitive inefficiencies in older adults are always permanent, progressive "dementing disorders" such as DAT, this is certainly not the case, and this notion represents a dangerous assumption. Indeed, some of the etiologies for cognitive impairment actually constitute disorders that are not truly "dementing disorders" at all but represent other important causes that must be addressed in lieu of such disorders. Some of the etiologies in both categories (i.e., true dementing disorders and other types of causes) are not only directly treatable, but are also reversible (e.g., Corey-Bloom et al., 1995; Devinsky, 1992). Clarfield (1988) reviewed a series of studies dealing with causes of dementia and concluded that 13.2% of 2,889 patients were determined to have potentially reversible causes of apparent dementia. It is also important to point out, of course, that combinations of etiological factors must always be considered.

Before addressing what could be considered true dementing disorders, we will briefly discuss some of the other etiologies for cognitive inefficiencies in older adults that can give a false impression that the individual is suffering from an actual dementia.

Sensory Changes and General Physical Health

Declines in visual and auditory acuity in the elderly are well-known phenomena (Storandt & VandenBos, 1994). Such changes can result in apparent, but not actual, cognitive impairment both in daily life and on formal testing. For example, hearing impairment is estimated to be present in 32% of individuals over 65 (Adams & Benson, 1992). A variety of changes in the visual system have been noted (Storandt & VandenBos, 1994). Such potentially confounding sensory variables must be considered when assessing the cognitive status of the elderly patient.

Further, decline in general physical health may contribute to poor cognitive test performance without a true underlying dementing disorder being present (Storandt & VandenBos, 1994). More than 80% of people over age 65 have at least one chronic condition, and many have more than one (Adams & Benson, 1992); arthritis, for example, being present in 48% of the sample of individuals 65 and older. Limitations in motor speed, increased fatigue, and discomfort can all play a part in poor test performance without the presence of a true underlying dementing disorder.

Psychiatric Conditions

Psychiatric disorders such as depression and anxiety are well-known causes of cognitive inefficiencies, including poor memory performance (Bajulaiye & Alexopoulous, 1994; Fleming, Adams, & Petersen, 1995; Storandt & Vandenbos, 1994). Depression was found to be the cause of intellectual dysfunction in 26% of patients suspected of having a dementing disorder in a series of studies reviewed by Clarfield (1988). Indeed, the very fear associated with the possibility of DAT has reportedly caused elderly individuals to perform poorly on standardized tests (Centofanti, 1998).

Delirium and Drug Toxicity

Delirium, also known as *acute confusional state,* is a common cause of cognitive impairment in the elderly (U.S. Department of Veterans Affairs, 1997). In this syndrome, the patient shows disturbance of consciousness and disturbances in cognition characterized by reduced attention and concentration, failure to register new information, and failure in tasks that require sustained attention (APA, 1994). One cannot address the question of an underlying dementia while the patient is experiencing a delirium. Further complicating matters is the fact that the patient with a true underlying dementia is also particularly vulnerable to delirium (Besidine, Dicks, & Rowe, 1992).

Delirium can be caused by a number of factors, such as febrile illness, metabolic abnormalities such as hyponatremia or hypoxemia secondary to cardiac or pulmonary disease, or medication effects. Larson, Reifler, Sumi, Canfield, and Chinn (1986) found that 5% of 200 elderly outpatients with suspected dementia had metabolic conditions that produced or contributed to their cognitive dysfunction. Metabolic conditions accounted for the cause of apparent dementia in data reviewed by Clarfield

(1988) in a subset of 1,051 patients. In one series, drug toxicity was responsible for cognitive changes in approximately 10% of patients thought to have dementia (Larson et al., 1986), and in another series, drugs were the etiological factor in 28% of the patients (Clarfield, 1988). The fact that many elderly individuals are taking large numbers of medications that might not be coordinated through one clinician adds to the likelihood that "polypharmacy" plays a role in what appears to be a developing cognitive decline. Again, many of these medication-related effects are reversible.

True Dementing Disorders

Having ruled out age effect alone, sensory limitations, psychiatric disorders, delirium, and the various other factors mentioned above as being sufficient explanations for what appears to be a clinically significant cognitive decline of sufficient severity to interfere with occupational and/or social functioning, the clinician must address a very long list of possible organic/physiological causes of the dementia. The list of causal entities has well over 50 categories of diseases/conditions, and from a historical perspective, this list continues to expand. For example, AIDS-related dementia and mental status changes associated with multiple sclerosis have been added to the list in recent years.

The differential diagnostic process involved in identifying the dementing disorder is typically the domain of the neurologist, geriatrician, or other medical practitioner. However, it is essential that behaviorally oriented health care providers understand the importance of pursuing the underlying biological/physiological cause of the dementia while also developing strategies to assist the patient in achieving maximum function. It should be emphasized again that there are many treatable and some reversible causes of true dementia, and virtually all of the causes are at least partially treatable if only in a palliative or collateral manner.

This diagnostic process involves careful analysis of the history, the presentation of the course of the dementia, the examination of the patient, and the results of various tests. The range of the tests that might be ordered extends from broad surveys of underlying factors such as blood studies and urinalysis to neuroimaging techniques, to very focused, invasive procedures such as brain biopsy. Again, the clinician is pursuing the possibility of a treatable or reversible cause of the dementia, such as thyroid disease, fungal infections, vitamin deficiencies, and structural lesions such as tumors, subdural hematomas, and hydrocephalus (Corey-Bloom et al., 1995).

DAT is a diagnosis by exclusion at this point, following the determination of a generalized progressive dementia with other more specific causes of dementia having been ruled out. This diagnosis by exclusion leads to a diagnosis of DAT in approximately 50% of cases. However, it is important to point out that in studies in which neuropathological confirmation was available (demonstrating the various pathological findings in brain tissue at autopsy, such as cortical Lewy bodies, abundant plaques, and neurofibrillary tangles), the accuracy rate of the diagnosis of DAT in life is only 80–90% (Corey-Bloom et al., 1995; Galasko et al., 1994; Mendez, Mastri, Sung, Zander, & Frey, 1991). In the future, DAT might be confirmed in life through various biological markers, which might also be used to identify individuals at risk for later development of DAT (Mayeux et al., 1992; Post et al., 1997; Saunders, Strittmatter, & Schmechel, 1976).

Vascular dementia affects about 5–10% of patients with dementia (Corey-Bloom et al., 1995). Symptoms appear as the patient has recurrent strokes in various locations throughout the brain. In this category the patient will frequently show focal or lateralizing signs on examination and on neuroimaging techniques and will also present with a stair-step progression of decline rather than the continuous decline seen in DAT. The accuracy of the diagnosis of vascular dementia in life varies considerably from 25% to 85% (Erkinjuntti, Haltia, Palo, Sulkava, & Paetau, 1988; Molsa, Paljarvi, Rinne, & Sako, 1985; Wade et al., 1987).

The coexistence of DAT and vascular dementia occurs in roughly 10% of patients, and this coexistence represents a significant challenge to the clinician as he or she attempts to determine whether one entity or both are contributing to the dementing process.

Several "dementing disorders" are neurological conditions in their own right, dementia being only one symptom of the disease process. Parkinson's disease represents an example of such a syndrome. Dementia is evident in approximately 50% of patients with Parkinson's (Mayeux et al., 1992).

Causes that have genetic implications, such as Huntington's disease (which typically presents in younger individuals), are important to identify not only in the process of ruling out other etiologies but also because of the implications for genetic counseling. Further, causes that are transmissible from human to human, such as Creutzfeldt-Jakob disease (CJD), must be identified to address risk to other patients and clinicians as well as the risks associated with organ donation and even the use of human brain tissue in the development of such processes as the production of human growth hormone (Fradkin et al., 1991; Geldmacher & Whitehouse, 1996; Leiderman, Decker, Borcich, & Choi, 1986; Tinter et al., 1986).

It should be noted that no matter how confident the clinician is in the diagnosis, there are demonstrable error rates in diagnosis even in carefully controlled studies (Corey-Bloom et al., 1995). Combinations of various factors must always be considered. These include multiple dementing disorders in the same patient, a dementing disorder and other chronic or acute medical problems, and a dementing disorder and another factor such as depression.

What Can Be Done About the Cause of the Cognitive Impairment?

It is clear that the clinician is confronted with a complicated task when evaluating a patient with suspected dementia. Once having ruled out age effects alone, the clinician addresses "other" causes of apparent dementia. If these have been ruled out, the clinician (while always being concerned about combinations of causes) addresses the etiological possibilities of a "true" dementing disorder.

Assuming that delirium and drug-related causes have been addressed, one is left with disorders that have as a primary element, or as one element in the syndrome, a true dementia. Having identified the cause(s), the clinician can embark on a course of intervention that is tied to the causal entity. This relationship can range from a direct treatment of the underlying cause to a palliative, indirect approach.

Treatable and reversible causes of dementia such as thyroid disease, certain infections, vitamin deficiencies, and certain structural lesions respond to direct medical or surgical treatment. The effect on the cognitive impairment can be total reversibility in some cases (U.S. Department of Veterans Affairs, 1997).

Medical treatments for DAT have traditionally been palliative in nature, attempting to treat anxiety and acting out. However, recent attempts have been made, with some success, to treat the condition more directly through pharmacological intervention based on the demonstrated central cholinergic hypofunction seen in DAT patients (Cummings et al., 1998; Morris et al., 1998). These efforts attempt to augment central cholinergic function through acetylcholine (ACh) precursors, ACh release facilitators, cholinergic receptor agonists, and, more recently, reversible inhibitors of the ACh degradative enzyme acetylcholinesterase. Efforts in this arena appear promising.

Vascular dementia can be addressed by attempting to decrease the likelihood of further infarction through the treatment of underlying hypertension and vascular disease through medication regimens, diet/exercise regimens, and/or surgical intervention such as carotid endarterectomy.

Conditions such as Parkinson's disease have, for several decades, had medication regimens guided by an understanding of the underlying biochemical process. These approaches, which address the underlying depletion of neurotransmitters such as dopamine, have contributed to the functional status of the patient but do not directly address the dementia per se. Various surgical techniques have also been used in an attempt to improve dopamine status or to interrupt the pathways involved in producing the motor symptoms. Again, the effect of these surgical techniques on the cognitive losses in Parkinson's disease is uncertain.

While direct treatments for such diseases as Huntington's are not yet available, the underlying genetic factors are becoming better understood with each passing decade, and this understanding has led to the possibility of earlier diagnosis and points to a possible eventual treatment that will have a direct scientific link to the underlying genetic causal element. Further, genetic counseling and early diagnosis can appreciably influence the incidence of this disease.

Research on conditions such as Creutzfeldt-Jakob disease (CJD) represent an exciting frontier in molecular biology. As viruses and prions are better understood (Glausiusz, 1998), direct treatments will emerge for what are now considered untreatable illnesses.

Nonetheless, even in conditions such as CJD one can provide comfort care and proper supervision of the declining patient, can treat the behavioral aspects of the condition, and can decrease risk of transmission to others. An accurate initial diagnosis of the cause of the dementia allows the clinician and the patient to design an appropriate response.

Conclusion

It is evident from the discussion above that regardless of the cause of the underlying dementia, there is now only a partial solution in most cases. Thus, there is essential work to be done in assisting the patient to achieve the maximal level of function possible given the patient's unique circumstance. The remaining chapters in Part IV address this aspect of patient care.

References

Adams, P. F., & Benson, V. (1992). *Current estimates from the National Health Interview Survey, 1991* (Vital and Health Statistics, Series 10, No. 184). Hyattsville, MD: National Center for Health Statistics.

Albert, M. L. (1994). Cognition and aging. In W. R. Hazzard, E. L. Bierman, J. P. Blass, W. H. Ettinger, & J. B. Halter (Eds.), *Principles of geriatric medicine and gerontology* (3rd ed., pp. 1013–1019). New York: McGraw-Hill.

American Psychiatric Association. (1994). *Diagnostic and statistical manual of mental disorders* (4th ed.; *DSM*-IV). Washington, DC: Author.

American Psychological Association. (1997). *What practitioners should know about working with older adults*. Washington, DC: Author.

Bajulaiye, R., & Alexopoulous, G. S. (1994). Pseudodementia in geriatric depression. In E. Chiu & D. Ames (Eds.), *Functional psychiatric disorders of the elderly* (pp. 126–141). Melbourne: Cambridge University Press.

Barona, A., Reynolds, C. R., & Chastain, R. (1984). A demographically-based index of premorbid intelligence for the WAIS-R. *Journal of Consulting and Clinical Psychology, 52*, 885–887.

Benton, A. L., & Sivan, A. B. (1984). Problems and conceptual issues in neuropsychological research in aging and dementia. *Journal of Clinical Neuropsychology, 6*, 57–64.

Besidine, R. W., Dicks, R., & Rowe, J. W. (1992). *Principles of geriatric neurology: Delirium in the elderly*. Philadelphia: F. A. Davis.

Bigler, E. D. (1988). *Diagnostic clinical neuropsychology*. Austin: University of Texas Press.

Blair, J. R., & Spreen, O. (1989). Predicting premorbid IQ: A revision of the National Adult Reading Test. *Clinical Neuropsychologist, 3*, 129–136.

Bolla, K. I., Lindgren, K. N., Bonaccorsy, C., & Bleecker, M. L. (1991). Memory complaints in older adults. *Archives of Neurology, 48*, 61–64.

Centofanti, M. (1998, June). Fear of Alzheimer's undermines health of elderly patients. *APA Monitor*, pp. 1, 33.

Clarfield, A. M. (1988). The reversible dementias: Do they reverse? *Annals of Internal Medicine, 109*, 476–486.

Corey-Bloom, J., Thal, L. J., Galasko, D., Folstein, M., Drachman, D., & Raskind, M. (1995). Diagnosis and evaluation of dementia. *Neurology, 45*, 211–218.

Corey-Bloom, J., Wiederholt, W. C., Edelstein, S., Salmon, D. P., Cahn, D., & Barrett-Connor, E. (1996). Cognitive and functional status of the oldest old. *Journal of the American Geriatrics Society, 44*, 671–674.

Cullum, C. M., & Rosenberg, R. N. (1998). Memory loss—When is it Alzheimer's disease? *Journal of the American Medical Association, 279*(21), 1689–1690.

Cummings, J. L., Cyrus, P. A., Bieber, F., Mas, J., Orazam, J., Gulanski, B., & the Metrifonate Study Group. (1998). Metrifonate treatment of the cognitive deficits of Alzheimer's disease. *Neurology, 50*, 1214–1221.

Devanand, D. P., Folz, M., Gorlyn, M., Moeller, J. R., & Stern, Y. (1997). Questionable dementia: Clinical course and predictors of outcome. *Journal of the American Geriatrics Society, 45*, 321–328.

Devinsky, O. (1992). *Behavioral neurology*. St. Louis: Mosby Year Book.

Dustman, R. E., Emmerson, R. Y., & Shearer, D. E. (1990). Electrophysiology and aging: Slowing, inhibition, and aerobic fitness. In M. L. Howe, M. J. Stones, & C. J. Brainerd (Eds.), *Cognitive and behavioral performance factors in atypical aging*. New York: Springer-Verlag.

Dustman, R. E., Shearer, D. E., & Emmerson, R. Y. (1991). Evoked potentials and EEG suggest

CNS inhibitory deficits in aging. In D. A. Armstrong (Ed.), *The effects of aging and environment on vision*. New York: Plenum Press.

Edelstein, B., Staats, N., Kalish, K. D., & Northrop, L. E. (1996). Assessment of older adults. In M. Hersen & V. B. Hasselt (Eds.), *Psychological treatment of older adults: An introductory text* (pp. 35–68). New York: Plenum Press.

Erkinjuntti, T., Haltia, M., Palo, J., Sulkava, R., & Paetau, A. (1988). Accuracy of the clinical diagnosis of vascular dementia: A prospective clinical and post-mortem pathological study. *Journal of Neurology, Neurosurgery and Psychiatry, 51*, 1037–1044.

Fleming, D. C., Adams, A. C., & Petersen, R. C. (1995). Dementia: Diagnosis and evaluation. *Mayo Clinic Proceedings, 70*, 1093–1107.

Fradkin, J. E., Schonberger, L. B., Mills, J. L., Gunn, W. J., Piper, J. M., & Wysowski, D. K. (1991). Creutzfeldt-Jakob disease in pituitary growth hormone recipients in the United States. *Journal of the American Medical Association, 265*, 880–884.

Galasko, D., Hansen, L. A., Katzman, R., Wiederholt, W., Masliah, E., & Terry, R. (1994). Clinical-neuropathological correlations in Alzheimer's disease and related dementias. *Archives of Neurology, 51*, 888–895.

Geldmacher, D. S., & Whitehouse, P. J. (1996). Evaluation of dementia. *New England Journal of Medicine, 335*, 330–336.

Glausiusz, J. (1998, January). Medicine 1997: Case closed. *Discovery*, pp. 56–57.

Graham, J. E., Rockwood, K., Beattie, B. L., Eastwood, R., Gauthier, S., & Tuokko, H. (1997). Prevalence and severity of cognitive impairment with and without dementia in an elderly population. *Lancet, 349*, 1793–1796.

Heaton, R. K., Grant, I., & Matthews, C. G. (1986). Differences in neuropsychological test performance associated with age, education, and sex. In I. Grant & K. M. Adams (Eds.), *Neuropsychological assessment of neuropsychiatric disorders* (pp. 100–120). New York: Oxford University Press.

Heaton, R. K., Grant, I., & Matthews, C. G. (1991). *Comprehensive norms for an expanded Halstead-Reitan battery: Demographic corrections, research findings, and clinical applications*. Odessa, FL: Psychological Assessment Resources.

Horn, J. L., & Cattell, R. B. (1967). Age differences in fluid and crystallized intelligence. *Acta Psychologica, 26*, 107–129.

Kaszniak, A. W. (1990). Psychological assessment of the aging individual. In J. E. Birren & K. W. Schaie (Eds.), *Handbook of the psychology of aging* (pp. 427–445). New York: Academic Press.

Katz, S., Ford, A., & Moskowitz, R. (1963). The index of ADL: A standardized measure of biological and psychosocial function. *Journal of the American Medical Association, 185*, 914–919.

Kaufman, A. S., Reynolds, C. R., & McLean, J. E. (1989). Age and WAIS-R intelligence in a national sample of adults in the 20–74 age range: A cross-sectional analysis with educational level controlled. *Intelligence, 13*, 235–253.

Kemper, T. (1984). Neuroanatomical and neuropathological changes in normal aging and in dementia. In M. L. Albert (Ed.), *Clinical neurology of aging* (pp. 9–52). New York: Oxford University Press.

Kuriansky, J. B., Gurland, B. J., & Fleiss, J. L. (1976). The assessment of self-care capacity in geriatric psychiatric patients by objective and subjective methods. *Journal of Clinical Psychology, 32*(1), 95–102.

Larrabee, G. J., Largen, J. W., & Levin, H. S. (1985). Sensitivity of age decline resistant ("Hold") WAIS subtests to Alzheimer's disease. *Journal of Clinical and Experimental Neuropsychology, 7*, 497–504.

Larson, E. B., Reifler, B. V., Sumi, S. M., Canfield, C. G., & Chinn, N. M. (1986). Diagnostic tests in the evaluation of dementia: A prospective study of 200 elderly outpatients. *Archives of Internal Medicine, 146,* 1917–1922.

Leiderman, D. B., Decker, K. P., Borcich, J., & Choi, D. W. (1986). Sporadic Creutzfeldt-Jakob disease in two coworkers. *Neurology, 36,* 835–837.

Lezak, M. D. (1995). *Neuropsychological assessment* (3rd ed.). New York: Oxford University Press.

Mayeux, R., Denaro, J., Hemenegildo, N., Marder, K., Tang, M., & Cote, L. J. (1992). A population-based investigation of Parkinson's disease with and without dementia: Relationship to age and gender. *Archives of Neurology, 49,* 492–497.

Mayeux, R., Stern, Y., & Ottman, R. (1993). The apolipoprotein epsilon4 allelle in patients with Alzheimer's disease. *Annals of Neurology, 34,* 752–754.

McFie, J. (1975). *Assessment of organic intellectual impairment.* London: Academic Press.

Mendez, M. F., Mastri, A. R., Sung, J. H., Zander, B. A., & Frey, W. H. (1991). Neuropathologically confirmed Alzheimer's disease: Clinical diagnoses in 394 cases. *Journal of Geriatric Psychiatry and Neurology, 4,* 26–29.

Metter, E. J. (1988). Positron tomography and cerebral blood flow studies. In M. S. Albert & M. B. Moss (Eds.), *Geriatric neuropsychology* (pp. 228–261). New York: Guilford Press.

Mittenberg, W., Seidenberg, M., O'Leary, D. S., & DiGiulio, D. V. (1989). Changes in cerebral functioning associated with normal aging. *Journal of Clinical and Experimental Neuropsychology, 11,* 918–932.

Molsa, P. K., Paljarvi, L., Rinne, J. O., Rinne, U. K., & Sako, E. (1985). Validity of clinical diagnosis in dementia: A prospective clinico-pathological study. *Journal of Neurology, Neurosurgery and Psychiatry, 48,* 1085–1090.

Morris, J. C., Cyrus, P. A., Orazam, J., Mas, J., Bieber, F., & Ruzicka, B. B. (1998). Metrifonate benefits cognitive, behavioral, and global function in patients with Alzheimer's disease. *Neurology, 50,* 1222–1230.

Morris, J. C., & McManus, D. Q. (1991). The neurology of aging: Normal versus pathologic change. *Geriatrics, 46*(8), 47–54.

Mortensen, E. L., Gade, A., & Reinisch, J. M. (1991). A critical note on Lezak's "best performance method" in clinical neuropsychology. *Journal of Clinical and Experimental Neuropsychology, 13,* 361–371.

Palmer, B. W., Boone, K. B., Lesser, I. M., & Wohl, M. A. (1998). Base rates of "impaired" neuropsychological test performance among healthy older adults. *Archives of Clinical Neuropsychology, 13*(6), 503–511.

Pfeifer, E. (Ed.). (1975). *Multidimensional functional assessment: The OARS Methodology.* Durham, NC: Duke University Center for the Study of Aging and Human Development.

Post, S. G., Whitehouse, P. J., Binstock, R. H., Bird, T. D., Eckert, S. K., & Farrer, L. A. (1997). The clinical introduction of genetic testing for Alzheimer disease: An ethical perspective. *Journal of the American Medical Association, 277*(10), 832–836.

Reitan, R. M., & Wolfson, D. (1985). *The Halstead-Reitan Neuropsychological Test Battery: Theory and clinical interpretation.* Tucson, AZ: Neuropsychology Press.

Rosenberg, I. H., & Miller, J. W. (1992). Nutritional factors in physical and cognitive functions of elderly people. *American Journal of Clinical Nutrition, 55,* 1237–1243

Rowe, J. W., & Kahn, R. (1987). Human aging: Usual versus successful. *Science, 237,* 143–149.

Rubenstein, L. Z., Schairer, C., Wieland, G. D., & Kane, R. (1984). Systematic biases in functional status assessment of elderly adults: Effects of different data sources. *Journal of Gerontology, 39*(6), 686–691.

Sager, M. A., Dunham, N. C., Schwantes, A., Mecum, L., Halverson, K., & Harlowe, D. (1992). Measurement of activities of daily living in hospitalized elderly: A comparison of self-report and performance-based methods. *Journal of the American Geriatrics Society, 40,* 457–462.

Saunders, A. A., Strittmatter, W. J., & Schmechel, D. (1976). Association of apolipoprotein E allele epsilon4 with late-onset familian and sporadic Alzheimer's disease. *Neurology, 76,* 1467–1472.

Schear, J. M. (1988). Attempt to cross-validate norm-based dysfunction scores in young and older neuropsychiatric patients. *Clinical Neuropsychologist, 2,* 57–66.

Scheibel, A. B. (1992). Structural changes in the aging brain. In J. E. Birren, R. B. Sloane, & G. Cohen (Eds.), *Handbook of mental health and aging* (pp. 147–173). New York: Academic Press.

Stebbins, G. T., Wilson, R. S., Gilley, D. W., Bernard, B. A., & Fox, J. H. (1990). Use of the National Adult Reading Test to estimate premorbid IQ in dementia. *Clinical Neuropsychologist, 4,* 18–24.

Storandt, M. (1990). Longitudinal studies of aging and age-associated dementias. In F. Boller & J. Grafman (Eds.), *Handbook of neuropsychology* (Vol. 4). Amsterdam: Elsevier.

Storandt, M., & VandenBos, G. R. (1994). *Dementia and depression in older adults.* Washington, DC: American Psychological Association.

Sweet, J. J., Moberg, P. J., & Tovian, S. M. (1990). Evaluation of the WAIS-R premorbid IQ formulas in clinical populations. *Psychological Assessment, 2,* 41–44.

Terry, R. D., DeTeresa, R., & Hansen, L. A. (1987). Neocortical cell counts in normal human adult aging. *Annals of Neurology, 21,* 530–539.

Tinter, R., Brown, P., Hedley-Whyte, E. T., Rappaport, E. B., Piccardo, C. P., & Gajdusek, D. C. (1986). Neuropathologic verification of Creutzfeldt-Jakob disease in the exhumed American recipient of human pituitary growth hormone: Epidemiologic and pathogenic implications. *Neurology, 36,* 932–936.

U.S. Department of Veterans Affairs. (1997). *Dementia identification and assessment: Guidelines for primary care practitioners* (U.S. Department of Veterans Affairs). Washington, DC: U.S. Government Printing Office.

Vanderploeg, R. D., & Schinka, J. A. (1995). Predicting WAIS-R IQ premorbid ability: Combining subtest performance and demographic variable predictors. *Archives of Clinical Neuropsychology, 10,* 225–239.

Wade, J. P. H., Mirsen, T. R., Hachinski, V. C., Fishman, M., Lau, C., & Merskey, H. (1987). The clinical diagnosis of Alzheimer's disease. *Archives of Neurology, 44,* 24–29.

World Health Organization (WHO). (1992). *The ICD-10 classification of mental and behavioral disorders. Clinical descriptions and diagnostic guidelines.* Geneva: World Health Organization.

12

Retrieval Strategies as a Rehabilitation Aid for Cognitive Loss in Pathological Aging

CAMERON J. CAMP

MICHAEL J. BIRD

KATIE E. CHERRY

Research on memory interventions for persons with dementia and other cognitive impairments is rapidly expanding, as the existence of this volume testifies. In this chapter, we will describe the use of active retrieval strategies as an aid in cognitive rehabilitation for pathological aging. More than 20 years have passed since the original research on which this chapter is based was published. In the late 1970s, Landauer and Bjork (1978) described a technique designed to allow new information, such as the name of a person in a photograph, to be learned efficiently. They called this phenomenon "spaced retrieval" (SR). Their study was published as a book chapter—part of the proceedings of the first Practical Aspects of Memory conference held in the United Kingdom. Today, SR is being implemented as a rehabilitation aid for cognitive loss associated with an increasingly diverse set of pathologies found in older adults. The SR technique described by Landauer and Bjork has been shown to allow persons with profound memory deficits characteristic of dementia to be able to learn new information and successfully recall it across clinically meaningful periods of time (days, weeks, months). Interventions using this approach, in combination with other techniques, can alleviate behavioral problems associated with dementia in real-world settings. Use of SR by therapists in different disciplines has recently been noted.

We will attempt to provide a historical background for the development of SR, including a brief review of early research utilizing SR as a memory intervention for persons with memory deficits. We focus primarily on research involving persons with dementia. We describe how the methods of applying SR as an intervention have evolved and are evolving. We then focus on two major topics: recent clinical applications of SR and recent efforts to determine the theoretical basis for effects produced by SR. We conclude the chapter with a case study and summary comments.

Historical Background

Landauer and Bjork's findings concerning SR were reported within the context of a movement within cognitive psychology: a drive to conduct research that would be more ecologically valid, addressing issues of everyday memory rather than lab-based phenomena. This movement has generated controversy regarding the efficacy of everyday memory research (see Baddeley, 1989; Banaji & Crowder, 1989, 1991; Landauer, 1989; Mook, 1989; Petrinovich, 1989; Tulving, 1991). Their study, in a sense, represented a bridging action. Their data were collected from a group of undergraduates in a university setting, but their findings had potential for application across a number of areas that could be explored by future investigators.

The Original Study

Landauer and Bjork's study (1978) was based on a line of research begun in the 1960s concerning the spacing effect. In essence, the spacing effect is the phenomenon in which spaced practice for learning and recalling new information results in better long-term retention than massed practice (see Landauer, 1989, for a description of the origins of spacing-effect research). Landauer and Bjork were interested in determining if one type of spacing schedule might be optimal for learning new information. Their results suggested that recall of information at successively longer intervals produced better long-term retention of new information than other schedules of recall practice. Though other schedules also produced good recall performance, such as multiple recall trials at fixed intervals, their data indicated that the expanding schedule worked best as a potential mnemonic intervention. They called their optimal technique "spaced retrieval."

It is informative to note the aspects of SR as originally implemented. Information about a person in a photograph, such as his or her name, was presented along with the photo. Then, a number of other photos were interspersed between this original presentation and later presentations of the target photo. For example, the initial photo might be shown, followed by a second photo and then another presentation of the original photograph. At this latter presentation of the target photo, recall of the name or other information presented at initial presentation of the photo was attempted. The number of photos interspersed between the original presentation of the target and latter presentations kept expanding in the SR condition. For example, Figure 12.1 shows a representation of a 1 : 5 : 10 expanding recall, or SR, schedule.

At the next Practical Aspects of Memory conference held about a decade later, Bjork (1988) described SR as a shaping technique applied to memory. Successful recall trials in this context represented closer and closer approximations to a desired goal, that is, retention and recallability of new information over time periods such as days or months or years. This reference to behavioral technology within the context of cognitive research is important, for it represents the acknowledgment that an eclectic approach to understanding cognitive phenomena and implementing potential interventions is both desirable and necessary. This approach to cognitive rehabilitation, which developed in the UK, has been clearly and forcefully described and contrasted with alternative approaches to cognitive rehabilitation, by Wilson (1997).

Time →

Initial Stimulus Presentation	Filler Item	First Recall of Associated Target Info (e.g., Name)	Filler Items (Spacing Effect)	Second Recall of Associated Target Info (e.g., Name)	Filler Items (Spacing Effect)	Third and Final Recall
Target Photo (First Presentation)	1 New Photo	Target Photo (Second Presentation)	5 New Photos	Target Photo (Third Presentation)	10 New Photos	Target Photo (Fourth Presentation)

Figure 12.1. Example of an expanded recall schedule.

First Uses of SR as a Rehabilitative Technique

Several years after the initial SR study, Dan Schacter and his colleagues (Schacter, Rich, & Stampp, 1985) described the use of SR as a cognitive intervention using a small sample of adults with a variety of etiologies and cognitive deficits. They used a procedure similar to that employed by Landauer and Bjork to create SR schedules (i.e., interspersing varying numbers of filler items between an initial target presentation and latter presentations of the target). Schacter's group found that persons with memory impairment could learn new information using SR, though attempts to train participants to spontaneously use a form of SR themselves when confronted with new information were not successful. They also reported that learning via SR appeared to be accomplished with relatively little expenditure of cognitive effort.

Several important points are exemplified in Schacter's use of SR as an aid to cognitive rehabilitation. First, this study was conducted within the context of a series of studies by Glisky and Schacter and their colleagues on cognitive remediation techniques designed to access implicit memory, which was assumed to be relatively spared in amnestic patients (see Glisky & Schacter, 1986, 1987; Glisky, Schacter, & Tulving, 1986; Schacter, 1992, 1994; Schacter & Tulving, 1994). Thus, the reference to cognitive effort is important. Since implicit memory is assumed to utilize relatively unconscious and automatic processes (i.e., those that should require little cognitive effort), a case was being made that SR might be accessing some aspect of implicit memory. Though the argument was based on rather anecdotal accounts of how effortful the SR procedure was to research participants, these accounts were seen as indirect evidence linking SR and implicit memory. In addition, Schacter's work had extended to the use of behavioral technologies such as fading cues as interventions for cognitive deficits (Glisky et al., 1986). These studies emphasized the need for eclectic approaches to designing cognitive rehabilitation aids, and they introduced the concepts of (low) cognitive effort and implicit memory in relation to the SR technique. Glisky and Schacter also emphasized the need to focus on training for retention of specific information rather than attempting to improve memory per se (see also Glisky & Schacter, 1986, 1987).

Moffat (1989) described the use of SR, which he referred to as "expanding rehearsal," to rehabilitate a man in his late 60s who had suffered cerebral anoxia as a result of a myocardial infarction. The targeted problem was his severe dysgraphia for letters and numbers. Moffat's study marked several important new features made available for the clinical use of SR as a rehabilitative technique. The target behavior was determined by the client, who was highly motivated to use the intervention. This intervention was implemented in a home setting, primarily by the client and the client's wife. Expanding intervals were determined by time periods rather than through interposing additional experimental stimuli. The retrieval schedule extended across hours and a large number of target stimuli. Learning acquired through SR was maintained through routinized practice schedules, and SR was implemented with a motor behavior rather than a verbal behavior.

Use of SR as an Intervention for Persons with Dementia

Moffat (1989) also described a case in which a woman diagnosed with Alzheimer's disease (AD) was trained using SR to relearn the names of objects. Impairment in naming ability is a common feature of dementia associated with AD and related disorders and is a source of frustration for those with this condition. Moffat set up a training regimen in the client's home, conducted by a nurse's aide. Names of 20 items displayed as pictures were targeted for training. At baseline, the client could not retain the name of any targeted item for any substantial length of time. Training for remembering the names of 20 common items involved giving her the name of a target item, checking its retention after a 2-minute interval, and then doubling the next recall interval after successful recall attempts and halving recall intervals after unsuccessful recall attempts. Again, here we see a shaping technology being applied to a cognitive ability. After an item was trained to a criterion level of recall, another item was initiated in an SR training sequence. Probed recall of all items was used every 2 weeks.

Several features of this case study add important information about SR. Moffat noted that the numbers of errors made for trained items and their latencies of response grew smaller across training sessions. The first few words, once learned to criterion, were always recalled immediately. These findings indicate that SR appears to be enabling learning to take place for trained stimuli, and that improvement in recall ability with practice is available for persons with AD via SR training.

Also, by the third session, only three words had been taught, but the majority of the 20 pictures were named accurately on the probe test. This finding poses some interesting questions. Does this finding mean that SR training produces a generalization of training effects (i.e., does the general ability to name objects improve after exposure to SR training for specific stimuli)? Alternatively, does the sheer act of giving practice at attempting recall as was done in the probe tests (especially if feedback is provided for failed attempts, but perhaps even if not) constitute an alternative SR schedule and result in enhanced recallability of probed items?

Landauer and Bjork (1978) tested several alternative recall intervals, of which expanding rehearsal was only one (but the most successful). Alternative spacing schedules can also be effective at enhancing recall (e.g., Foss, 1994; Landauer & Bjork, 1978). What if probes to determine whether nontrained items can be recalled constitute an alternative form of SR training or, at the very least, increase likelihood of recall over multiple probe sessions? If such is the case, this result creates challenges to researchers seeking to create control conditions for determining the efficacy of the SR intervention as a rehabilitation technique.

Further Use of SR for Persons with Dementia: Camp's Research

Camp and his colleagues (Abrahams & Camp, 1993; Brush & Camp, 1998, in press; Camp, 1989, 1996; Camp & Foss, 1997; Camp & Schaller, 1989; Camp & Stevens, 1990; Camp et al., 1993, 1996a, 1996b; Hayden & Camp, 1995; McKitrick, 1993; McKitrick & Camp, 1993; McKitrick, Camp, & Black, 1992; Stevens, O'Hanlon, & Camp, 1993) also began using SR as an intervention for persons with dementia, using a free recall format. In initial pilot studies, he found that the expanding interval schedule used by Moffat (i.e., doubling the previous recall interval) was producing high error rates. Instead, he switched to the use of a more gradual recall interval expansion rate: 5 sec, 10 sec, 20 sec, 40 sec, 60 sec, 90 sec, 120 sec, and so on, in which intervals were increased by 30 sec once a 60-sec successful recall interval had been attained. A participant who failed in an attempt at recall was provided the answer and immediately asked to recall it. The next recall interval was shortened to that of the last successful recall interval.

This schedule was used in a number of studies in which persons with dementia were trained to remember names of persons or objects, locations of objects, motor activities, and even a strategy (remembering to look at a calendar to learn about daily appointments and other personally relevant information). A portable computer, in most instances, was used to record recall successes and failures and controlled the timing of recall intervals. A musical cue informed researchers when to institute the next recall trial. Use of this schedule was somewhat serendipitous, since Camp's initial pilot participants were more advanced in their dementia than the person trained by Moffat. Still, this approach proved successful across a variety of both levels of dementia, as assessed by measures such as the Mini-Mental State Exam (MMSE), and types of dementia.

One important finding in this research was that if participants with dementia were able to successfully recall information over a critical recall interval, perhaps 6–8 min, they could retain information across training sessions (Camp et al., 1996b). In other words, if persons with dementia could be trained by SR to retain new information across a critical interval within a training session, that information seemed to be consolidated into long-term memory and could be recalled across days. Though other researchers have reported that a longer retention interval (15 minutes or 1 hour) is required to predict long-term retention (see Bird's research, described later in this chapter), the finding that such a critical recall interval may exist has several important implications. First, training effects of SR can extend beyond the training session and thus can be brought to bear on clinically meaningful targets. Second, if the critical interval needed to place information in long-term memory can be determined for a particular individual (and the interval may vary across individuals, levels of dementia, etc.), this information will be helpful in predicting when to expect long-term retention of information outside training sessions. Third, this knowledge can be used to determine when SR training sessions are ready to be terminated and long-term maintenance of trained information can be instituted.

Extending the Use of SR: Implementation by Caregivers and Therapists

Most of this research involved persons living at home, the intervention being implemented by researchers. Some of the studies were conducted in home settings. Some were conducted in adult day care centers attended by persons with dementia. McKitrick (1993; McKitrick & Camp, 1993) extended this line of research by having family caregivers implement the training, similar to the approach taken by Moffat (1989). Other researchers likewise trained caregivers to implement SR as an intervention for persons with dementia, (Arkin, 1991; Riley, 1992). Riley (1992) also reported a case study in which a man in the initial stages of dementia was able to train himself to remember new information by utilizing SR. Brush and Camp (1998, in press) reported the use of SR by speech-language pathologists to reach clinical goals in persons with dementia, most of whom were living in a long-term care facility. Carruth (1997) reported the use of SR within the context of a music therapy session as a means of training nursing-home residents to remember names of staff members.

In these contexts, timing of recall intervals was not controlled by computer. For example, caregivers in McKitrick's studies used a hand-held digital timer and a non-electrical tracking device to track and determine recall intervals (see McKitrick, 1993, for a detailed description of apparatus and procedures). In the case of speech-language pathologists, recall trials occurred during breaks between therapeutic activities conducted during speech therapy sessions (Brush & Camp, 1998, in press). Though this approach creates less precision than would be the case using more lab-based experimental procedures, SR appears to produce robust effects when applied in these real-world contexts. Furthermore, SR can be implemented by therapists while conducting billable procedures. Thus, it is more likely to be implemented on a large scale than if training effects were attainable only under more tightly controlled conditions, and/or only when applied by researchers.

Further Clinical Applications: Bird's Research

SR also has been implemented as a clinical intervention by Bird and his associates. His research using SR evolved from a more lab-based research paradigm, though it has taken a relatively direct route to using SR in clinical applications. As already noted, the work of Camp and associates has clear clinical implications, for example, in training dementia sufferers in daily calendar use (Camp et al., 1996b). Bird and Kinsella (1996) expanded the field in a more overtly clinical direction, attempting to add to the repertoire of well-researched psychosocial techniques that can be used to lessen behavior problems in dementia. The predominant experimental memory paradigm in dementia has been traditional verbal learning using word lists that are arguably low in ecological validity. But the major problem for many dementia sufferers and their caregivers is behavior that is far from trivial, such as violence, continuous screaming, repetitive questions, and incontinence (Patterson & Whitehouse, 1994; Teri et al., 1992). The basic research question, therefore, was whether it was possible to use SR to train persons with dementia to associate more adaptive behavior with a cue or cues so that on encountering the cue in common problem situations, they might respond differently.

The basic model is presented in Figure 12.2. The theoretical and experimental rationale that suggested such an operation might be possible drew mainly from the dementia list-learning literature, which has used a three-stage model of learning and memory: initial learning of new information (acquisition), storage of information in accessible form (retention), and accessing stored material when required (retrieval).

There were three findings of particular relevance in the literature. First, there is evidence that there are severe deficits at both acquisition and retrieval, at least in AD and vascular dementia. The provision of structured support at both these points on the processing continuum is essential to maximize learning, though performance still remains well below that of matched controls (Bird & Luszcz, 1991, 1993; Cherry & Plauche, 1996; Diesfeldt, 1984; Tuokko & Crockett, 1989). Second, a few studies that have provided extensive acquisition assistance and then strong support at retrieval in the form of forced choice recognition have shown that there can be substantial savings over clinically significant intervals (Hart, Kwentus, Taylor, & Harkin, 1987; Kopel-

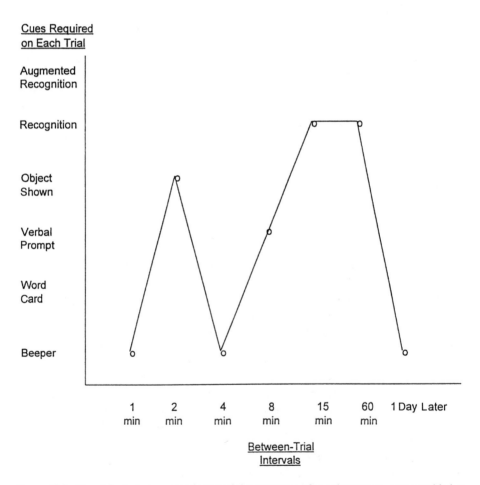

Figure 12.2. Example from one experiment of the sequence of supplementary cues provided at each trial where failure occurred. Sequence worked through until the participant was successful.

man, 1985). Third, the frequently found learning advantage for behavioral tasks also seems to apply in dementia (e.g., Herlitz, Adolfsson, Bäckman, & Nilsson, 1991).

From these findings, it was assumed that behavioral responses would be easier to learn than verbal material for older adults with dementia. In addition, so long as sufficient assistance was provided at acquisition and retrieval, these persons might be able to retain the information over periods long enough for such retention to be clinically relevant. However, the key to this type of intervention would be the cue, as a retrieval aid in itself, and also to ensure that retrieval occurred at the required time and/or place.

University students (Intons-Peterson & Fourner, 1986) as well as cognitively intact elderly persons (Dobbs & Rule, 1987; Einstein & McDaniel, 1990) use external cues extensively to prompt retrievals in ecologically relevant situations such as prospective memory operations; they are absolutely critical for persons with dementia. The cue thus has two roles at retrieval: determining whether the behavior is recalled at all and determining when it is recalled.

Acquisition Assistance and Use of Cues

The use of environmental cues has long been advocated in care for persons with dementia (e.g., painting toilet doors a different color), but there is little evidence other than the anecdotal of their efficacy in dementia. Unfortunately, texts advocating use of environmental cues in dementia seldom address the problem of acquisition. Yet, if the patient cannot spontaneously work out the association between the cue and the to-be-remembered information and is not assisted to acquire the association, the cue is of little value. Classic ward orientation studies (Gilleard, Mitchell, & Riordan, 1981; Hanley, 1981) showed that even signposts—for example, "Toilet"—were ineffective for persons with dementia in the absence of systematic assistance in learning what they related to.

A number of methods are known to assist acquisition of material in dementia, most commonly by inducing active processing. Two examples are requiring participants to decide about the taxonomic category of the item (e.g., Bird & Luszcz, 1991; Tuokko & Crockett, 1989) and about where it might be found (Martin, Brouwers, Cox, & Fedio, 1985). For the work under discussion, SR effect was used as the primary acquisition aid, for four reasons.

First, a preliminary study (Bird, 1995) showed that a single retrieval trial was as effective as presenting the material in a way that guaranteed active processing. That is, this study confirmed experimentally that the act of retrieval has a mnemonic effect in dementia; a successful recall increases the chance of subsequent recall. Second, Camp and his associates had already shown that learning and retention of nontrivial material over clinically significant intervals was possible by the use of SR. Third, the advantage of a series of retrieval trials over all other methods is that each presentation, as well as being a fresh learning trial, is also by definition a memory probe, enabling the experimenter or clinician to monitor progress and adjust the procedure to the patient's learning rate. Finally, Hanley (1981, 1984) used something analogous to retrieval trials in successful ward orientation studies. Rather than being repeatedly told the information (the method used by most caregivers and health professionals), persons with dementia had to provide the answer themselves in response to cues such as "Mrs. Smith, show me the dining room please"; "Show me where you have your meals"; and "Look, the tables are set for tea. What room is this, Mrs. Smith?" (Hanley, 1984).

Two main experiments reported in Bird and Kinsella (1996) were part of a series where retrieval was used to teach cue/task associations to samples with either probable AD and/or vascular dementia. Trivial experimental tasks were used, for example, putting a card in an envelope or opening a box and reading a message. As shown in Figure 12.3, cues were primarily auditory alarms or words presented visually.

Level	Cue [a]
1	Beeper.
2	Card showing the word *Box*.
3	Experimenter: "You have to do something with this box when you hear this sound."
4	Experimenter: "Something to do with this box" (object indicated).
5	Forced-choice recognition (one plausible distracter).
6	Forced-choice recognition with the correct task heavily emphasized.

[a] Assume the task is opening a box and reading a card.

Acquisition

Retrieval effect used to teach patient to associate a cue with behavior or information that will prompt behavior (e.g., picture of cat on door = this is my room; beeper = it's time to visit the toilet).

Retrieval

Patient encounters or is presented with the cue in the environment. Recalls and acts on associated information (e.g., enters correct room).

Figure 12.3. Number of cues required by a female subject (MMSE = 18) to retrieve a task (opening a box and reading a card) on each trial, and at a final recall trial 1 day later.

The acquisition technique was an adaptation of SR; it was combined with the method of fading cues. Initial presentations were quite similar to the process described earlier in this chapter, with the first trial occurring immediately after first presentation of the material, for example:

- "This beeper (alarm sounds) is to remind you to put the card in the envelope."
- (Short pause). "So what will this beeper remind you to do?"

Participants had their first delayed trial after 30 seconds. If failure occurred, they were given a series of extra cues, each successively providing more information, until they successfully retrieved the task. The provision of supplementary cues where required also applied at all subsequent trials.

In the SR procedure described earlier in the chapter, the intertrial intervals are tailored to the subject's individual learning rate to ensure that successful retrieval will take place on most trials. If failure occurs, the intervals are reduced. For the experiments currently under discussion, it was the level of cued support that was tailored to individual needs. This method permitted standardization of intervals, which were roughly doubled for each successive trial (see Figure 12.3).

It also provided the outcome measure, tested 1 day after learning. That is, the dependent variable was not the number of items recalled from a list (the predominant experimental learning paradigm for more than a century), but the number of cues required to retrieve a single item. Single-task learning merits much more attention with this severely impaired population; it is more relevant to the clinical situation, where highly specific problems have to be addressed one at a time. Combining SR with fading cues also has the potential to significantly reduce the number of learning trials required for effective learning, because it increases the chances of successful retrieval occurring on any one trial.

At this stage, however, it is not known whether SR alone or the combined method has any other advantage, for example, in consolidation of the memory trace. In the clinical situation, there is the flexibility to use both, though the number of learning trials illustrated in Figure 12.3 is not recommended except with very mildly impaired persons with dementia. Nevertheless, despite the very limited number of trials used in the experimental work, two thirds of two separate samples, each of 24 participants (MMSE range 7–24) had retrievable memory for a task a day after learning it. Like the participant in Figure 12.3, a substantial proportion required only the primary cue and no subsidiary cues at final recall. Primary findings of this research can be summarized as follows:

- A substantial proportion of participants with mild to moderate dementia could be trained, by SR, to associate a cue with a behavioral task so that the cue had specific recallable meaning after a delay of 1 day—a retention interval that indicates these findings can have clinical utility.
- Participants who could recall the task after a delay of 1 hour were usually able to recall it 1 day later. Capacity to remember after a 15-minute delay was a less reliable marker.
- Confirming anecdotal clinical accounts (e.g., McEvoy & Patterson, 1986) and experimental work in dementia by Bäckman and associates (for review, see Bäckman, 1992), there was a mnemonic effect of actually performing a task on each trial, as opposed to observing it. It was equivalent to SR effects. That is, motor performance alone, in

the absence of retrieval on each trial, and retrieval alone on each trial, in the absence of motor performance, were equally effective.

- Motor performance combined with retrieval on each trial added nothing to the ability to verbally recall the task when tested after 1 day. However, actually performing a task made it much more likely that participants, having verbally recalled the task, would then spontaneously perform the task—again a minimum requirement for clinical utility.

Research on the Basis of the SR Effect

One issue that has received scant attention in prior research concerns the potential mechanisms underlying the memorial benefit of SR. While most researchers emphasize the pragmatic implications (or clinical utility) of SR as a memory intervention technique, turning attention toward theoretical mechanisms of SR effects is an important challenge for at least two reasons. First, conceptual frameworks for research with special populations, such as persons with neurological impairment, are often borrowed from mainstream cognitive psychology. This is an advantageous practice in that findings from studies with special populations may yield important evidence regarding the theoretical constructs under investigation (Butters, 1984). For example, evidence showing that certain aspects of memory are affected in AD, while others seem unaffected, at least initially, provides convergent validity for several conceptual distinctions, including episodic/semantic memory and implicit/explicit memory (see Heindel, Salmon, Shults, Walicke, & Butters, 1989, for discussion). In principle, research on SR effects in cognitively impaired older adults may contribute to the evolution of theoretical constructs in cognitive psychology. As a second point, knowledge derived from basic research on the component processes that underlie SR effects may aid in the design of broad-based applications of the SR technique for improving retention in the daily lives of older persons with probable AD.

Accounts of Factors Underlying Spacing Effects in Normal Populations

Greene (1992) gave two accounts of the general spacing effect based on research primarily conducted with normal young adults. The first he called *deficient-processing theories*. By this account, information is not processed as fully when it is encountered in a massed versus a spaced presentation. One variation of this account states that persons engaged in spaced practice of items engage in more rehearsal for such items than for similar items presented in a massed-practice situation. Another variation is that more attention or cognitive effort, in general, is paid to items presented in a spaced presentation compared to a massed presentation, resulting in better recall of spaced items.

The second general account Greene (1992) gave for the spacing effect he called *encoding-variability theories*:

> Multiple traces formed by spaced repetitions are likely to differ from each other more in some way than are the multiple traces formed by massed repetitions. This can then be used to explain the spacing effect if one goes on to assume that the probability of retriev-

ing at least one of two traces increases as a function of the differences between the traces. (p. 150)

Greene noted that encoding variability would best account for spacing effects found in free recall tasks, since factors facilitating retrieval such as encoding variability should have large effects in free recall. He also speculated, however, that spacing effects found in recognition tasks might best be accounted for by processing-deficit hypotheses, where access to memory traces is facilitated more than recall, and thus, the informativeness of traces is a critical component for successful recognition. Greene concluded that a dual-processing approach best explains the spacing effect, and that the underlying cause of the spacing effect seems to be task-specific.

Attempts to Determine the Locus of SR Effects in Persons with Dementia

Repetition alone does not seem to satisfactorily account for the success of SR in inducing new learning. In a study with patients diagnosed with AD, alcholomastic disorder, major depression, and normal elderly volunteers, Weingartner et al. (1993) found that persons with AD were the only group that was insensitive to repetition effects. Their AD subjects were unable to make use of multiple presentations to encode to-be-remembered words in either recognition or recall testing conditions. These researchers concluded that persons with Alzheimer's disease are unable "to generate an explicit semantically appropriate context that can be used to rehearse and encode stimuli" (p. 393). The effects of repetition alone, therefore, cannot explain the success of the SR technique in facilitating the learning of new information in AD and related disorders.

Bird (1995), working with a sample of persons with AD, compared effects of a form of SR with a condition he labeled "baseline recall." This baseline recall condition was used to control for repetition effects and was similar to SR procedures (in this case, asking participants to name an object in a picture) except that participants were not required to retrieve information from memory, since the required information was kept visible at all times. Bird's results indicated that it is neither repetition alone nor the use of intervals alone that causes improved memory; the combination of recall practice across intervals is necessary for SR to function successfully. The problem of determining why SR should be effective for persons with dementia still remains.

Accessing an Implicit Memory System as an Explanation for SR Effects

The efficacy of SR for cognitively impaired older adults has been attributed to implicit memory processes that are thought to be spared until the later stages of AD (see Camp et al., 1993; Camp & McKitrick, 1992; Camp et al., 1996a, 1996b). Implicit memory is inferred when task performance is facilitated by previous exposure to test materials, without awareness of prior learning episodes at test (Lewandowsky, Dunn, & Kirsner, 1989). Bäckman (1992), among others, noted that under some testing conditions, implicit memory may be relatively spared in older adults with cognitive impairment associated with early stages of dementia (see Cherry & Plauche, 1996, for a review), and there is evidence that for some abilities, this sparing may be seen in late stages of dementia as well (Bologna & Camp, 1995, 1997).

Much of the evidence behind the assumption that SR accesses implicit memory is either indirect or anecdotal. For example, levels of recall performance in persons with dementia trained with SR are generally not correlated with performance on standard (i.e., explicit) memory measures (Camp et al., 1996b; Foley, 1996; McKitrick et al., 1992; but also see Bird & Kinsella, 1996). Therefore, it is assumed that some mechanism other than explicit memory (such as implicit memory) must be involved in SR effects.

It was also reasoned that SR could be a form of errorless learning, in which persons with memory impairment acquire new information if they are not allowed to make errors at initial presentation and on subsequent training trials (Baddeley, 1992; Wilson, Baddeley, Evans, & Shiel, 1994). Errorless learning is assumed to access implicit memory and is effective for rehabilitation because external controls prevent errors and thus allow error-free learning to take place (Baddeley, 1992; Wilson et al., 1994). Without such controls, persons with explicit memory disorders cannot generally self-correct (i.e., they do not have conscious access to previous learning episodes) and thus may experience drift and inclusion of faulty information in learning trials over time. Since SR provides high rates of successful recall and any errors made are corrected and followed by an immediate (and therefore successful) recall trial, it would appear that SR is a type of errorless learning procedure.

Camp et al. (1996b) report anecdotal evidence of source amnesia in persons with dementia regarding use of an external memory aid (an appointment calendar). Participants would forget who had trained them or where the calendars had come from but could still remember and use the strategy of looking at the calendar to remember important information. Source amnesia is an indication of impaired explicit memory function. When seen in combination with successful SR training, an implication is that SR is utilizing an alternative memory system, implicit memory being the likely candidate.

Foss (1994) conducted an initial attempt to gather more direct evidence on the underlying basis for the effects produced by SR in persons with dementia. In her study, older adults with probable AD were trained to learn new face-name associations. The interval between retrieval trials was filled with a second activity that varied in the amount of cognitive effort required to do that activity (the Trail Making Task, Forms A and B). In Foss's study, recall intervals were fixed at 60 seconds, and eight trials were given to each participant for each face-name pair, to ensure that all participants would be expending comparable amounts of effort over comparable time periods between recall trials. Foss found that all older adults in her study were able to demonstrate near-perfect levels of learning and retention of face-name associations independent of the level of cognitive effort required to complete the Trail Making Task between recall trials.

Foss assumed that if efforts to manipulate cognitive effort on a task completed between recall trials had no effect on recall performance, then face-name learning could be taking place effortlessly and unconsciously between recall trials. Her findings were interpreted as evidence that implicit memory might be accessed via SR to enable new learning to take place in persons with dementia. This conclusion was reached based on the assumption made by Camp and his colleagues, among others (e.g.,

Schacter, Rich, & Stampp, 1985) that recall attempts in SR training do not require great expenditure of cognitive effort on the part of persons with dementia (see also the description by Moffat, 1989).

Foley (1996) noted that other studies using normal participants found that long-term retention is actually improved when a difficulty task is placed between repetitions of information to be remembered (Bjork & Allen, 1970; Tzeng, 1973). This finding suggests that, at least in normal adults, recall can be influenced during SR training by manipulation of cognitive effort. There was a similar trend is Foss's data regarding better recall performance when the interpolated task required the highest cognitive effort, though small sample size and near ceiling effects for recall precluded a conclusive test to see if a similar pattern is found in persons with dementia. Clinically, we have found that when intervals between recall trials are filled with meaningful, attention-focusing activity in order to prevent rehearsal, the effectiveness of SR training seems to be enhanced. Foley (1996) concluded that this finding is evidence that learning, at least in the sense of effortful processing, cannot be occurring between trials during SR training. This was the conclusion reached by Foss and by Camp et al. (1996a), which led them to assume that the locus of the SR effect could be automatic consolidation between recall trials stimulated by the pattern of recall attempts used in SR.

It is interesting to note that Cermak, Verfaellie, Lanzon, Mather, and Chase (1996) found that amnestics could benefit from spaced repetition in a recall task, and that spacing effects found in amnestics were similar in magnitude to those found in normal controls. They speculated that in recall tasks, spacing effects found in amnestics are the result of automatic activation of associates of studied words.

While the work of Cermak et al. (1996) and Foss (1994) might militate against an explanation of SR being based on active rehearsal of items, at least in persons with dementia, other variations of Greene's deficient-processing account might still apply. For example, Magliero (1983) found that pupil dilation in persons studying word lists found greater dilation for items presented in a spaced-practice than in a massed-practice format, indicating greater processing of information in the spaced-practice format.

Cherry, Simmons, and Camp (in press) reported preliminary evidence consistent with the notion that implicit memory contributes to SR effects in cognitively impaired older adults. In the study by Cherry et al., the SR method was used to improve recall of everyday objects in four older persons with probable AD (ages 73, 86, 83, and 88). Three training sessions were administered at a local adult day care center on alternate days over 1 week. On each training trial, participants selected a designated item from an array of nine common household objects that were positioned on a flat 3×3 matrix. The items were exemplars of different taxonomic categories (e.g., carrot—a vegetable; see Cherry & Park, 1993, for a description). A different object served as the target item in each training session.

To demonstrate implicit retention of the target items trained via SR, Cherry et al. (in press) used an adapted category exemplar generation task modeled after Light and Albertson (1989). They assumed that a category exemplar generation task would provide a sensitive measure of implicit memory because there is some evidence to indicate that category structures remain largely intact in AD (see Nebes, 1993, for discussion). Prior to SR training, a category exemplar generation pretest was given where participants were asked to name items that belonged to the same taxonomic category as the to-be-trained target item. The purpose of the pretest was to obtain baseline information to aid in the interpretation of the category exemplar generation posttest data. The SR training trials followed. After the last trial, array items were removed from sight, and participants named items that belonged to the same taxonomic category as the target item. On the assumption that implicit memory contributes to SR effects, Cherry et al. expected to observe repetition-priming effects for the target items trained via SR. That is, a repetition-priming effect is observed when a target item is named in the category exemplar generation posttest, but not in the pretest.

As expected, SR training enhanced retention of the target items for all participants both within and across sessions. These findings provide further evidence of the mnemonic benefit of SR and the maintenance of SR effects over time. Importantly, each participant showed a repetition priming effect for the target item in at least one of the three training sessions, an outcome providing modest evidence of the contribution of implicit memory to SR. A limitation of this study was that one target item was never named in the posttest, while another item was named in the pretest by two of the four participants, so that repetition-priming effects for that item could not be interpreted unequivocally for those participants. Consequently, the two problematic target items were replaced with two new objects selected for training in the follow-up study described next.

Cherry and her associates have since conducted a second study to examine the reliability and generality of their earlier findings. They tested four persons with probable AD (ages 96, 84, 82, and 83 years) who were enrolled in the local adult day care program. The materials and general procedures were the same as those used in Cherry et al. (in press), except that two target items were replaced with new objects to increase the sensitivity of the category exemplar generation task as a measure of implicit retention. They also added a two-letter word-stem completion task as a second measure of implicit retention of the trained objects. The word-stem completion task was administered immediately after the category exemplar generation posttest in each training session.

Table 12.1 presents the longest retention interval achieved by each participant in each of the three training sessions. As can be seen in Table 12.1, all participants were able to continue the training for a longer period of time and showed larger performance gains in the second session than in the first. Moreover, three of the four participants reached a substantially longer retention interval in the third session than in the first. For example, on the last day of training, S2 had successfully reached a retention

Table 12.1 Longest Retention Interval Achieved, in Minutes, by Participants Across Training Sessions

Participant	Training session		
	Session 1	Session 2	Session 3
S1	4.0	6.5	2.5
S2	3.0	7.0	10.0
S3	5.0	9.5	8.5
S4	5.5	9.0	10.0

interval that represented over a threefold increase in duration, relative to the first training session. Whether further gains in performance would occur if more than three training sessions are included is a potentially important direction for future research. Camp's research would indicate that further gains with increased training would be likely.

One participant named the target item jacket, two participants named the item bracelet, and one participant named the item carrot after SR training in Sessions 1–3, respectively. These repetition-priming effects can be interpreted unequivocally as evidence of implicit retention, insofar as none of these items were named as exemplars of their respective taxonomic categories in the pretest. Interestingly, repetition-priming effects were not found in the word-stem completion task. In addition, these same participants showed extreme deficits in external memory functioning, as expected. Future research could be directed toward developing other methods of assessing implicit retention in persons with probable AD.

Accessing the Explicit Memory System as an Explanation for SR Effects

Bird and Kinsella (1996) directly addressed the issue of effortful versus automatic processing underlying SR for persons with dementia. They concluded that while some SR trials seemed to elicit automatic processing, their participants also seemed to consciously attempt retrieval with SR tasks on other occasions. In addition, they noted that memory for the target information could at least fleetingly be made consciously available at recall. As a result, they speculated that expenditure of conscious effort may take place in SR, and that repeated practice in recalling stimuli could make retrieval eventually automatic. The implication of this line of argument is that SR is engaging an explicit memory system and requires expenditure of cognitive effort in order to succeed.

Foley (1996) further investigated the possible locus of the SR effect. She conducted a study comparing effects of SR and three other conditions (spaced reminding, massed retrieval, and massed reminding) on face-name recall in older adults with dementia. In her study, SR produced superior performance compared to all other conditions. In fact, training in the other conditions did not appear to assist memory performance in these participants. Thus, there was strong evidence that SR effects in persons with dementia require both active recall attempts and the spacing of such attempts.

In addition, Foley wished to determine whether the locus of SR effects might be due to the amount of effort expended when persons with dementia attempt recall. She used an SR training task involving cued recall, rather than free recall. In addition, she looked at the number of cues necessary to correctly recall target information, at the time taken between cue presentation and subsequent recall, and at the amount of time necessary to retrieve target information after a cue was given. She hypothesized that at least in a cued-recall paradigm, SR effects are due to effortful processing, and that the provision of cues enables an impaired explicit memory system to utilize experimentally provided compensations and operate more effectively. She further hypothesized that greater amounts of time are needed to successfully recall information after long recall intervals (i.e., 4 min) than after short recall intervals. Such an outcome would indicate that recall in a SR paradigm is actually an effortful process, and that the amount of effort expended is a function of recall intervals.

Replicating the results of Camp et al. (1996b), Foley found that SR performance is not related to other measures of explicit memory. While the number of retrieval cues needed to elicit correct recall was smaller for persons in the SR condition than in the other conditions, as described earlier, an average of at least three cues was needed to elicit correct recall. In addition, as in the findings of Bird and Kinsella (1996), some individuals in the SR condition needed substantial amounts of time to correctly recall information at the longest time interval, but others required little time. Foley, like Greene, concluded that it seems unlikely that any single factor or process is adequate to explain SR effects.

The Problem of Defining Implicit and Explicit Memory: Task Versus Memory System

A problematic feature in discussing the nature of SR effects is that the terms *implicit memory* and *explicit memory* are sometimes used to describe both experimental tasks (e.g., defining recognition memory as an implicit memory task and recall as an explicit memory task, as was done by Cermak et al., 1996) as well as memory systems and processes (e.g., an implicit memory system or an explicit memory system, as was done by Schacter, 1994, and Squire, 1994). If a recall task such as successful recall of newly learned information is accomplished by an individual with dementia, researchers are faced with a dilemma. To claim that recall is an explicit memory task, one is faced with the need to describe a form of explicit memory that is not devastated by dementia. Since conscious/effortful process is damaged in dementia, one must decide that there are automatic/effortless/unconscious aspects of explicit memory tasks. Thus, one is faced with using the classification system shown in Figure 12.4 to describe memory research outcomes.

For example, Ostergaard, Heindel, and Paulsen (1995) found that they could induce biasing effects in a recognition task for ambiguous figures in persons with AD by labeling figures at encoding. (In contrast to Cermak et al., 1996, these researchers categorized their recognition task as an explicit memory task, exemplifying further complexities of the classification problem in this type of research.) This biasing was

Memory Task

	Explicit	Implicit
	Conscious/ Effortful	Automatic/ Effortless
Type of Processing		
	Automatic/ Effortless	Conscious/ Effortful

Figure 12.4. Classification system to describe memory research outcomes.

shown after a 30-minute delay, even though conscious recognition of these stimulus items was at chance levels in persons with AD. Yet researchers often feel that if recall or recognition tasks are employed in a study in which priming takes place, explicit memory is critically involved. As a result, Ostergaard et al. concluded that "seemingly unconscious cognitive processes can bias the *explicit* [italics theirs] memory performance of AD ... patients, whose explicit memory is otherwise severely compromised" (p. 279).

In this model, recall training using SR might be classified as an explicit memory task in which persons with dementia and other memory disorders utilize automatic/unconscious processing to successfully learn and retain new information. Alternatively, as Foley (1996) suggested, SR might be classified as an explicit memory task that requires effortful/conscious processing at initial encoding to be successful. It remains to be seen whether a model that focuses on tasks or a model that focuses on hypothesized underlying memory systems is most fruitful in generating research that will help discover the underlying locus of SR effects. We will discuss this issue further in our final summary. The following case study also illustrates a number of points germane to the discussion of the complexities involved in ascertaining the locus of SR effects.

A Case Study

Mrs. D was an 83-year-old woman with vascular dementia. Her MMSE score was 19. She had been admitted a few weeks previously to a hostel following failure to self-care at home and was referred for "paranoid delusions and violence." In practice, this meant accusing staff of stealing her personal possessions and outbursts of temper, including physical aggression to caregivers and property. Detailed assessment demonstrated that the most parsimonious and clinically useful explanation was not the language of psychiatric illness, but that Mrs. D was simply making a mistake. Prior to admission to the hostel, she had given most of her property away, but the dementing process meant that she had no easily retrievable memory for this action. Early in her stay, nursing staff could successfully remind her of what had happened when she asked about her possessions, but as the memory of her property distribution became more remote, she ceased to believe them. This made some staff irritable, and heated discussions ensued. The situation escalated from there.

Hypotheses about how Mrs. D saw the world are an essential requirement of assessment with problems of this sort. Our hypotheses suggested that she was living in a place she didn't know; furthermore, she was being told, with increasing acerbity, by people she didn't know, that she had given all her possessions away. Accordingly, she arrived at what was, to her, the most parsimonious explanation: They had stolen her things, and she had a right to be furious.

The intervention involved, first, a session with Mrs. D and the family member who had assisted in disposal of her personal effects, using multiple situational cues to assist her to recall these events. A list was produced in large print, with a prominent, colored "Smiley" face in the corner, and posted in her wardrobe (she refused to have it on public display in her room). Over a 2-hour period, she was trained, by use of the retrieval effect and motor performance, to associate anxiety about her things with going to the wardrobe and looking at the list.

Thus, after the notice was posted with some ceremony (to make the posting more memorable), learning was initiated with questions such as "What will help you remember what happened to your things?" "How do you find out who you gave your sewing machine to?" and "Tell me what happened to your things before you came here." Intertrial intervals increased as the memory consolidated.

If failure occurred on any trial, Mrs. D was given graded cues as required, for example, "Isn't there a notice somewhere that will tell you?" "Isn't there a notice somewhere with a smiley face?" "Isn't there a notice somewhere that looks like this?" (blank notice with smiley face presented). On each trial after the first closely spaced few, she was encouraged to actually go and look at the notice.

Staff were subsequently trained to use graded cues to help Mrs. D remember to use the notice. Demands had dropped from a mean of 35–40 demands daily to 5 after 1 week, and they soon ceased entirely. Mrs. Ds' mistake had been corrected by her being given access to information she could not retrieve for herself. At 5-month follow-up, there were still no problems. Though there were other factors in this case, the memory intervention played a critical role. The behavior dropped off immediately after training, and on testing 2 weeks postintervention, Mrs. D still knew all about the smiley-face notice in her wardrobe and what it was there for.

Comments and Caveats

First, a particular feature of this and many similar cases is that the change in behavior was maintained. This is consistent with the mnemonic effects of SR. Each naturalistic encounter with the cue in which its meaning is retrieved becomes a fresh spaced-learning trial, which may maintain the association.

Second, it should be noted that the cue was an anxious thought, not a tangible auditory or visual prompt. The notice was simply the means by which anxiety was allayed. A similar case can be found in Bird, Alexopoulos, and Adamowicz (1995) with a patient who asked obsessively for her bowel medication. This type of clinical application of SR clearly extends the experimental findings significantly, as well as further challenging myths held by many health professionals and researchers about the learning capacities of people with dementia. In other cases, participants have managed to internalize cue/behavior associations (Camp & Foss, 1997; Camp et al., 1996a, 1996b; Woods & Bird, in press), with no need for external prompting. Such findings generate an argument for more memory research addressing real-life problems and capacities of people with dementia.

Third, this intervention was multifaceted, both clinically and theoretically. Equally important clinical facets of this case were building up rapport and trust with a very suspicious and angry patient and working sensitively with the exasperated caregivers, not only to ensure that they would continue to cue Mrs. D, but to change their responses from confrontation to empathy.

Theoretically, the active ingredients of the intervention are multiple and difficult to disentangle. The initial training was critical to induce use of the notice, but apart from the maintenance of memory by repeated naturalistic retrievals, operant conditioning probably helped equally in maintaining use of the notice because of its role as an anxiety reducer. Further, as staff responses changed, trust and rapport built up between them and Mrs. D, so that it was less likely that staff would be perceived as thieves. Staff change was easier to accomplish because they now had a concrete memory-prompting procedure to follow instead of acrimonious and futile argument with Mrs. D. That is, it is futile to regard cued recall of adaptive behavior or any other psychosocial technique in isolation; it is not equivalent to a pill, which, if taken will fix the situation by itself.

Finally and more generally, SR is not a panacea for behavior problems in dementia. In many cases, as here, it will form only part of the intervention, which may require many therapeutic modalities. In yet other cases, it will be inappropriate or ineffective, or the patient will not cooperate. As discussed elsewhere in this volume, the idiosyncratic and multifaceted nature of each case profile requires detailed assessment and careful selection of the most appropriate techniques. Training in cued recall of adaptive behavior as described here is simply something that, like all other techniques (including sensitive use of medication), will assist some persons with dementia in some situations some of the time.

Summary

The use of SR as an intervention for dementia is still relatively new, though it is hoped that readers of this chapter will see that there is considerable cause for optimism about its utility as a clinical/rehabilitative intervention. Large-scale studies of the effects of SR, and the parameters that influence its effectiveness and clinical utility are yet to be performed. Within the two areas of clinical application and theoretical explanations of the locus of SR effects, a number of areas suggest themselves for future research.

Clinical Application Issues in SR

Camp (1989) listed a number of clinical application issues in SR that needed (and still need) to be addressed. One issue is the amount of information that can be trained and retained by use of SR. To date, most research has focused on a single target or, at most, up to three targets (Brush & Camp, 1998, in press; McKitrick et al., 1992). SR has the potential to train a large number of items of information, but we simply don't know the limits (such as potential interference effects) that dementia will place on this potential. For example, though McKitrick et al. (1992) reported little problem with interference effects in their study, this topic has yet to be adequately explored.

In related areas, we don't understand the forgetting functions of information learned by means of SR, nor do we know about how to best maintain information once it has been learned. We also do not know how to create individualized optimal expansion schedules. Similarly, given that in many instances standard measures of memory performance do not predict how well individuals with dementia will succeed during SR training, it would be extremely useful to develop predictors of which persons will learn most readily in an SR training paradigm.

Theoretical Explanations of the Locus of SR Effects

The attempt to determine the theoretical locus of SR effects has been hampered by a variety of problems. Is it best to assume that SR accesses one and only one type of memory in free recall and/or cued recall and/or recognition tests? Is it possible for a single memory system to be involved across multiple tasks? That is, is it best to conceptualize any memory success seen in persons with dementia as being supported by a single memory system, such as implicit memory, and to ascribe any memory failures to a declining explicit memory system? Is it best to view each system as capable of generating memory failures and successes, though at generally different rates, depending on the specific training context?

An ultimate resolution to this discussion may await the use of on-line measures of brain functioning such as PET used in conjunction with SR training to determine which areas of the brain are being activated in SR. If memory systems' functions show anatomical correlates with areas of brain activation, the basis for SR's success across a variety of experimental contexts (e.g., recall, cued recall, recognition) may be addressed more directly through brain imaging.

Of course, much of the research in this area has taken the approach that an implicit-explicit memory dichotomy is the appropriate perspective from which to view SR training in particular and memory functioning in general. The utility of such a dichotomy in studying memory functioning is not universally shared. Rovee-Collier (1997), in reviewing research on the development of implicit and explicit memory during infancy, made the following comments:

> Evidence amassed from a large number of studies that were conducted over the past 25 years . . . disputes claims that implicit and explicit memory follow different developmental lines and challenges the utility of conscious recollection as the defining characteristic of explicit memory. It seems unlikely that any simple dichotomy could adequately characterize a process as complex as memory, even during the infancy period. (pp. 467–468)

Adults with dementia usually learn new associations when trained with SR. Some learn associations quickly, with few errors, while others learn more slowly, and it appears possible that some individuals may not learn at all. Some individuals with dementia seem to expend cognitive effort when attempting to recall information trained with SR, and others don't, and the amount of cognitive effort expended by an individual may change over time. Some retain new information learned via SR over long periods, and in others, the memory seems to fade more quickly. Why such diversity of SR effects occurs has both clinical and theoretical significance. Current theoretical formulations have proven unsatisfactory in providing a general explanation for the locus of SR effects, much less in addressing the issues of variability in SR training outcomes just described. Perhaps the studies conducted thus far have not been adequate in their efforts to design critical tests of theory. More likely, in our opinion, current theory is inadequate to deal with outcomes generated by SR training paradigms for persons with dementia. It is our hope that attempts to explain such outcomes will spur further theoretical development, which is always an important contribution of applied research to a developing science.

References

Abrahams, J. P., & Camp, C. J. (1993). Maintenance and generalization of object naming training in anomia associated with degenerative dementia. *Clinical Gerontologist, 12,* 57–72.

Alexopoulos, P. (1994). Management of sexually disinhibited behaviour by a demented patient. *Australian Journal on Ageing, 13,* 119.

Arkin, S. M. (1991). Memory training in early Alzheimer's disease: An optimistic look at the field. *American Journal of Alzheimer's Care and Related Disorders and Research, 6,* 17–25.

Bäckman, L. (1992). Memory training and memory improvement in Alzheimer's disease: Rules and exceptions. *Acta Neurologica Scandinavica, 84,* 84–89.

Baddeley, A. D. (1989). Finding the bloody horse. In L. W. Poon, D. C. Rubin, & B. A. Wilson (Eds.)., *Everyday cognition in adulthood and late life* (pp. 104–115). New York: Cambridge University Press.

Baddeley, A. D. (1992). Implicit memory and errorless learning: A link between cognitive theory and neuropsychological rehabilitation? In L. R. Squire & N. Butters (Eds.), *Neuropsychology of memory* (2nd ed., pp. 309–314). New York: Guilford Press.

Banaji, M. R., & Crowder, R. G. (1989). The bankruptcy of everyday memory. *American Psychologist, 44,* 1185–1193.

Banaji, M. R., & Crowder, R. G. (1991). Some everyday thoughts on ecologically valid methods. *American Psychologist, 46,* 78–79.

Bird, M. (1995). *Aids to acquisition in senile dementia: Retrieval and effortful processing.* Unpublished manuscript.

Bird, M., Alexopoulos, P., & Adamowicz, J. (1995). Success and failure in five case studies: Use of cued recall to ameliorate behaviour problems in senile dementia. *International Journal of Geriatric Psychiatry, 10,* 5–11.

Bird, M., & Kinsella, G. (1996). Long-term cued recall of tasks in senile dementia. *Psychology and Aging, 11,* 45–56.

Bird, M. J., & Luszcz, M. A. (1991). Encoding specificity, depth of processing, and cued recall in Alzheimer's disease. *Journal of Clinical and Experimental Neuropsychology, 13,* 508–520.

Bird, M. J., & Luszcz, M. A. (1993). Enhancing memory performance in Alzheimer's disease: Acquisition assistance and cue effectiveness. *Journal of Clinical and Experimental Neuropsychology, 15,* 921–932.

Bjork, R. A. (1988). Retrieval practice and the maintenance of knowledge. In M. M. Gruneberg, P. Morris, & R. Sykes (Eds.), *Practical aspects of memory* (Vol. 2, pp. 396–401). London: Academic Press.

Bjork, R. A., & Allen, T. W. (1970). The spacing effect: Consolidation or differential encoding? *Journal of Verbal Learning and Behavior, 9,* 567–572.

Bologna, S. M., & Camp, C. J. (1995). Self-recognition in Alzheimer's disease: Evidence of an implicit/explicit dissociation. *Clinical Gerontologist, 15,* 51–54.

Bologna, S. M., & Camp, C. J. (1997). Covert versus overt self-recognition in late stage Alzheimer's disease. *Journal of the International Neuropsychological Society, 3,* 195–198.

Brush, J. A., & Camp, C. J. (1998). Using spaced retrieval as an intervention during speech-language therapy. *Clinical Gerontologist, 19,* 51–64.

Brush, J. A., & Camp, C. J. (in press). Using spaced retrieval to treat dysphagia in a long-term care resident with dementia. *Clinical Gerontologist.*

Butters, N. (1984). The clinical aspects of memory disorders: Contributions from experimental studies of amnesia and dementia. *Journal of Clinical Neuropsychology, 6,* 17–36.

Camp, C. J. (1989). Facilitation of new learning in Alzheimer's disease. In G. C. Gilmore, P. J. Whitehouse, & M. L. Wykle (Eds.), *Memory, aging, and dementia* (pp. 212–225). New York: Springer.

Camp, C. J. (1996). The return of Sherlock Holmes: A pilgrim's progress in memory and aging research. In M. R. Merrens & G. G. Brannigan (Eds.), *The developmental psychologists* (pp. 217–232). New York: McGraw-Hill.

Camp, C. J., & Foss, J. W. (1997). Designing ecologically valid memory interventions for persons with dementia. In D. G. Payne & F. G. Conrad (Eds.), *Intersections in basic and applied memory research* (pp. 311–325). Mahwah, NJ: Erlbaum.

Camp, C. J., Foss, J. W., O'Hanlon, A. M., & Stevens, A. B. (1996a). Memory interventions for persons with dementia. *Applied Cognitive Psychology, 10,* 193–210.

Camp, C. J., Foss, J. W., Stevens, A. B., & O'Hanlon, A. M. (1996b). Improving prospective memory task performance in Alzheimer's disease. In M. A. Brandimonte, G. O. Einstein, & M. A. McDaniel (Eds.), *Prospective memory: Theory and applications* (pp. 351–367). Mahwah, NJ: Erlbaum.

Camp, C. J., Foss, J. W., Stevens, A. B., Reichard, C. C., McKitrick, L. A., & O'Hanlon, A. M. (1993). Memory training in normal and demented elderly populations: The E-I-E-I-O model. *Experimental Aging Research, 19,* 277–290.

Camp, C. J., & McKitrick, L. A. (1992). Memory interventions in Alzheimer's-type dementia populations: Methodological and theoretical issues. In R. L. West & J. D. Sinnott (Eds.), *Everyday memory and aging: Current research and methodology* (pp. 155–172). New York: Springer-Verlag.

Camp, C. J., & Schaller, J. R. (1989). Epilogue: Spaced-retrieval memory training in an adult day care center. *Educational Gerontology, 15,* 81–88.

Camp, C. J., & Stevens, A. B. (1990). Spaced retrieval: A memory intervention for Dementia of the Alzheimer's Type (DAT). *Clinical Gerontologist, 10,* 58–61.

Carruth, E. K. (1997). The effects of singing and the spaced retrieval technique on improving face-name recognition in nursing home residents with memory loss. *Journal of Music Therapy, 34,* 165–186.

Cermak, L. S., Verfaellie, M., Lanzoni, S., Mather, M., & Chase, K. A. (1996). Effect of spaced repetitions on amnesia patients' recall and recognition performance. *Neuropsychology, 2,* 219–227.

Cherry, K. E., & Park, D. C. (1993). Individual difference and contextual variables influence spatial memory in younger and older adults. *Psychology and Aging, 8,* 517–526.

Cherry, K. E., & Plauche, M. F. (1996). Memory impairment in Alzheimer's disease: Findings, interventions, and implications. *Journal of Clinical Geropsychology, 2,* 263–296.

Cherry, K. E., Simmons, S. S., & Camp, C. J. (in press). Spaced-retrieval enhances memory in older adults with probable Alzheimer's disease. *Journal of Clinical Geropsychology.*

Diesfeldt, H. F. A. (1984). The importance of encoding instructions and retrieval cues in the assessment of memory in senile dementia. *Archives of Gerontology and Geriatrics, 3,* 51–57.

Dobbs, A. R., & Rule, B. G. (1987). Prospective memory and self-reports of memory abilities in older adults. *Canadian Journal of Psychology, 41,* 209–222.

Einstein, G. O., & McDaniel, M. A. (1990). Normal aging and prospective memory. *Journal of Experimental Psychology, Learning Memory and Cognition, 16,* 717–726.

Foley, L. C. (1996). *Spaced retrieval as a mnemonic in dementia: Its efficacy and the role of cognitive effort.* Unpublished master's theses, Australian National University, Department of Psychology, Canberra.

Foss, J. W. (1994). *Cognitive effort: Effects of spaced-retrieval on learning in AD.* Unpublished master's thesis, University of New Orleans, Department of Psychology.

Gilleard, C., Mitchell, R. G., & Riordan, J. (1981). Ward orientation training with psychogeriatric patients. *Journal of Advanced Nursing, 6,* 95–98.

Glisky, E. L., & Schacter, D. L. (1986). Remediation of organic memory disorder: Current status and future prospects. *Journal of Head Trauma Rehabilitation, 1,* 54–63.

Glisky, E. L., & Schacter, D. L. (1987). Aquisition of domain-specific knowledge in organic amnesia: Training for computer-related work. *Neuropsychologia, 25,* 893–906.

Glisky, E. L., Schacter, D. L., & Tulving, E. (1986). Learning and retention of computer-related vocabulary in amnestic patients: Method of vanishing cues. *Journal of Clinical and Experimental Neuropsychology, 8,* 292–312.

Greene, R. L. (1992). Repetition paradigms. In R. L. Greene (Ed.), *Human memory: Paradigms and paradoxes* (pp. 132–152). Hillsdale, NJ: Erlbaum.

Hanley, I. G. (1981). The use of signposts and active training to modify ward disorientation in elderly patients. *Journal of Behavioural Therapy and Experimental Psychology, 12*, 241–247.

Hanley, I. (1984). Theoretical and practical considerations in reality orientation therapy with the elderly. In I. Hanley & J. Hodge (Eds.), *Psychological approaches to the care of the elderly* (pp. 164–191). London: Croom Helm.

Hart, R. P., Kwentus, J. A., Taylor, J. R., & Harkin, S. W. (1987). Rate of forgetting in dementia and depression. *Journal of Consulting and Clinical Psychology, 55*, 101–105.

Hayden, C. M., & Camp, C. J. (1995). Spaced-retrieval: A memory intervention for dementia in Parkinson's disease. *Clinical Gerontologist, 16*(3), 80–82.

Heindel, W. C., Salmon, D. P., Shults, C. W., Walicke, P. A., & Butters, N. (1989). Neuropsychological evidence for multiple memory systems: A comparison of Alzheimer's, Huntington's, and Parkinson's disease patients. *Journal of Neuroscience, 9*, 582–587.

Herlitz, A., Adolfsson, R., Bäckman, L., & Nilsson, L.-G. (1991). Cue utilization following different forms of encoding in mildly, moderately, and severely demented patients with Alzheimer's disease. *Brain and Cognition, 15*, 119–130.

Intons-Peterson, M. J., & Fourner, J. (1986). External and internal memory aids: How often do we use them? *Journal of Experimental Psychology, 115*, 267–280.

Kopelman, M. D. (1985). Rates of forgetting in Alzheimer-type dementia and Korsakoff's syndrome. *Neuropsychologia, 23*(5), 623–638.

Landauer, T. K. (1989). Some bad and good reasons for studying memory and cognition in the wild. In L. W. Poon, D. C. Rubin, & B. A. Wilson (Eds.), *Everyday cognition in adulthood and late life* (pp. 116–125). New York: Cambridge University Press.

Landauer, T. K., & Bjork, R. A. (1978). Optimal rehearsal patterns and name learning. In M. M. Gruneberg, P. E. Harris, & R. N. Sykes (Eds.), *Practical aspects of memory* (pp. 625–632). New York: Academic Press.

Lewandowsky, S., Dunn, J. C., & Kirsner K. (1989). *Implicit memory: Theoretical issues.* Hillsdale, NJ: Erlbaum.

Light, L. L., & Albertson, S. A. (1989). Direct and indirect tests of memory for category exemplars in young and older adults. *Psychology and Aging, 4*, 487–492.

Magliero, A. (1983). Pupil dilations following pairs of identical and related to-be-remembered words. *Memory and Cognition, 11*, 609–615.

Martin, A., Brouwers, P., Cox, C., & Fedio, P. (1985). On the nature of the verbal memory deficit in Alzheimer's Disease. *Brain and Language, 25*, 323–341.

McEvoy, C., & Patterson, R. (1986). Behavioral treatment of deficit skills in dementia patients. *Gerontologist, 26*, 475–478.

McKitrick, L. A. (1993). *Caregiver participation in word-retrieval training with anomic Alzheimer's disease patients.* Unpublished doctoral dissertation, University of New Orleans, Department of Psychology.

McKitrick, L. A., & Camp, C. J. (1993). Relearning the names of things: The spaced-retrieval intervention implemented by a caregiver. *Clinical Gerontologist, 14*, 60–62.

McKitrick, L. A., Camp, C. J., & Black, F. W. (1992). Prospective memory intervention in Alzheimer's Disease. *Journal of Gerontology: Psychological Sciences, 47*, 337–343.

Moffat, N. J. (1989). Home-based cognitive rehabilitation with the elderly. In L. W. Poon, D. C. Rubin, & B. A. Wilson (Eds.), *Everyday cognition in adulthood and late life* (pp. 659–680). New York: Cambridge University Press.

Mook, D. G. (1989). The myth of external validity. In L. W. Poon, D. C. Rubin, & B. A. Wilson (Eds.), *Everyday cognition in adulthood and late life* (pp. 25–43). New York: Cambridge University Press.

Nebes, R. D. (1993). Cognitive dysfunction in Alzheimer's Disease. In F. I. M Craik & T. A.

Salthouse (Eds.), *The handbook of aging and cognition* (pp. 373–446). Hillsdale, NJ: Erlbaum.

Ostergaard, A. L., Heindel, W. C., & Paulsen, J. S. (1995). The biasing effect of verbal labels on memory for ambiguous figures in patients with progressive dementia. *Journal of the International Neuropsychological Society, 1,* 271–280.

Patterson, M. B., & Whitehouse, P. J. (1994). Behavioral symptoms in dementia. *Alzheimer Disease and Associated Disorders, 8*(Suppl. 3), 1–3.

Petrinovich, L. (1989). Representative design and the quality of generalization. In L. W. Poon, D. C. Rubin, & B. A. Wilson (Eds.), *Everyday cognition in adulthood and late life* (pp. 11–24). New York: Cambridge University Press.

Riley, K. P. (1992). Bridging the gap between researchers and clinicians: Methodological perspectives and choices. In R. L. West & J. D. Sinnott (Eds.), *Everyday memory and aging: Current research and methodology* (pp. 182–189). New York: Springer-Verlag.

Rovee-Collier, C. (1997). Dissociations in infant memory: Rethinking the development of implicit and explicit memory. *Psychological Review, 104,* 467–498.

Schacter, D. L. (1992). Understanding implicit memory. *American Psychologist, 47,* 559–569.

Schacter, D. L. (1994). Priming and multiple memory systems: Perceptual mechanisms in implicit memory. In D. L. Schacter & E. Tulving (Eds.), *Memory systems 1994* (pp. 233–268). Cambridge, MA: MIT Press.

Schacter, D. L., Rich, S. A., & Stampp, M. S. (1985). Remediation of memory disorders: Experimental evaluation of the spaced-retrieval technique. *Journal of Clinical and Experimental Neuropsychology, 7,* 70–96.

Schacter, D. L., & Tulving, E. (1994). What are the memory systems of 1994? In D. L. Schacter & E. Tulving (Eds.), *Memory systems 1994* (pp. 1–38). Cambridge, MA: MIT Press.

Squire, L. R. (1994). Declarative and nondeclarative memory: Multiple brain system supporting learning and memory. In D. L. Schacter & E. Tulving (Eds.), *Memory systems 1994* (pp. 203–232). Cambridge, MA: MIT Press.

Stevens, A. B., O'Hanlon, A. M., & Camp, C. J. (1993). Strategy training in Alzheimer's Disease: A case study. *Clinical Gerontologist, 13,* 106–109.

Teri, L., Truax, P., Logsdon, R., Uomoto, J., Zarit, S., & Vitaliano, P. P. (1992). Assessment of behavioral problems in dementia: The revised memory and behavior problems checklist. *Psychology and Aging, 7,* 622–631.

Tulving, E. (1991). Memory research is not a zero-sum game. *American Psychologist, 46,* 41–42.

Tuokko, H., & Crockett, D. (1989). Cued recall and dementia. *Journal of Clinical and Experimental Neuropsychology, 11,* 278–294.

Tzeng, O. J. L. (1973). Stimulus meaningfulness, encoding variability, and the spacing effect. *Journal of Experimental Psychology: General, 99,* 162–166.

Weingartner, H., Eckhardt, M., Grafman, J., Molchan, S., Putnam, K., Rawlings, R., & Sunderland, T. (1993). The effects of repetition on memory performance in cognitively impaired patients. *Neuropsychology, 7,* 385–395.

Wilson, B. A. (1997). Cognitive rehabilitation: How it is and how it might be. *Journal of the International Neuropsychological Society, 5,* 487–496.

Wilson, B. A., Baddeley, A., Evans, J., & Shiel, A. (1994). Errorless learning in the rehabilitation of memory impaired people. *Neuropsychological Rehabilitation, 4,* 307–326.

Woods, B., & Bird, M. (in press). Non-pharmacological approaches to treatment. In G. Wilcock, R. Bucks, & K. Rockwood (Eds.), *Diagnosis and management of dementia: A manual for memory disorders teams.* Oxford: Oxford University Press.

13

Psychosocial Rehabilitation for Problems Arising From Cognitive Deficits in Dementia

MICHAEL BIRD

According to most definitions, rehabilitation aims at the restoration of normal everyday functioning, for example, "The process of restoring the person's ability to live and work as normally as possible after a disabling injury or illness" (Miller & Keane, 1987, p. 826). With the dementias, a group of illnesses that cause progressive deterioration and have no known cure, further qualification is required. This chapter concerns psychosocial interventions whose express target is serious clinical problems arising from cognitive deficits in dementia.

A first section addresses attempts, based on a cure or recovery model, to compensate for or restore lost cognitive function. The consistent failure of this line of research to demonstrate generalization to the problems of everyday life means, however, that most of the chapter has a more overt clinical focus. A second section outlines research on generic or standard strategies—primarily manipulations of the social and physical environment, which seek to ameliorate difficulties dementia sufferers experience in negotiating the world. The final section, moving from the generic to the specific, presents four case studies to illustrate the idiosyncratic nature of clinical work.

The Quest for Generalized Improvement

Mnemonics

There was, briefly, enthusiasm for the idea that mnemonic strategies, many known to the ancient Greeks, might generalize across memory problems for persons suffering cognitive damage, including dementia (e.g., Hill, Evankovich, Sheikh, & Yesavage,

1987; Yesavage, Sheikh, Friedman, & Tanke, 1990). Enthusiasm quickly waned; mnemonic procedures such as imagery or the method of loci do not appear to be an option. They require that the dementia sufferer remember the procedure, and even if this were possible, they require self-initiation and flexibility to be generalized to new situations. These requirements have normally proved beyond the capacity of persons suffering brain insults (Bäckman, Josephsson, Herlitz, Stigsdotter, & Viitanen, 1991; Godfrey & Knight, 1987; Herrman, Rea, & Andrzejewski, 1988).

Reality Orientation

The basic reality orientation (RO) method, summarized by Drummond, Kirchoff, and Scarbrough (1978), is to orient confused patients to their present circumstances in all relevant interactions. Most RO research and clinical application, however, has been based on "classroom" sessions, where information such as personal history or ward orientation is repeatedly presented. The rationale appears to be a hope that this approach will lead to generalized improvement in functioning. Though plagued by methodological problems (Greene, 1984; Woods & Britton, 1985) and inclusion of a diverse range of different procedures under the RO rubric (Hanley, 1984; Powell-Procter & Miller, 1982), there is a fairly consistent finding. Limited information may sometimes be learned, but it is not maintained and does not generalize to everyday life (Downes, 1987; Godfrey & Knight, 1987; Götestam, 1987; Hanley & Lusty, 1984).

The ineffectiveness of reality orientation as most commonly applied in improving orientation to reality has not entirely diminished its appeal, perhaps because the semblance of doing something therapeutic is known to improve staff morale and therefore probably patient care in what is often an unstimulating, low-status work environment (Ferrario, Cappa, Molaschi, Rocco, & Fabris, 1991; Hanley, 1984; Powell-Procter & Miller, 1982). In my home country, Australia, RO boards can still be seen displaying the (often wrong) date and other irrelevant facts, even in nursing homes where crucial information such as the location of toilets is not marked.

Research studies also still appear, for example, Zanetti et al. (1995), who gave patients repeated cycles of classroom RO. Though a slight gain in scores on the Mini-Mental State Exam (MMSE; Folstein, Folstein, & McHugh, 1975) was reported against a loss for matched controls, the study nicely illustrates problems in inferring the clinical utility of these exercises. Some sessions contained MMSE orientation items, raising the possibility that subjects were unwittingly trained to "pass" the MMSE. Further, there was a decline in scores roughly equivalent to the control group loss during rest cycles. There were no significant differences between experimental subjects and controls on any other cognitive or affective measure and, of most relevance to the thrust of this chapter, no differences in activities of daily living (ADLs). That is, even supposing the MMSE advantage was valid, no effect was demonstrated on everyday functioning, presumably the ultimate goal of the exercise.

Cognitive Training and Stimulation

Zanetti et al. (1995) included memory, attention and visuospatial components as well as orientation in their study, reflecting a trend toward applying to dementia sufferers the type of repetitive cognitive exercises that have gained currency in the brain injury literature. Again, the rationale appears to be that mental exercise or stimulation may lead to generalized improvement in everyday life, though little evidence has been gathered in support of this approach. For example, Beck, Heacock, Mercer, Thatcher, and Sparkman (1988) found a small significant effect on recall of digits following repetitive training on cognitive tasks but no effect on any other neuropsychological test. No attempt was made to investigate whether this outcome alleviated everyday difficulties. Other studies have also shown small gains (Bach, Bach, Böhmer, Frühwald, & Grilc, 1995; Breuil et al., 1994), but even these have not investigated whether such outcomes have had any practical effect.

Breuil et al. (1994) and Zanetti et al. (1995) have suggested that ADL scales may not be sensitive enough to reflect gains in everyday functioning. However, this suggestion places the onus of proof on investigators who are serious about providing rehabilitation for real-life difficulties, rather than simply adding a few points to the odd neuropsychological test. At present, the most parsimonious explanation is that the multiple cognitive, behavioral, and affective problems associated with dementing illnesses are impervious to the kind of small improvements occasionally shown following cognitive stimulation.

Some of the best evidence that regular cognitive exercise affects real-life difficulties in dementia comes from Quayhagen, Quayhagen, Corbeil, Roth, and Rodgers (1995), who trained family members to provide such exercise at home. There were small but significant cognitive differences between experimental and control subjects with dementia at follow-up and significantly fewer behavioral problems in the experimental group. However, a third, "placebo" group equaled the experimental subjects on some cognitive measures and on the behavioral measure. A plausible explanation is that the active factor in the most important clinical outcome (fewer behavioral problems) was not cognitive stimulation per se, but the daily interaction of carer and patient in meaningful activity, which occurred in both experimental and placebo conditions. A subsequent paper (Quayhagen & Quayhagen, 1996) supports this hypothesis by reporting improved communication and relationships for couples who took part.

Summary

Despite what sometimes appears to be a cargo-cult mentality with RO and a curious belief that the brain is analogous to a muscle, there is slight evidence that small improvements in some cognitive scores can sometimes be obtained by persons with dementia following cognitive stimulation. Nevertheless, there is still no convincing evidence that it translates into everyday benefits. Placed alongside whether the patient can find the toilet, can inhibit a desire to sexually assault others, or is suicidal because of a recognition of his or her deteriorating cognitive status, a slight increase in MMSE scores is clinically meaningless.

The idea of a standard cognitive treatment, applicable across a range of cases, is very attractive. Clearly, this line of research will continue. However, despite a 30-year history, data on the efficacy of repetitive cognitive exercise in ameliorating the real-life problems of dementia sufferers and, by extension, of their carers are still not in—a caveat that applies equally to drug therapies (Davis & Powchik, 1995; Kelly & Hunter, 1995).

Accordingly, the conceptual foundation for the remainder of this chapter is an assertion made by Woods and Britton (1985):

> We need to break away from our pre-occupation with treatment in the sense of cure and recovery, and be aware of the different types of goal that are feasible, and the value of some of the more limited goals in improving the patient's quality of life. (p. 217)

The remaining two sections describe attempts not to produce cognitive improvement in dementia, but to ameliorate the effects of cognitive decline, that is, the reduction of "excess disability" (Body, Kleban, Lawton, & Silverman, 1971). The scientific as opposed to the anecdotal literature is, in the main, minuscule. Nevertheless, it appears to indicate clinical and research directions for cognitive and behavioral scientists whose definition of rehabilitation in dementia means assisting the patient to cope more adaptively with its effects.

Generic Strategies to Ameliorate Difficulties Arising From Cognitive Impairment

This section addresses attempts to produce standardized strategies, that is, programs or methods generally applicable by a range of health professionals across a range of clinical problems. What are these problems? They are primarily behavioral and can range from low-level difficulties like not being able to find the dining room to extreme disturbance, such as violence or continuous screaming.

Though such disturbances are sometimes called noncognitive symptoms of dementia (e.g., Patterson & Whitehouse, 1994), impaired cognitive function plays a major role in the interaction of factors that produce them (Ballard & Oyebode, 1995; Cohen-Mansfield, Werner, Marx, & Lipson, 1993; Morriss, Rovner, & German, 1995; Rapp, Flint, Herrmann, & Proulx, 1992; Zandi, 1994). An example may be found in chapter 12 in the case study of a patient referred for "paranoid delusions" and violence associated with her perceived thievery of her possessions. The behavior was largely due to impaired memory of events surrounding her recent move to residential care.

A secondary group of problems, notionally separate from behavioral difficulties but actually intimately linked to them, is the patient's affective response to cognitive loss and/or the difficulties of negotiating the world because of that loss. The violent "paranoid" reaction of the patient described in chapter 12 is a typical example. Unfortunately, the subjective response of the person with dementia has been almost completely ignored by serious research until recently (Kitwood, 1997). Emotional distress in dementia and research into means of alleviation are beyond the ambit of this chapter, but they are not without relevance. Anxiety and/or depression is common throughout the course of dementia and causes excess cognitive and functional disability, which is often treatable (Ballard, Patel, Solis, Lowe, & Wilcock, 1996; Reifler & Larson, 1990; Teri, 1994; Teri et al., 1991). For a brief discussion of these issues, see Woods and Bird (1998).

Environmental Strategies

Broad-based strategies, applicable across a range of patient profiles to alleviate problems associated with cognitive deficits in dementia, fall mostly under the rubric of adjustments to the physical and social environment. This includes, most critically, the behavior and characteristics of carers.

Social/Care Environment

EDUCATION AND SUPPORT OF HOME CARERS   There is a large literature on strain among people who care for a relative with dementia (see Gilhooly, Sweeting, Whittick, & McKee, 1994, for review). In the current context, this is of relevance only where attempts to relieve carer distress have also produced measurable effects in the patient with dementia. Unfortunately, only a minority of studies reporting benefits of various interventions for carers provide objective evidence, and of that minority, only a tiny proportion also attempt assessment of outcome for the dementia sufferer.

Where the primary focus has been support for carers, provision of general coping strategies, and general education on dementia, results have been equivocal. For example, Winogrund, Fisk, Kirsling, and Keyes (1987) and Zarit, Anthony, and Boutselis (1987) found no effect on patient behavior problems following such a program. On the other hand, 3-year follow-up after an intensive 2-week residential program for home carers that also included behavior management training showed not only that morbidity in the carers was reduced, but also that they were able to care for the patient at home for longer, and that there were fewer deaths among the patients (Brodaty, McGilchrist, Harris, & Peters, 1993). Assuming that continued care at home and staying alive may be called normal life, this program had a marked rehabilitative effect.

Other programs that have been proactive in directly training carers in management techniques have had positive results. Hinchliffe, Hyman, Blizard, and Livingston (1995) trained home carers in a variety of psychosocial methods for dealing with difficult behaviors, though medication was used in some cases. Problems ranged from repetitive questions to violence. There was a significant reduction in problem behavior in 75% of cases, maintained at 4-month follow-up, and a significant improvement in mental health among carers.

INSTITUTIONAL STAFF   By contrast with home carers, the characteristics of nursing and ancillary staff who care for patients with dementia have been almost unmapped until recently. However, it is known that workers in residential care for the elderly often suffer low morale, burnout, and stress (Baillon, Scothern, Neville, & Boyle, 1996; Karuza & Feather, 1989). The precise contribution to stress levels of caring for patients with dementia is difficult to determine, but it is known to have an effect (Berg, Hansson, & Hallberg, 1994; MacPherson, Eastley, Richards, & Mian, 1994).

As with home carers, emotional states and attitudes amongst nurses are only of relevance here if it can be shown that they cause excess disability in patients, and that addressing these states and attitudes reverses the process. There is a small literature supporting both propositions. Baltes, Neumann, and Zank (1994) found that staff behaviors can increase dependence (a directly counterrehabilitative process), and it has been shown that staff characteristics affect the quality of care (Block, Boczhowski, Hansen, & Vanderbeck, 1987; Edberg, Nordmark Sandgreen, & Hallberg, 1995; Hallberg, Holst, Nordmark, & Edberg, 1995). Conversely, sustained support/education programs for staff have shown improvements in morale and care attitudes. Patient benefits have included increases in carer-patient communication (Kihlgren et al., 1992; Ripich, 1994) and decreases in use of psychotropic drugs and restraint (Levine, Marchello, & Totolos, 1995; Ray et al., 1993; Rovner, 1994).

Assuming that not being socially isolated, tied up, or medicated with neuroleptics or hypnotics approximates more "normal life," these programs have had a clear rehabilitative effect. Further, a few studies have reported measurable improvements in patients themselves, including reductions in behavior problems and depressed mood (Bråne, Karlsson, Kihlgren, & Norberg, 1989; Hagen & Sayers, 1995; Rovner, Steele, & Folstein, 1996).

What should be the goal of residential care staff programs? Hallberg and Norberg (1995) asserted that what is required is the development of a less authoritarian, more sensitive and mutually cooperative relationship between carer and patient. This claim was backed by a 1-year support and education program for nurses that improved attitudes toward the patients, reduced staff stress, improved the quality of care, and reduced difficult patient behavior (Edberg, Hallberg, & Gustafson, 1996; Berg et al., 1994). That is, there is evidence that packages that assist staff to deliver more informed and humane care have, in themselves, a rehabilitative effect for persons with dementing illnesses. This is far from the concept of rehabilitation defined in the narrow sense of restoring lost function. It is rehabilitative in the sense that carers who are helped to understand and empathize with the effects of the disorder can significantly alleviate the extreme difficulties patients encounter in making sense of and coping adaptively with the world. For example, most incidents of "aggression" by patients take place during personal care (Bridges-Parlet, Knopman, & Thompson, 1994; Nilsson, Palmstierna, & Wistedt, 1988). More informed and sensitive handling can often significantly reduce it (for example, see Case C, discussed later).

In summary, excellent qualitative and quantitative research into dementia nursing is at last taking place, but like much other applied clinical research in dementia it is in its infancy. The scope for further careful research by cognitive and behavioral scientists in the nursing home to improve the quality of dementia care is almost limitless (Burgio & Bourgeois, 1992).

SUMMARY: CARE ENVIRONMENT   There is a small but emerging body of evidence in support of treatment approaches that provide home and institutional carers with methods not only to deal with their own emotional state, but also to understand and cope with the problems facing the dementia sufferer. It is scarcely surprising that this research indicates that such interventions can produce rehabilitative effects for both the carer and the dementia sufferer. Most persons with dementia live in dependent dynamic and interactive relationships (Pruchno, Peters, & Burant, 1995; Qureshi & Walker, 1989), with the behavior of carers affecting the patient and the behavior of patients affecting the carers (Edberg et al., 1996; Morriss, Rovner, & German, 1996; Rahman, 1993). It follows that attempts to ameliorate problems by applying a psychosocial "treatment" to the patient in isolation are unlikely to be efficacious. Carers are an integral part of the case profile, and few psychosocial interventions will succeed without carer involvement. In many cases, the carers are cotherapists (Bird, Alexopoulos, & Adamowicz, 1995; Hinchliffe et al., 1995; McEvoy & Schonfeld, 1989;

Teri, 1994). In others cases, carers are part of the problem. An intervention in Bird et al. (1998) nicely illustrates these interactions. A female carer's exasperation at her husband's obsessive toilet visits was exacerbating them because it increased his anxiety. The problem was directly due to the patient's memory impairment overlaid onto a lifelong belief in the necessity of daily bowel movements. "Treatment of the behavior" actually involved educating the carer to respond with empathic assertion rather than angry confrontation. There were rehabilitative effects for both patient and carer: a reduction in toilet visits to manageable levels and a significant improvement in the carer's mental health.

Physical Environment

Though several decades have passed since Lindsley (1964) coined the term *prosthetic environment* in arguing that declining competence with age can be assisted by a more supportive physical environment, many anecdotal accounts but remarkably little evidence have been produced with respect to dementia. In fact, important though rarely cited studies of confused elderly ward patients by Gilleard, Mitchell, and Riordan (1981) and Hanley, McGuire, and Boyd (1981) showed that environmental cues to improve spatial orientation are ineffective without active training in their use. (See also the argument on the use of environmental cues in chapter 12.)

Nevertheless, there has been a surge in development of dementia-specific facilities, often termed *special care units* (SCU) in the United States. They represent a move away from the acute nursing model, which, inexplicably, still informs much residential dementia care, and they typically incorporate features that clinical experience or belief suggests may reduce excess disability (Cohen & Day, 1994; Leon, 1994). Examples are breaking up long corridors and large facilities into small units, providing areas for safe wandering, and eliminating glare (Mintzer et al., 1993). Specialized dementia nursing-care programs are usually also incorporated; in some cases, an SCU is defined by the programming (Leon, 1994). There are similar trends elsewhere, for example, the units for confused and disturbed elderly (CADE) in Australia (Atkinson, 1995; Fleming, Bowles, & Mellor, 1989) and group-living units in Sweden (Wimo, Asplund, Mattsson, Adolfsson, & Lundgren, 1995).

Despite the proliferation of these units, there is still only anecdotal evidence that they are more effective than traditional care (Cohen & Day, 1994; Maslow, 1994; Weisman, Calkins, & Sloane, 1994). Wimo et al. (1993) found that patients given a well-informed and well-implemented special care regime actually deteriorated behaviorally compared with a control group. Conversely, Turner, Willden, Halpin, and Patrick (1997) found a significant decrease in behavioral problems following the combination of a dementia-specific care regime and the redesign of a psychogeriatric ward into smaller units that permitted safe wandering and clear access to facilities.

One problem highlighted in reviews by Teresi, Powell Lawton, Ory, and Holmes (1994) and Weisman et al. (1994) is difficulty of measurement. Issues in this regard include ill-defined concepts and ill-defined treatment goals. Others include the problem that there is often a concentration of difficult residents in these units, making fair comparisons with traditional care problematic, and that special care is often globally different from traditional care, with multiple potentially active variables.

Nevertheless, it is possible to measure the effects of certain discrete aspects of the physical environment, and though tiny in number by comparison with the anecdotal literature, empirical studies are beginning to emerge. Weisman et al. (1994) summarized evidence from some SCU programs in the United States, including reductions in incontinence when toilets were visible and less time required by residents to find their rooms when personal memorabilia were displayed by the door. A much-cited study by Hussian and Brown (1987), who utilized a grid pattern to reduce wandering, actually failed on replication (Chafetz, 1990), but there is now other evidence in support of the general principle of utilizing visuoperceptual impairments of the patients, in juxtaposition with ambiguous visual barriers, for this common problem (Chafetz, 1990; Namazi, 1989).

Recent work investigating manipulations in the sensory environment have also begun to show a shift from the enthusiastically anecdotal to the empirical. In a carefully constructed study, Burgio, Scilley, Hardin, Hsu, and Yancey (1996) showed that seascape sounds reduced disruptive vocalizations by nine severely dementing nursing-home residents, despite noncompliance by nurses. Several studies have found that music at strategic times reduced various problem behaviors (Gerdner & Swanson, 1993; Goddaer & Abraham, 1994; Helmes & Wiancko, 1997). Similarly, some authors have produced data suggesting that structured administration of bright light significantly reduces problems associated with disrupted sleep-wake patterns and sundowning (Lovell, Ancoli, & Gervitz, 1995; Mishima, Okawa, Hishikawa, Hori, & Takahashi, 1994; Satlin, Volicer, Ross, Herz, & Campbell, 1992).

A major point about these studies, which provide details of clinical procedure and quantitative outcome data, is their rarity. This is perhaps the reason for the frequent citing of Hussian and Brown's procedure despite its (rarely cited) failure on replication. However, though small in volume, the work outlined in this section shows that determined clinical researchers committed to the scientific method can collect clean data at the very messy and unpredictable clinical level, where manifold confounders such as staff noncompliance (e.g., Burgio et al., 1996) make the tightly controlled laboratory conditions of traditional cognitive research appear alien and even irrelevant.

Summary: Environmental Adjustments

When the environment is broadly defined to include the physical, the sensory, and the social context, there is a potentially large scope for a rehabilitative effect on dementia sufferers. Possibilities range from adjustments to the many situations where the environment is directly causing excess disability to creation of dementia-friendly environments which are less stressful for the patient to negotiate. There are encouraging signs of a move from anecdotes and unsupported assertions to empirical research in this area, which covers such diverse adjustments as reducing home carer stress and increasing management skills, changing nurse's attitudes, and developing prosthetic features of the environment. Nevertheless, the number of scientific studies is still at a derisory level, and many methodological difficulties remain. The opportunities for contributions by cognitive and behavioral scientists prepared to work in the clinical setting are almost infinite.

Working Directly with the Patient

Operant Conditioning

A number of texts describe the use of behavior modification principles to alleviate problems in dementia (e.g., Rabins, 1994), and clearly, adjustments to the environment could be labeled *stimulus control procedures* within the *antecedent-behavior-consequence model*. However, the huge and diverse complex of interacting environmental factors with the potential to produce change—ranging from reducing carer stress to reducing glare in the lounge—makes attempts to understand environmental manipulations in terms of such a global label largely useless, or even pernicious. With naive or inflexible behavioral clinicians, use of labels such as stimulus-control is likely to restrict analysis to immediate antecedents of the behavior. On the other hand, the *consequence* component of the model and the use of reinforcement may most usefully be discussed separately.

Unfortunately, texts extolling operant conditioning either are general (e.g., Cohen-Mansfield et al., 1993; Rabins, 1994) or give case descriptions that only involve adjustments to the environment, including more informed and sensitive nursing care (McGovern & Koss, 1994; Rapp et al., 1992). Clearly, operant principles are involved in many aspects of dementia care (for example, low staff morale in an unrewarding work environment) and are an integral part of some interventions (e.g., Bird et al., 1995). Nevertheless, there are almost no cases reported in the literature of differential reinforcement being used specifically to change the maladaptive behavior of patients with dementia (though see Cases A and B below). Studies by Vaccaro (1988) and Pinkston, Linsk, and Young (1988), sometimes cited in support of the utility of reinforcement schedules in dementia, involved, respectively, samples who did not have dementia or that mixed frail aged. The two cases described in detail by Pinkston et al. involved depressed, not dementing, patients.

Major problems include poor application of behavioral principles by health professionals who mistakenly assume they understand them (Burgio & Bourgeois, 1992) and inconsistent application in nursing homes (see Case A below). A more fundamental difficulty is that operant conditioning requires, by definition, new learning. The patient must learn and act upon the association between the behavior and the consequence, even if the learning is implicit. To date, there has been little evidence other than the anecdotal that such learning is possible. One intrusive nursing-home patient described by Bird et al. (1995) was enduring the aversive consequences, including violence, of entering other residents' bedrooms many times a day without these consequences' changing her behavior.

Despite these caveats, investigation of operant conditioning to reduce excess behavioral disability in dementia is probably worth pursuing, given the paucity of direct behavior change techniques in dementia that have been subjected to even the most cursory empirical investigation. Like much else in this area, the experimental and clinical work remains to be done. The possibilities will remain speculative until systematic studies are undertaken to investigate the conditions under which persons with dementia are able to associate consequences with a behavior and act on those consequences and/or until many detailed clinical case series are published showing the effectiveness of differential reinforcement in dementia.

Use of Residual Memory Capacity

It has been clear since verbal-learning retention studies in the 1980s (e.g., Hart, Kwentus, Taylor, & Harkin, 1987; Kopelman, 1985) that under certain conditions, persons with mild to moderate dementia can remember limited amounts of new information over clinically significant intervals. More recent experimental and clinical work is presented in Chapter 12, including the finding that patients can be assisted to learn and retain the association between a cue and a behavior. For example, the intrusive nursing-home resident alluded to above was taught to associate a large "stop" sign with stopping and walking away. Intrusive incidents dropped from 40 a day to nil when the sign was displayed in no-go areas (Bird et al., 1995). This and similar interventions (see also the case study in Chapter 12) can best be conceptualized as helping the patient to remember information that will cue more adaptive behavior.

The Case-Specific Approach: Four Studies

Two pairs of case studies are presented here to illustrate some clinical and research issues. They have been chosen because of the apparent similarity of the behavior in each pair, and because every case is an example of cognitive impairment interacting with other factors to produce excess behavioral disability. All took place in excellent facilities with a good understanding of dementia. Figure 13.1 shows the frequency of each problem behavior prior to the intervention and at follow-up.

Repetitive Questions

Case A

Mrs. A, 81 years old, with probable Alzheimer's disease, lived in a dementia-specific unit. Her MMSE score was 9, and she was dependent in most personal care. She delivered her repertoire of questions up to 150 times per hour on occasion, though the mean was about 45. The problem had at least an 18-month history. Some questions concerned her mother; others were helpless inquiries to which she knew the answer. Replies would briefly satisfy her, but then she would forget and ask again, often attaching herself to staff like a limpet. Only somebody who has not experienced this common phenomenon could regard it as a minor irritation. Previous failed interventions had included antidepressants and low-dose antipsychotics (producing a severe drug reaction), and frequent validation therapy (Feil, 1993) on the grounds that unresolved issues about her mother were responsible.

Assessment suggested that during a life of deprivation and insecurity, Mrs. A had developed a sophisticated verbal repertoire for gaining emotional reassurance. The referred behavior appeared to be the remnants of this technique, reduced by cognitive decline to a few questions, and exacerbated by inability to remember that she had just asked one. Behavioral experimentation showed that reassurance could be provided by holding and stroking Mrs. A's hand, and the questions could be ignored. They would rise to a crescendo in an extinction burst, then cease, with Mrs. A often calm enough to be left. This was the basis of the intervention, and though there was noncompliance by some staff, there was a maintained reduction in questions to manageable proportions (Figure 13.1).

Case B

Mr. B, 72 years old, with probable Alzheimer's disease, lived in a dementia-specific unit. He refused cognitive testing but was assessed in the moderate range on the Clinical Dementia

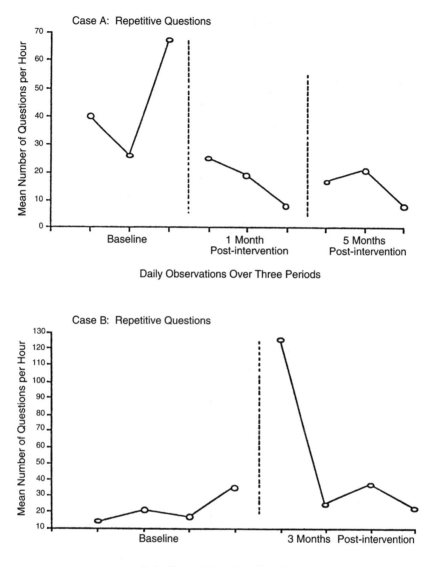

Figure 13.1. Graphical depictions of four case studies where cognitive impairment interacts with behavioral disability.

Rating (CDR; Morris, 1993). Mr. B's repertoire was more diverse than Mrs. A's but, equally, appeared due to a chronic need for reassurance.

Assessment revealed wartime service in Lancaster bombers and, ever since, high anxiety and low tolerance of noise. A number of interventions were tried. Relocating him to a quiet wing produced a dramatic decrease in questions, but his anxiety and behavior eventually affected other residents, and the wing became severely disrupted and noisy. Attempts to preempt common questions—for example, providing a continuous supply of his favorite

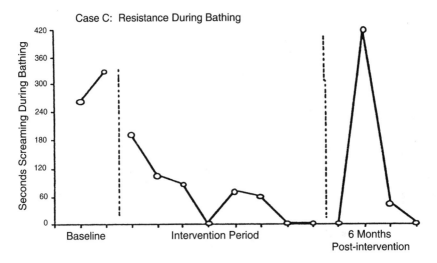

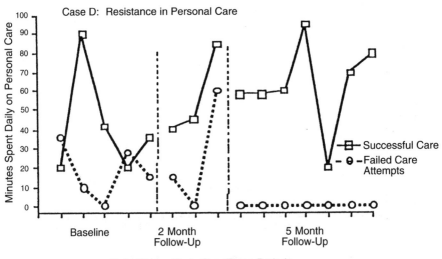

Figure 13.1. *Continued.*

Lancaster bomber shirts—had no discernible effect. Following Case A, differential reinforcement was also attempted. His questions were systematically ignored, but he was given verbal reinforcement and company when quiet, though, unlike Mrs. A, he did not like physical touch. Figure 13.1 shows the total failure of these efforts. Mr. B finally medicated with antipsychotics. This severely reduced his self-care skills, but it also reduced his anxiety. It was probably the optimum outcome. He died, a relatively calm man, 8 months later.

Resistance in Personal Care

Case C

Mrs. C, 82 years old, with probable Alzheimer's disease, lived in a dementia-specific facility. She was untestable and was assessed in the severe category on the CDR. She was referred for violent resistance and screaming during bathing, which was necessary at least weekly because of incontinence. Showering was even more dangerous. The problem had continued for more than 6 months.

Observation suggested that what many staff were interpreting as stubbornness or fierce independence was actually panic. Family information revealed lifelong avoidance of exposure of her body because of unsightly birthmarks and lifelong avoidance of aquatic leisure activities. A family story of a near-drowning as a girl had resonance with some of her screamed words during bathing. Consistent with many phobias, anticipatory anxiety appeared to be worse than exposure; once she was in the bath, her screaming would gradually diminish. However, it would then rise to unstoppable levels when her hair was washed.

Experimentation showed that Mrs. C's hair could be washed without incident at a hair salon. Thereafter, reducing prebath cues to a minimum (e.g., undressing her in her bedroom) and inducing calm before entering the bathroom virtually eliminated resistance. Noncompliance by some staff led to rereferral at 6 months, when the intervention still proved to retain its effect (Figure 13.1). The failure in the second week of follow-up monitoring (7 minutes' screaming) happened when a nurse unfamiliar with the procedure attempted bathing Mrs. C, making this a de facto ABAB design.

Case D

Mrs. D, 87 years old, had progressive dementia of unknown etiology and lived in a hostel. She had no intelligible expressive speech and was dependent in most self-care, falling in the moderate category on the CDR. She was massively incontinent, and the problem was violent resistance to intimate personal care, which had been escalating over 6 months. Mrs. D. would consistently allow only two familiar nurses to toilet or shower her, and only after skilled manipulation of bribes, assertion, and persuasion. The result was pressure on the two favored staff and also Mrs. D's often remaining in soiled and soaked clothing until one of them came on duty. Other staff, distressed by repeated traumatic failures, were demoralized. Antipsychotic medication quieted Mrs. D but produced severe side effects.

In this case, the resistance *was* due to fierce independence. Assessment revealed a history of mild obsessive-compulsive disorder (OCD) related to cleanliness. Mrs. D had coped by doing everything for herself, including during her early years in the hostel, but declining cognitive function had now compromised self-care. The goal here, therefore, was not to reduce her fear of surrendering control—probably an impossible task—but to empower more staff to attempt intimate personal care and develop the necessary blend of skills. Information was provided to all staff about Mrs. D's past and about OCD to put her behavior into context, and the two favored nurses were encouraged to provide hands-on and emotional support as others tried to shower Mrs. D. Staff motivation "to do something" was assisted serendipitously by a serious fall suffered by Mrs. D when she was still on anti-psychotic medication preintervention.

Figure 13.1 shows little reduction in time taken to shower and toilet Mrs. D, but this was not the object of the exercise. The figure also shows the eventual cessation of unsuccessful attempts to do so; all nurses were now able to perform these tasks.

Comment

These few cases are sufficient to raise some important clinical and research issues. The effect on staff of Mrs. D's drug-induced fall shows the frequent difficulty of attributing the cause of an outcome to any specific component of the intervention, especially when there is delay before change is apparent. Case B illustrates the need for more honesty in the literature; failures are almost never reported. It is possible that psychosocial intervention success rates are higher than the success rates for drugs (Burgio & Bourgeois, 1992), but we will never know until it becomes commonly accepted that reporting failure is as important in advancing scientific knowledge as reporting success. The need for long-term follow-up is clearly demonstrated by these cases. Had we assessed outcome 1 week after moving Mr. B to the quiet area, we could have reported a miracle cure. Conversely, Case D shows that some interventions need time to take effect; staff had gradually to build up skill and confidence.

The simple before-and-after graphs in Figure 13.1 illustrate the fact that more sophisticated quasi-experimental designs are not always possible. All these cases were referred because carers could no longer cope and needed immediate help. Further, when an intervention is in place, carers or the patient (e.g., Bird et al., 1995) are rarely willing to reverse it for the sake of methodological rectitude.

At a more global level, these cases illustrate the profoundly idiosyncratic nature of problems suffered by persons with dementia and, by extension, by their carers. It follows that attempts to classify them in a kind of *DSM-ization* enterprise must, at this stage, be treated with caution. This is true whether the classification is based on manifested behavior (e.g., Patel & Hope, 1992), behavior clustered into pseudopsychiatric syndromes (e.g., Sultzer, Berisford, & Gunay, 1995), or presumed environmental etiology (Cohen-Mansfield & Werner, 1997). Though preferable to the common practice of labeling absolutely everything as agitation (e.g., Finkel et al., 1995), present classification systems have severely limited heuristic value. They may even be pernicious, leading to assumptions that standard treatments for named syndromes like "repetitive questions" or "noncompliance" exist or can be found.

Yet, in each pair of cases, though the manifested behavior was almost identical, the treatment was not. In Cases A and B, even the etiology was similar, but the technique successfully used for Case A was completely ineffective when adapted for Case B. An alternative method of providing reassurance could be found for Mrs. A; probably only one-to-one attention all day would have sufficed for Mr. B. Where etiology is different, as in Cases C and D, it is usually the most salient factor that informs treatment choice. Nevertheless, there are many others. These include the nature and resources of the physical environment, the emotional resources and competence of the carers, and the patient's level and nature of cognitive impairment—including insight. Even the clinical goal will vary: In Case C, it was to reduce the behavior by reducing the trauma of bathing; in Case D, it was to empower more nurses to cope with a behavior that was never likely to change.

Profound idiosyncracy case to case in both etiology and intervention options means that psychosocial studies that attempt to apply a standard treatment for a named syndrome—for example, operant conditioning for "repetitive questions"—are unlikely to yield much fruit. The syndrome remains an illusive concept at this stage of the research enterprise; the standard treatment is, accordingly, a chimera. Until vastly more case studies appear following the lead of investigators like Hussian and Brown (1987) in reporting the exact technique or combination of techniques used and objective measures of outcome—including *all* failures—it will not be possible to identify which tools are more likely to fit particular case profiles.

At present, in most cases, the hypothesis-testing, case-specific method remains the approach of choice. What health workers require in any given case is access to an extensive tool kit of techniques, including pharmacological methods, that have been scientifically validated and that can be flexibly applied to each idiosyncratic case profile. As is apparent throughout this chapter, empirically validated techniques are astonishingly few in number.

Summary and Conclusion

When rehabilitation in dementia is defined as partial cure or recovery, there is little evidence, despite 30 years of valiant effort, that this is possible by cognitive means. There is no evidence at all that gains, if any, translate to the amelioration of problems encountered in everyday life, surely the minimum goal. When rehabilitation is defined as minimizing the emotional and behavioral sequelae of cognitive loss and maximizing the potential of the social, physical, and sensory world to make it less confusing and confronting, there appears to be considerable scope. Overlaid are potential methods of directly reducing excess behavioral disability. Unfortunately, the evidence for the efficacy of techniques in this area remains limited because the hard research simply has not been done. Nevertheless, more than 90 years after Alzheimer's original patient was referred for behavioral problems (Alzheimer, 1907), the situation at last is changing. Careful scientific studies are beginning to emerge and to produce promising findings.

The overall conclusion is that the top-down approach that has driven the quest for a generalized cognitive or drug treatment needs to be supplemented by an equal or larger amount of effort that chips away at the clinical level. Much more research is required that focuses not on delaying or reversing the dementing process, but on methods for ameliorating the everyday behavioral and affective consequences of progressive cognitive loss. These problems are common (Cohen-Mansfield et al., 1993) and are a major source of burden to family members and the major reason for transfer to full-time residential care (Donaldson, Tarrier, & Burns, 1997; Morriss et al., 1996), where they also cause significant distress to professional carers (Hallberg & Norberg, 1995; MacPherson et al., 1994).

Unfortunately, the findings of cognitive science remain largely peripheral to the concerns of carers dealing with these problems. Reading many cognitive texts, one could be forgiven for believing that the worst difficulty likely to be faced by a patient with dementia is inability to remember appointments or find the lounge. Yet the severe problems alluded to in this chapter cannot be separated from the cognitive aspects of dementia. Profound cognitive impairment, in interaction with diverse within-patient and environmental characteristics, plays a major role in etiology. For this reason, cognitive science has the potential to make a major contribution to management, not only in the development or adaptation of specific techniques (e.g., the work in Chapter 12), but also more generally. A sophisticated understanding of the cognitive sequelae and retained learning possibilities in dementia is a critically needed adjunct in such diverse research areas as the rehabilitative effects of changes in the physical environment, use of reinforcement, and education to develop or change attitudes and skills in nursing-home staff.

What is required is the difficult and methodologically unappealing business of identifying individual problems suffered by persons with dementia, devising interventions to ameliorate them, and devising valid ways of measuring the outcome of such interventions. A large body of such work, informed by direct consumer need rather than laboratory-based assumptions, would eventually provide data to feed back into more generic research. Much of this generic work could then be done in controlled laboratory conditions, so long as findings were then tested again in the clinical setting.

Until this happens, psychosocial work on dementia at the clinical level will be based primarily on unsupported assertion. It is safe to assume that many more texts, written with information unsupported by evidence, will assert that environmental cues are essential in dementia care, but providing no details about what types of cues have proven efficacy and how one gets patients to notice them, learn what they mean, or, having done so, act on them. The scientific vacuum means that there is no way for consumers, often desperate for answers, to separate the wheat from the chaff. In at least one major Australian university, a technique of proven inefficacy (classroom RO) and one of unproven efficacy (validation therapy; Feil, 1993) are taught in nursing courses as evidence-based practices. Such phenomena are by no means rare.

In 1979, Edgar Miller, a pioneer in the application of the information-processing framework to memory in dementia, observed, "Psychologists have not so far been very forthcoming in trying to apply their skills and knowledge to the amelioration of the disturbances in memory and other functions that occur in the elderly" (p. 144). There is a strong tradition of commitment to the scientific method in cognitive psychology. Until we start coming to grips with applying it to the analysis and amelioration of the difficult individual behavioral and affective problems suffered as a result of cognitive impairment by this frail, unstable, vulnerable, and highly heterogeneous population, Miller's claim will continue to resonate. The fact that extreme methodological difficulties are involved is no excuse for not trying.

References

Alzheimer, A. (1907). A characteristic disease of the cerebral cortex. In E. Schultze & O. Snell (Eds.), *Allegemeine Zeitschrift für Psychiatrie und psychisch-gerichtliche Medizin* (pp. 146–148). Berlin: Georg Relmer.

Atkinson, A. (1995). Managing people with dementia: CADE units. *Nursing Standards, 9,* 29–32.

Bach, D., Bach, M., Böhmer, F., Frühwald, T., & Grilc, B. (1995). Reactivating occupational therapy: A method to improve cognitive performance in geriatric patients. *Age and Ageing, 24,* 222–226.

Bäckman, L., Josephsson, S., Herlitz, A., Stigsdotter, A., & Viitanen, M. (1991). The generalizability of training gains in dementia: Effects of an imagery based mnemonic on face-name retention duration. *Psychology and Aging, 6,* 489–492.

Baillon, S., Scothern, G., Neville, P. G., & Boyle, A. (1996). Factors that contribute to stress in care staff in residential homes for the elderly. *International Journal of Geriatric Psychiatry, 11,* 219–226.

Ballard, C., & Oyebode, F. (1995). Psychotic symptoms in patients with dementia. *International Journal of Geriatric Psychiatry, 10*, 743–752.

Ballard, C. G., Patel, A., Solis, M., Lowe, K., & Wilcock, G. (1996). A one-year follow-up study of depression in dementia sufferers. *British Journal of Psychiatry, 168*, 287–291.

Baltes, M. M., Neumann, E.-M., & Zank, S. (1994). Maintenance and rehabilitation of independence in old age: An intervention program for staff. *Psychology and Aging, 9*, 179–188.

Beck, C., Heacock, P., Mercer, S., Thatcher, R. N., & Sparkman, C. (1988). The impact of cognitive skills retraining on persons with Alzheimer's disease or mixed dementia. *Journal of Geriatric Psychiatry, 21*, 73–88.

Berg, A., Hansson, U. W., & Hallberg, I. R. (1994). Nurses' creativity, tedium and burnout during one year of clinical supervision and implementation of individually planned nursing care: Comparisons between a ward for severely demented patients and a similar control ward. *Journal of Advanced Nursing, 20*, 742–749.

Bird, M., Alexopoulos, P., & Adamowicz, J. (1995). Success and failure in five case studies: Use of cued recall to ameliorate behavior problems in senile dementia. *International Journal of Geriatric Psychiatry, 10*, 5–11.

Bird, M., Llewllyn-Jones, R., Smithers, H., Andrews, C., Cameron, I., Cottee, A., Hutson, C., Jenneke, B., & Kurrle, S. K. (1998). Challenging behaviors in dementia: A project at Hornsby/Ku-ring-gai Hospital. *Australasian Journal on Ageing, 17*, 10–15

Block, C., Boczhowski, J., Hansen, N., & Vanderbeck, M. (1987). Nursing home consultation: Difficult residents and frustrated staff. *Gerontologist, 27*, 443–446.

Body, E., Kleban, M., Lawton, P., & Silverman, H. (1971). Excess disability of mentally impaired aged; Impact of individualized treatment. *Gerontologist, 11*, 124–133.

Bråne, G., Karlsson, I., Kihlgren, M., & Norberg, A. (1989). Integrity-promoting care of demented nursing home patients: Psychological and biochemical changes. *International Journal of Geriatric Psychiatry, 4*, 165–172.

Breuil, V., de Rotrou, J., Forette, F., Tortrat, D., Ganansia-Ganem, A., Frambourt, A., Moulin, F., & Boller, F. (1994). Cognitive stimulation of patients with dementia: Preliminary results. *International Journal of Geriatric Psychiatry, 9*, 211–217.

Bridges-Parlet, S., Knopman, D., & Thompson, T. (1994). A descriptive study of physically aggressive behavior in dementia by direct observation. *Journal of the American Geriatrics Society, 42*, 192–197.

Brodaty, H., McGilchrist, C., Harris, L., & Peters, K. (1993). Time until institutionalisation and death in patients with dementia: Role of caregiver training and risk factors. *Archives of Neurology, 50*, 643–650.

Burgio, L., & Bourgeois, M. (1992). Treating severe behavioral disorders in geriatric residential settings. *Behavioral Residential Treatment, 7*, 145–168.

Burgio, L., Scilley, K., Hardin, J., Hsu, C., & Yancey, J. (1996). Environmental "White Noise": An intervention for verbally agitated nursing home residents. *Journal of Gerontology: Psychological Sciences, 51B*, P364–P373.

Chafetz, P. K. (1990). Two-dimensional grid is ineffective against demented patients exiting through glass doors. *Psychology and Aging, 5*, 146–147.

Cohen, U., & Day, K. (1994, January/February). Emerging trends in environments for people with dementia. *American Journal of Alzheimer's Care and Related Disorders and Research*, pp. 3–11.

Cohen-Mansfield, J., & Werner, P. (1997). Typology of disruptive vocalizations in older persons suffering from dementia. *International Journal of Geriatric Psychiatry, 12*, 1079–1091.

Cohen-Mansfield, J., Werner, P., Marx, M. S., & Lipson, S. (1993). Assessment and management of behavior problems in the nursing home. In L. Z. Rubenstein & D. Wieland (Eds.),

Improving care in the nursing home: Comprehensive reviews of clinical research (pp. 275–313). London: Sage.

Davis, K. L., & Powchik, P. (1995). Tacrine. *Lancet, 345,* 625–630.

Donaldson, C., Tarrier, N., & Burns, A. (1997). The impact of the symptoms of dementia on caregivers. *British Journal of Psychiatry, 170,* 62–68.

Downes, J. J. (1987). Classroom reality orientation and the enhancement of orientation: A critical note. *British Journal of Clinical Psychiatry, 26,* 147–148.

Drummond, L., Kirchoff, L., & Scarbrough, D. R. (1978). A practical guide to reality orientation: A treatment approach for confusion and disorientation. *Gerontologist, 18,* 568–573.

Edberg, A.-K., Hallberg, I. R., & Gustafson, L. (1996). Effects of clinical supervision on nurse-patient cooperation quality. *Clinical Nursing Research, 5,* 127–149.

Edberg, A.-K., Nordmark Sandgreen, Å., & Hallberg, I. R. (1995). Initiating and terminating verbal interaction between nurses and severely demented patients regarded as vocally disruptive. *Journal of Psychiatric and Mental Health Nursing, 2,* 159–167.

Feil, N. (1993). *The validation breakthrough: Simple techniques for communicating with people with Alzheimer's-type dementia.* Baltimore: Health Professions Press.

Ferrario, E., Cappa, G., Molaschi, M., Rocco, M., & Fabris, F. (1991). Reality orientation therapy in institutionalized elderly patients: Preliminary results. *Archives of Gerontology and Geriatrics,* pp. 139–142.

Finkel, S. I., Lyons, J. S., Anderson, R. L., Sherrell, K., Davis, J., Cohen-Mansfield, J., Schwartz, A., Gandy, J., & Schneider, L. (1995). A randomized, placebo-controlled trial of thiothixene in agitated, demented nursing home patients. *International Journal of Geriatric Psychiatry, 10,* 129–136.

Fleming, R., Bowles, J., & Mellor, S. (1989). Some observations on the first fifteen months of the first C.A.D.E. unit. *Australian Journal on Ageing, 8,* 29–32.

Folstein, M. F., Folstein, S. E., & McHugh, P. R. (1975). Mini-mental state: A practical method for grading the cognitive state of patients for the clinician. *Journal of Psychiatric Research, 12,* 189–198.

Gerdner, L., & Swanson, E. (1993). Effects of individualized music on confused and agitated elderly patients. *Archives of Psychiatric Nursing, 7,* 284–291.

Gilhooly, M. L. M., Sweeting, H. N., Whittick, J. E., & McKee, K. (1994). Family care of the dementing elderly. *International Review of Psychiatry, 6,* 29–40.

Gilleard, C., Mitchell, R. G., & Riordan, J. (1981). Ward orientation training with psychogeriatric patients. *Journal of Advanced Nursing, 6,* 95–98.

Goddaer, J., & Abraham, I. (1994). Effects of relaxing music on agitation during meals among nursing home residents with severe cognitive impairment. *Archives of Psychiatric Nursing, 8,* 150–158.

Godfrey, H. D. B., & Knight, R. G. (1987). Interventions for amnesiacs: A review. *British Journal of Clinical Psychology, 26,* 83–91.

Götestam, K. (1987). Learning versus environmental support for increasing reality orientation in senile demented patients. *European Journal of Psychiatry, 1,* 7–12.

Greene, J. G. (1984). The evaluation of Reality Orientation. In I. Hanley & J. Hodge (Eds.), *Psychological approaches to the care of the elderly* (pp. 192–212). London: Croon Helm.

Hagen, B., & Sayers, D. (1995). When caring leaves bruises: The effects of staff education on resident aggression. *Journal of Gerontological Nursing, 21,* 7–16.

Hallberg, I. R., Holst, G., Nordmark, A., & Edberg, A.-K. (1995). Cooperation during morning care between nurses and severely demented institutionalized patients. *Clinical Nursing Research, 4,* 78–104.

Hallberg, I. R., & Norberg, A. (1995). Nurses' experiences of strain and their reactions in the care of severely demented patients. *International Journal of Geriatric Psychiatry, 10,* 757–766.

Hanley, I. (1984). Theoretical and practical considerations in reality orientation therapy with the elderly. In I. Hanley & J. Hodge (Eds.), *Psychological approaches to the care of the elderly* (pp. 164–191). London: Croom Helm.

Hanley, I. G., & Lusty, K. (1984). Memory aids in reality orientation: A single case study. *Behavior Research and Therapy, 22,* 709–712.

Hanley, I. G., McGuire, R. J., & Boyd, W. D. (1981). Reality orientation and dementia: A controlled trial of two approaches. *British Journal of Psychiatry, 138,* 10–14.

Hart, R. P., Kwentus, J. A., Taylor, J. R., & Harkin, S. W. (1987). Rate of forgetting in dementia and depression. *Journal of Consulting and Clinical Psychology, 55,* 101–105.

Helmes, E., & Wiancko, D. (1997). Effects of music in reducing disruptive behavior in a general hospital. *Ageing Beyond 2000: Proceedings of the 16th Congress of the International Association of Gerontology.* Adelaide, Australia.

Herrman, D., Rea, A., & Andrzejewski, S. (1988). The need for a new approach to memory training. In P. E. Morris, M. M. Gruneberg, & R. N. Sykes (Eds.), *Practical aspects of memory: Current research and issues: Vol. 2. Clinical and educational implications* (pp. 415–420). Chichester, UK: Wiley.

Hill, R., Evankovich, K., Sheikh, J., & Yesavage, J. (1987). Imagery mnemonic training in a patient with primary degenerative dementia. *Psychology and Aging, 2,* 204–205.

Hinchliffe, A. C., Hyman, I. L., Blizard, B., & Livingston, G. (1995). Behavioral complications of dementia—Can they be treated? *International Journal of Geriatric Psychiatry, 10,* 839–847.

Hussian, R. A., & Brown, D. C. (1987). Use of a two dimensional grid pattern to limit hazardous ambulation in demented patients. *Journal of Gerontology, 5,* 558–560.

Karuza, J., & Feather, J. (1989). Staff dynamics. In P. R. Katz & E. Calkins (Eds.), *Principles and practice of nursing home care* (pp. 82–90). New York: Springer.

Kelly, C., & Hunter, R. (1995). Current pharmacological strategies in Alzheimer's disease. *International Journal of Geriatric Psychiatry, 10,* 633–646.

Kihlgren, M., Kuremyr, D., Norberg, A., Bråne, G., Engström, B., Karlson, I., & Melin, E. (1992). *Nurse-patient interaction after training in integrity promoting care at a long-term ward: Analysis of videorecorded morning care sessions.* Ph.D. thesis, University of Umea.

Kitwood, T. (1997). The experience of dementia. *Aging and Mental Health, 1,* 13–22.

Kopelman, M. D. (1985). Rates of forgetting in Alzheimer-type dementia and Korsakoff's syndrome. *Neuropsychologia, 23*(5), 623–638.

Leon, J. (1994). The 1990/1991 National Survey of special care units in nursing homes. *Alzheimer Disease and Associated Disorders, 8*(Suppl. 1), S72–S85.

Levine, J. M., Marchello, V., & Totolos, E. (1995). Progress toward a restraint-free environment in a large academic nursing facility. *Journal of the American Geriatric Society, 43,* 914–918.

Lindsley, O. R. (1964). Geriatric behavioral prosthetics. In R. Kastenbaum (Ed.), *New thoughts on old age,* pp. 41–60. New York: Springer.

Lovell, B., Ancoli, I., & Gervitz, R. (1995). Effect of bright light treatment on agitated behavior in institutionalized elderly subjects. *Psychiatry Research, 29,* 7–12.

MacPherson, R., Eastley, R. J., Richards, H., & Mian, I. H. (1994). Psychological distress among workers caring for the elderly. *International Journal of Geriatric Psychiatry, 9,* 381–386.

Maslow, K. (1994). Current knowledge about special care units: Findings of a study by the U.S. Office of Technology Assessment. *Alzheimer Disease and Associated Disorders, 8*(Suppl. 1), S14–S40.

McEvoy, C., & Schonfeld, L. (1989). Family treatment in Alzheimer's disease. *Clinical Gerontologist, 9,* 58–61.

McGovern, R. J., & Koss, E. (1994). The use of behavior modification with Alzheimer patients: Values and limitations. *Alzheimer Disease and Associated Disorders, 8,* 82–91.

Miller, B. F., & Keane, C. B. (1987). *Encyclopedia and dictionary of medicine, nursing, and allied health* (4th ed.). Philadelphia: Saunders.

Miller, E. (1979). Memory and ageing. In M. M. Gruneberg & P. E. Morris (Eds.), *Applied problems in memory* (pp. 127–149). London: Academic Press.

Mintzer, J. E., Lewis, L., Pennypaker, L., Simpson, W., Bachman, D., Wohlreich, G., Meeks, A., Hunt, S., & Sampson, R. (1993). Behavioral intensive care unit (BICU): A new concept in the management of acute agitated behavior in elderly demented patients. *Gerontologist, 33,* 801–806.

Mishima, K., Okawa, M., Hishikawa, Y., Hori, H., & Takahashi, K. (1994). Morning bright light therapy for sleep and behavior disorders in elderly patients with dementia. *Acta Psychiatrica Scandanavica, 89,* 1–7.

Morris, J. C. (1993). The Clinical Dementia Rating (CDR): Current version and scoring rules. *Neurology, 43,* 2412–2414.

Morriss, R. K., Rovner, B. W., & German, P. S. (1995). Clinical and psychosocial variables associated with different types of behavior problem in new nursing home admissions. *International Journal of Geriatric Psychiatry, 10,* 547–555.

Morriss, R. K., Rovner, B. W., & German, P. S. (1996). Factors contributing to nursing home admission because of disruptive behavior. *International Journal of Geriatric Psychiatry, 11,* 243–249.

Namazi, K., Rosner, T., & Calkins, M. (1989). Visual barriers to prevent ambulatory Alzheimer's patients from exiting through an emergency door. *Gerontologist, 29,* 699–702.

Nilsson, K., Palmstierna, T., & Wistedt, B. (1988). Aggressive behavior in hospitalized psychogeriatric patients. *Acta Psychiatrica Scandinavica, 78,* 172–175.

Patel, V., & Hope, R. A. (1992). A rating scale for aggressive behavior in the elderly—The RAGE. *Psychological Medicine, 22,* 211–221.

Patterson, M. B., & Whitehouse, P. J. (1994). Behavioral symptoms in dementia. *Alzheimer Disease and Associated Disorders, 8*(Suppl. 3), 1–3.

Pinkston, E., Linsk, N., & Young, R. (1988). Home-based behavioral family treatment of the impaired elderly. *Behavior Therapy, 19,* 331–344.

Powell-Procter, L., & Miller, E. (1982). Reality Orientation: A critical appraisal. *British Journal of Psychiatry, 140,* 457–463.

Pruchno, R. A., Peters, N. D., & Burant, C. J. (1995). Mental health of coresident family caregivers: Examination of a two-factor model. *Journal of Gerontology: Psychological Sciences, 50B,* P247–P256.

Quayhagen, M. P., & Quayhagen, M. (1996). Discovering life quality in coping with dementia. *Western Journal of Nursing Research, 18,* 120–135.

Quayhagen, M. P., Quayhagen, M., Corbeil, R. R., Roth, P. A., & Rodgers, J. A. (1995). A dyadic remediation program for care recipients with dementia. *Nursing Research, 44,* 153–159.

Qureshi, H., & Walker, A. (1989). *The caring relationship: Elderly people and their families.* Basingstoke, UK: Macmillan.

Rabins, P. V. (1994). The phenomenology of behavior: An overview of behavioral principles. *Alzheimer Disease and Associated Disorders, 8,* 61–65.

Rahman, N. (1993). Conflict and caregiving: Testing a social-psychological model. *Australian Journal on Ageing, 12,* 16–19.

Rapp, M. S., Flint, A. J., Herrmann, N., & Proulx, G.-B. (1992). Behavioral disturbances in the demented elderly: Phenomenology, pharmacotherapy and behavioral management. *Canadian Journal of Psychiatry, 37,* 651–657.

Ray, W., Taylor, J., Meador, K., Lichtenstein, M., Griffin, M., Fought, R., Adams, M., & Blazer, D. (1993). Reducing antipsychotic drug use in nursing homes: A controlled trial of provider education. *Archives of Intern Medicine, 22,* 713–721.

Reifler, B., & Larson, E. (1990). Excess disability in dementia of the Alzheimer's type. In E. Light & Lebowitz (Eds.), *Alzheimer's disease treatment and family stress* (pp. 363–382). New York: Hemisphere.

Ripich, D. N. (1994). Functional communication with AD patients: A caregiver training program. *Alzheimer Disease and Associated Disorders, 8,* 95–109.

Rovner, B. W. (1994). What is special about special care units? The role of psychosocial rehabilitation. *Alzheimer Disease and Associated Disorders, 8*(Suppl. 1), S355–S358.

Rovner, B., Steele, C., & Folstein, M. (1996). A randomized trial of dementia care in nursing homes. *Journal of the American Geriatrics Society, 44,* 7–13.

Satlin, A., Volicer, L., Ross, V., Herz, L., & Campbell, S. (1992). Bright light treatment of behavioral and sleep disturbances in patients with Alzheimer's disease. *American Journal of Psychiatry, 148,* 1028–1032.

Sultzer, L., Berisford, M., & Gunay, I. (1995). The neurobehavioral scale: Reliability in patients with dementia. *Journal of Psychiatry Research, 29,* 185–191.

Teresi, J., Powell Lawton, M., Ory, M., & Holmes, D. (1994). Measurement issues in chronic care populations: Dementia special care. *Alzheimer Disease and Associated Disorders, 8*(Suppl. 1), S144–S183.

Teri, L. (1994). Behavioral treatment of depression in patients with dementia. *Alzheimer Disease and Associated Disorders, 8,* 66–74.

Teri, L., Reifler, V. B., Keith, R. C., Barns, R., White, E., McLeon, P., & Roskind, M. (1991). Imipramine in the treatment of depressed Alzheimer's patients: Impact on cognition. *Journal of Gerontology, 46,* P372–377.

Turner, J., Willden, K., Halpin, R., & Patrick, G. (1997). Structural changes and the effect on behavior. *Proceedings of Australian Psychological Society Annual Conference.* Cairns, Australia.

Vaccaro, F. J. (1988). Application of operant procedures in a group of institutionalized aggressive geriatric patients. *Psychology and Aging, 3,* 22–28.

Weisman, G. D., Calkins, M., & Sloane, P. (1994). The environmental context of special care. *Alzheimer Disease and Associated Disorders, 8*(Suppl. 1), S308–S320.

Wimo, A., Asplund, K., Mattsson, B., Adolfsson, R., & Lundgren, K. (1995). Patients with dementia in group living: Experiences 4 years after admission. *International Psychogeriatrics, 7,* 123–127.

Wimo, A., Nelvig, A., Nelvig, J., Adolphsson, R., Mattsson, B., & Sandman, P. O. (1993). Can changes in ward routines affect the severity of dementia? *International Psychogeriatrics, 5,* 169–180.

Winogrund, I. R., Fisk, A. A., Kirsling, R. A., & Keyes, B. (1987). The relationship of caregiver burden and morale to Alzheimer's disease patients and function in a therapeutic setting. *Gerontologist, 27,* 336–339.

Woods, B., & Bird, M. (1998). Non-pharmacological approaches to treatment. In G. Wilcock, R. Bucks, & K. Rockwood (Eds.), *Diagnosis and management of dementia: A manual for memory disorders teams.* Oxford: Oxford University Press.

Woods, R. T., & Britton, P. G. (1985). *Clinical psychology with the elderly.* London: Croom-Helm.

Yesavage, J. A., Sheikh, J. I., Friedman, L., & Tanke, E. (1990). Learning mnemonics: Roles of aging and subtle cognitive impairment. *Psychology and Aging, 5,* 133–137.

Zandi, T. (1994). Understanding difficult behaviors of nursing home residents: A prerequisite for sensitive clinical assessment and care. *Alzheimer Disease and Associated Disorders, 8*(Suppl. 1), S345–S354.

Zanetti, O., Frisoni, G., De Leo, D., Buono, M., Bianchetti, A., & Trabucchi, M. (1995). Reality Orientation therapy in Alzheimer's disease: Useful or not? *Alzheimer's Disease and Associated Disorders, 9,* 132–138.

Zarit, S. H., Anthony, C. R., & Boutselis, M. (1987). Interventions with caregivers of dementia patients: A comparison of two approaches. *Psychology and Aging, 2,* 2225–2232.

14

Strategies for the Rehabilitation of Cognitive Loss in Late Life Due to Stroke

CLIVE SKILBECK

The Importance of Cognitive Deficits Following Stroke

Increasingly, the importance of cognitive rehabilitation is being recognized as a key factor in the outcome of general rehabilitation following stroke. Most areas of rehabilitation rely upon the patient's learning, and if cognitive deficits are frustrating this learning process, then all aspects of the rehabilitation program will be frustrated to some degree. For example, Lincoln, Drummond, and Berman (1997), in a multiple regression study of 315 inpatients, found that a main predictor of activities-of-daily-living (ADL) outcome at 12 months poststroke was a measure of visual organization (Rey figure copy score; Lezak, 1995) on admission.

Calvanio, Levine, and Petrone (1993) also addressed this issue, pointing out that deficits in perception, memory, and executive functions are central to ADL failures. Similarly, Galski, Bruno, Zorowitz, and Walker (1993) found that cognitive deficits after stroke were associated with longer inpatient stays and higher rates of referral for outpatient therapy or domiciliary services. In a retrospective investigation, Carter, Oliveira, Duponte, and Lynch (1988) found significantly better ADL scores in stroke patients who had received cognitive remediation in addition to the routine rehabilitation programs from physiotherapists, speech therapists, and occupational therapists, than in those who received only the routine programs. The cognitive retraining included visual scanning, spatial perception, and time judgment exercises. These authors went on to carry out a prospective study of the relationships between cognitive remediation and ADL, which is discussed in the section titled "Strategies for Other Areas of Attention/Spatial Deficit."

In a prospective study, Moroney and Desmond (1996) followed 242 older stroke patients to research the risk of stroke recurrence. They noted that cognitive status independently predicted a subsequent recurrence, a finding that underlines the importance of cognitive deficits after stroke.

General Strategies for Remediating Cognitive Deficits

Introduction

Wilson (1987) described four basic strategies used when attempting cognitive rehabilitation:

1. *Those focusing on drills or exercises,* the underlying assumption being that it is possible to remediate cognitive deficits by stimulation and practice (analogous to physical exercise to improve muscle tone). The work of Sohlberg and Mateer (1989) and of Diller and colleagues (e.g., Diller & Riley, 1993), reported later, would be classified under this strategy.
2. *Those drawing upon models from cognitive neuropsychology.* The cognitive model is used to identify and characterize the deficit so that the dysfunctional elements can be isolated and treated. Often, however, remediation employs the methods outlined above. This strategic approach is favored in reading, language, and visual attention. This strategy is reviewed in Riddoch and Humphreys (1994).
3. *Those combining theory and practice elements from cognitive psychology, neuropsychology, and learning theory.* This approach draws upon the behavioral and neuropsychological traditions, which are included in clinical psychology training, and combines these with cognitive psychology elements. The work of Robertson provides examples of this approach, as does the case study described by von Cramon and Matthes-von Cramon (1994); both are discussed later.
4. *Those providing a holistic treatment strategy,* which addresses noncognitive aspects, including emotional and motivational factors in thepatient. Important in this conceptualization is the patient's own experience of their illness (Prigatano, 1997).

The strengths and limitations of these strategies will be returned to in the discussion, following descriptions of a variety of applications. Sohlberg and Mateer (1989) provided a wealth of practical information on cognitive retraining using their process-specific approach. This approach aims to identify specific deficits and then provides targeted rehabilitation input. It utilizes theory and is similar to the cognitive neuropsychology approach, although the level of detail in the model is lower. Other aspects of the process-specific approach are the repetitive presentation of retraining tasks, the use of a hierarchy of therapy goals, and the use of generalization data as measures of outcome.

In general terms, approaches to the process of cognitive rehabilitation can be divided into:

1. *Internal approaches,* where the rehabilitative effort is focused upon improving patients' impaired cognitive behavior, or on developing alternative appropriate skills. Examples include training of visual scanning in remediation of neglect, and the use of mnemonics in memory impairment.
2. *External approaches,* in which appropriate aids are provided to reduce the effects of the cognitive deficit (e.g., prosthetic language device). These can include designing environments for patients on the basis of their cognitive deficits.

Personal computers (PCs) have been used often in cognitive rehabilitation, in ways that may embody the principles of either of the above strategies. Two different approaches have been employed in using PCs to assist cognitive functioning in elderly people. The more popular is to use the PC as the vehicle for delivering cognitive retraining routines. This strategy has evolved since the late 1970s and has been applied to a wide range of cognitive deficits (see Skilbeck, 1991) with variable success, as indicated below. Sohlberg and Mateer (1989) viewed PC-based cognitive retraining as being highly consistent with their process-specific approach to rehabilitation. In their study, Finkel and Yesavage (1990) compared the learning by elderly people of a mnemonic device (method of loci) using either a traditional teaching or computer-aided instruction (CAI). The CAI approach proved as effective as the traditional training (14 hours of basic skills training and classroom teaching) on a word-learning task using the method of loci, even though CAI participants were significantly older and had lower initial pretraining scores on the task.

Although the assumption may be made that older people will be more anxious and resistant to change where the use of PCs is concerned, there is evidence that their attitudes and responses to new technology are similar to those of younger age groups. For example, in their survey research, Ansley and Erber (1988) observed that older adults (aged 55–86) held attitudes toward computer applications that were not significantly different from those of undergraduates. These authors also noted no differences between these two participant groups on subsequent tasks involving PC interaction, in either time taken or number of errors made.

An approach using the PC as a prosthetic device (e.g., Chute & Bliss, 1994) has been introduced as an external approach to rehabilitation. It is not designed to remediate the cognitive deficits of stroke patients; rather, it seeks to augment their impaired functioning within their particular environment. The strengths and weaknesses of this prosthesis strategy are illustrated in the section on applications to language difficulties.

Whichever strategic approach is implemented, Kurlychek and Levin (1987) suggested a number of core elements that maximize cognitive gains in use of a PC in cognitive retraining:

1. Present tasks in sequence from simple to complex.
2. Select the initial task difficulty level to ensure a high success rate.
3. Move to more a difficult level only after high success at a current one.
4. Emphasize the rate/speed of the response, not just accuracy.
5. Provide frequent positive or corrective feedback.
6. Gradually reduce/fade the cues.
7. Gradually increase required initiative and endurance.

Evaluation of Outcome

Calvanio et al. (1993) considered three indices when judging the success of a cognitive intervention, namely, efficacy, generality, and utility. *Efficacy* refers to the amount of change produced by the intervention on the training tasks. *Generality* (or generalization) is the index reflecting the degree to which beneficial effects of the intervention can be demonstrated beyond the training tasks themselves (the transfer-of-training effect). The intervention's *utility* is its ability to produce clinically significant (not just statistically significant) improvement that is lasting. Utility is of particular importance to the patient who is seeking a meaningful change in his or her condition.

Many studies still do not address the issue of generalization from the cognitive retraining task to related objective neuropsychological assessment and real life, and those that do often fail to observe an appropriate generalization effect. For example, McClure (1997) carried out iconic memory training with 12 brain-injured patients, noting significant improvements in iconic memory skills, but no evidence of generalization to a parallel real-life task (reading speed). Bradley, Welch, and Skilbeck (1993) discussed the issue of generalization in some detail, stressing that the most desirable outcome of cognitive retraining is an improvement in functional status. Their research investigated the use of PCs in a number of neurological groups, including stroke patients. They concluded that gains obtained during retraining generalized to neuropsychological test scores, and self-report questionnaire measures suggested generalization to real-life contexts as well. The retraining software proved useful with stroke patients.

An important measure of utility is long-term outcome, which has received little attention in the cognitive retraining literature. One such investigation was carried out by Kelly, Skilbeck, Welch, Bradley, and Britton (1993), using PC-based retraining. These researchers followed up the patients studied by Bradley et al. (1993) more than 2 years after completion of the retraining. They noted that on most PC tasks, the gains made during training were maintained at the long-term follow-up.

Summary

Cognitive deficits following stroke are important because they can interfere with attempts at rehabilitation. General strategies to remediate such deficits include the use of practice and strategies based upon cognitive neuropsychology, cognitive psychology, and/or learning theory. The approach adopted may attempt to improve the patient's cognitive deficits or may employ external aids to help limit the effects of the deficits. PCs have been used to deliver the cognitive retraining, though their involvement as prosthetic devices is a recent development. In evaluating the success of an intervention to improve cognition, efficacy, generality, and utility are important in judging outcome.

Perceptual and Attentional Deficits

Strategies for Neglect

Remediation of perceptual impairment is the neuropsychological area with the longest history of rehabilitation research following stroke. Although much of the research undertaken in this domain has not had a strong basis in theory, most used the exercise approach outlined in the previous section. This literature began in the early 1970s and is characterized by the work of Diller and his colleagues, whose research focused on remediating perceptual disorders acquired in right-hemisphere stroke, particularly visual neglect (reviewed by Diller & Riley, 1993). The strategy behind this research was to directly address impaired visual scanning, viewed as a major factor in spatial dysfunction, and several techniques were described that attempted to remediate the dysfunction in scanning:

1. *Anchoring*—use of strong cues to fix the initial point for scanning.
2. *Pacing*—introducing a method to aid steady search.
3. *Feedback*—confirmation of the accuracy of responses.
4. *Density*—increasing distance between targets, and use of larger targets, to reduce errors.
5. *Awareness*—encouraging engagement in the task.
6. *Repetition*—practice to convert a new strategy into a habit.
7. *Platforms*—combining acquired behaviors into new skills.

The results obtained from this research demonstrated significant gains on target and relevant nontarget tasks in the experimental group, but not in the control group. The findings showed both *generality* and *utility* and a severity effect (patients with the more severe deficits improved most). Details of these studies are available elsewhere (e.g., Gordon et al., 1985; Weinberg et al., 1977, 1979). Diller and Riley (1993) provided a historical review of the concept of visual neglect and its rehabilitation.

However, impressive as the early findings from visual scanning research were, it is clear that there are difficulties in the generalization of improvement beyond the training tasks themselves (Robertson, Halligan, & Marshall, 1993). For example, Wagenaar et al. (1992), using five single cases, observed significant improvement for four patients after scanning training, but these gains did not generalize beyond the task specifically trained.

Ladavas, Menghini, and Umilta (1994) adopted the cognitive neuropsychology strategy and reviewed the theoretical basis of visual neglect (arousal, representational, and orientating hypotheses), favoring the orientating explanation. They carried out a PC-based rehabilitation study that attempted to manipulate the orienting aspects of spatial attention and to address the question of whether spatial attention is controlled by one central mechanism, or by a number of modular processes. Although the left-sided visual neglect remained stable during baseline, the training intervention, based upon visual cuing of attention (both covert and directed), led to significant reductions in neglect. An untreated control group did not show improvement. The findings indicated that covert orienting was as effective as overt cuing, an outcome that argues against the position that neglect results principally from biased gaze direction. Ladavas et al.'s findings, too, provided support for the modular view of control of attention. This study is helpful in determining which strategies might be applied to the remediation of neglect, although evidence of generalization was not sought, as is frequently the case in the cognitive neuropsychology approach.

Another treatment strategy for neglect is limb activation. Joanette, Brouchon, Gauthier, and Samson (1986) noted that neglect was reduced when the limb contralateral to the lesion, compared with the ipsilateral limb, was used to indicate target stimuli. This finding accords with the theory of Rizzolatti and Camarda (1987) that spatial attention is associated with a range of motor planning circuits. In a number of studies (see Robertson et al., 1993), Robertson and his colleagues have investigated the use of contralateral limb activation to reduce neglect. These studies offer strong support for Rizzolatti and Camarda's position, demonstrating that it is the activation of the left limb itself (rather than the use of the arm as a visual anchor cue) that produces the therapeutic effect. Similarly, Robertson and North (1992) showed that producing motor activation in the left extrapersonal space by *right arm movements* yields no beneficial effect.

Robertson et al. (1993) reviewed a number of additional techniques for reducing neglect, each of which had an underlying rationale. However, as there is little evidence that they produced effects that generalized to the real world of ADL, some of them might better be regarded as minor environmental, or external, aids. For example, Butters and his coworkers proposed placing an eye patch over the right eye in left visual neglect (as retinal projection to the right and left superior colliculi is primarily from the contralateral eye). Reduction in neglect was noted, but only for the time that the eye patch was in place. The same technique was investigated by Walker, Young, and Lincoln (1996), who also concluded that eye patching was unlikely to be of general value when attempting to treat neglect. Similarly, attachment of Fresnel prisms, which displace a retinal image to the right or the left according to prism orientation, to the glasses of stroke patients yielded gains on perceptual tasks (compared with the outcome in a control group), but not on ADL tasks (Rossi, Kheyfets, & Reding, 1990).

However, Seron, Deloche, and Coyette (1989) employed an external aid (a buzzer) to assist in the reduction of neglect. The buzzer was placed in the patient's left shirt pocket and emitted its sound at random 5- to 20-second intervals. The task was to locate the buzzer and switch it off, and the result was significant gains in ADL functioning.

Strategies for Other Areas of Attention/Spatial Deficit

Beyond the area of neglect, there are a number of often ill-defined cognitive problems following stroke that appear to arise due to spatial/attentional deficits. Although this field is less popular than neglect, some literature exists on attempts at remediation for these problems, and Sohlberg and Mateer (1989) provided both a clinically relevant classification of attentional deficits and a range of tasks that might be employed in remediation. In their study of 58 patients in the first 12 months poststroke, Egelko et al. (1989) noted improvements in visual neglect and affect comprehension in the right-hemisphere group, but not in the left-hemisphere group. In addition, reaction time (RT) did not improve in the right-hemisphere group between initial assessment and the 10-month follow-up, an outcome leading the authors to advocate more intensive remediation in this cognitive area.

Following the recommendations of Egelko et al. (1989), Sturm and Willmes (1991) provided RT training for both right- and left-hemisphere stroke patients. These authors reviewed evidence that specific aspects of attention may be differentially affected, according to the hemisphere of damage (right-hemisphere lesions particularly disrupting sustained attention, or vigilance, and left-hemisphere damage being associated more with reduced speed and accuracy in choice RT). Sturm and Willmes employed a PC-based approach, along cognitive neuropsychology lines, utilizing training-program routines that included comparisons of stimulus configurations with a multiple-choice array to detect matches. Stimulus material was varied according to complexity, employing letters, digits, geometric figures, and nonsense patterns. Rate of presentation and spatial rotation of material were also used to manipulate complexity. The results demonstrated significant attention-training effects, except for vigilance, although there

was no evidence of generalization to other cognitive tasks. Gains in attentional performance were maintained over a 6- to 9-week period of no training.

In a subsequent PC-based study, Sturm, Willmes, Orgass, and Hartje (1997) used
single-case methodology to separate out different components of attention and found
specific training effects according to the targeted component of the intervention: "In
patients with localised vascular lesions, specific attention disorders need specific training" (p. 97). Patients (27 with left-hemisphere damage, 8 with right-hemisphere lesions) completed 14 sessions of 30 minutes each, over 3 weeks, and training outcome
was assessed on a battery of 10 psychometric tests. Evidence in support of the "lateral-
ization" of different aspects of attention was obtained. Significant gains in performance over the training period were noted on tasks that closely resembled the training
tasks, though the number of significant improvements fell as similarity to the training
task decreased. Overall, training gains were lower in the right-hemisphere stroke patients, though a lack of improvement in vigilance was apparent in both groups.

Carter et al. (1988) carried out a prospective study of the relationships between
cognitive functioning and ADL outcome in 21 stroke patients, 17 of whom had right-
hemisphere damage. They noted a significant correlation ($r = +0.59$; $p < .01$) between
pretraining cognitive skills and (posttraining) ADL outcome. The single best predictor
of outcome ADL was an auditory vigilance attention task, which correlated significantly with five out of six ADL indices (correlation range: +0.49 to +0.71). Visuospatial ability was the next best predictor of posttraining ADLs, correlating significantly
with three activities (including dressing and personal hygiene, which replicated earlier
findings from these researchers). Carter and her colleagues advocated that auditory
vigilance attention should receive further attention as a cognitive remediation task,
given its importance in their studies. This study is important as it specifically bears
upon the critical question of carryover, or generalization, of cognitive retraining gains
into real life.

Another investigation focusing upon real-life application was that of Klavora et al.
(1995). These authors employed a specific apparatus (Dynavision) to retrain a number
of attentional/information-processing abilities considered important in driving ability
(including reaction time, anticipation, movement time, scanning, and endurance).
Their study involved 10 patients who were 6–18 months poststroke and who had
demonstrable attentional deficits sufficient to render them unsafe to drive. The retraining program used three sessions per week, each of approximately 20 minutes, for
6 weeks. Subjects underwent pre- and posttraining assessment, including follow-up
assessment at 3 months. Of nine cognitive variables examined, seven showed significant improvement, the exceptions being choice visual reaction time and anticipation
time. The gains on these seven variables were maintained at follow-up. As a consequence of the cognitive remediation program, 6 of the 10 patients moved from "unsafe
to drive" to "safe to resume driving and/or to receive on-road driving lessons."

Hajek, Kates, Donnelly, and McGree (1993) adopted a PC-based retraining strategy
for visuospatial impairment in an attempt to augment routine rehabilitation. They
failed to observe generalization of PC training (using the seven visuospatial exercises
of Bracy, 1982) to the Rey-Osterrieth Complex Figure test, Raven's Coloured PM
test, and the Benton line orientation test, although significant improvement in (WAIS-
R) Block Design (see Lezak, 1995) score was noted in male patients. The study involved 20 right-hemisphere patients, half of whom received the usual rehabilitation

program from physiotherapists and occupational therapists (control group), and half of whom also received additional PC visuospatial exercises, delivered as three 30-minute sessions each week for 4 weeks. Most patients were less than 3 months posts-troke. Gains were noted in both groups.

In their PC-based study, Bradley et al. (1993) included five stroke patients who were 4–72 months poststroke. Improvements on retraining tasks involving visual attention, speed of information processing, and performance on the WAIS-R Digit Symbol task were noted over the 12-week (24-session) rehabilitation period. Follow-up more than 2 years after retraining indicated that task and WAIS-R Digit Symbol gains were still significant.

Summary

There is along history of attempts to remediate neglect in elderly patients following stroke. Diller and his colleagues have researched the rehabilitation of visual scanning with considerable success, although achieving generalization to real life has proved problematic. Theories of visual neglect have been based on arousal, representation, or orientation. Treatments employing cuing or limb activation have yielded promising results, though eye patching appears to be ineffective. Attempts to address other areas of attentional/spatial impairment following stroke have also been researched, the work often involving PCs in the retraining intervention.

Memory Impairment

Strategies

Harris (1992) offered a classification of strategies for improving memory deficits arising from acquired brain damage. He divided internal strategies, which have some basis in theory, into those naturally learned (e.g., primacy and recency) and those employing artificial mnemonics, and he divided external strategies into those based upon a storage of useful information and those offering cues. Harris also included repetitive practice (exercise) and drugs as being of potential benefit. The strategy adopted should also take into account a number of factors. For example, the tasks selected for remediation attempts should be have practical and personal importance to the patient, should include other cognitive skills that the patient does possess, and should be capable of being manipulated in terms of level of difficulty (Moffat, 1992). Feedback is also important as a way of demonstrating to the stroke patient that progress is being made. In this regard, the use of graphs may better illustrate improvement to patients.

When deciding on an appropriate level of task difficulty, an entry point in the retraining should be selected to minimize the patient's errors. This minimization can be manipulated via amount or complexity of material, by the learning strategies offered to the patient, by duration of the retention required, and by the retrieval cues provided (Moffat, 1992). Short, frequent training sessions are preferred, as these usually yield greater learning, and thought should be given to providing the patient with maintenance mechanisms to preserve the gains achieved.

External Aids

Although use of external aids to memory is natural, developing across the life span, these aids usually lack theoretical underpinning. Harris (1992) provided a brief review of two types of possible external aids for those with damaged memories. The first relates to the external storage of required information, for example, (a) use of a diary to remind the person of important dates, such as birthdays, and (b) use of a shopping list to assist recall at the supermarket. More sophisticated examples include the employment of a pocket dictaphone to assist future recall or a pocket computer upon which very large quantities of personal information can be stored (e.g., names and phone numbers). Unfortunately, operation of the latter is often beyond the competence of a stroke patient.

The second class of external memory aid provides a reminder, or cue, for the patient that she or he has to do something. This cue often takes the form of an auditory signal, such as a wristwatch alarm. The difficulty with this form of aid is that usually little information is provided by the cue that connects it with the to-be-remembered activity. For example, although the buzzer may remind the patient that he or she should do *something,* it may not be clear what the something is. The recent development (the Neuropager; Wilson, Evans, Emslie, & Malinek, 1997) of a more comprehensive reminder system may offer a solution to this problem; that is, not only is the patient cued that it is time to do something, but specific information is also provided with the cue that informs the patient what has to be done. This type of external aid is in the early stages of development for clinical use, but it appears to offer a good combination of cue and specific information for the patient. Existing alternative devices to both cue and offer some information include electronic diaries and display alarm watches (Harris, 1992; Kapur, 1995).

Exploiting external devices to their full extent may result in manipulating the environment to provide cues. For example, reality orientation (RO) therapy (Woods, 1996) aims to help the orientation of patients in terms of time, place, and person. This therapy includes the color coding of doors to overcome topographical difficulties (e.g., to allow independent use of bathroom and sitting room). RO is based upon a number of principles (Moffatt, 1992):

1. Provision of information in a range of formats
2. Correction of confused behavior
3. Reinforcement of appropriate cognitive behavior
4. Use of cues, prompts, and rehearsal
5. Use of memory aids as prostheses

Skilbeck and Robertson (1992) reported case study material that indicated improvement in patient orientation when RO was delivered by a PC that included graphics software to enhance the clarity and interest of the presented material. In this study, PC-based RO was as effective in promoting orientation as when the same treatment was provided by a therapist. This latter finding is important, given that the provision of RO therapy is very labor-intensive.

Glisky, Schacter, and Butters (1994) specifically considered the issue of transfer, or generalization, of learning, pointing out that too often the acquired learning is closely associated with the learning context and not responsive to different cues. These authors concluded that retraining routines should try to build upon the patient's prior preserved knowledge and should include considerable overlearning to facilitate generalization to other tasks and settings, coupled with elaborated task material designed to link with the patient's infrastructure of knowledge.

Internal Strategies

Moffatt (1992) listed a variety of internal approaches to remediating memory deficits, including the use of visual imagery, in which, for example, the patient is taught to link a specific feature of a person with a visual image in order to remember that person's name. Visual imagery's effectiveness has been demonstrated in clinical studies (e.g., Wilson, 1987). Peg mnemonics were also considered by Moffatt (1992), a strategy whereby a rhyming mnemonic is combined with a visual image to aid retrieval. The technique may be particularly helpful with lists of material, such as shopping lists. The rhyming component might be "One-is-a-bun, two-is-a-shoe, three-is-a-tree," and so on, and a visual image can be provided to link an item of shopping with one of the pegs.

Glasgow, Zeiss, Barrera, and Lewinsohn (1977) addressed the issue of improving recall for written material by using a structured study method. They taught their patient the following (PQRST) structure:

*P*review: Skim the text and establish its general order.

*Q*uestion: Devise the main questions to ask of the text.

*R*ead: Read the text slowly and carefully.

*S*tate: State aloud the material that has been read.

*T*est: Test whether the material has been understood and the questions posed have been answered.

Wilson (1987) carried out a number of studies using the PQRST strategy, reporting that it proved superior to rehearsal alone for both immediate recall and retrieval after a delay. In their research, Downes et al. (1997) employed the concept of *preexposure,* which may be regarded as a brief version of the *P* and *Q* elements in the strategy. These authors aimed to teach 25 memory-impaired patients 10 face-name associations, using imagery, preexposure, or a combination of both. In the preexposure condition, subjects were initially shown each face for 6 seconds, and 10 questions were prepared, of which 2 or 3 were presented for each of the faces to be learned (e.g., "Does he/she look friendly/intelligent/honest?"). The results were clear: Preexposure enhanced learning significantly by itself and also boosted the effects of imagery (which alone was also effective).

The vanishing cues strategy involves providing prompts for an area of memory failure and gradually increasing the number of cues until reliable recall is established. Over succeeding sessions, the number of cues required diminishes until cues vanish. The approach is ideal for PC administration. In acquiring recall for the name *Chloe,* during Session 1 the following sequence may occur:

Trial	Cues	No. of cues
1	——	0
2	C——	1
3	CH——	2
4	CHL——	3
5	CHLO—	4
6	CHLOE	5

Session 2 might require only four cues (CHLO), and by Session 4, a single cue might suffice (C).

Wilson (1992) suggested a number of general principles to follow when attempting to remediate memory impairments:

1. Simplify the information you wish the patient to remember.
2. Reduce the amount to be remembered.
3. Ensure that the material has been understood.
4. Link the material to information already available to the patient.
5. Schedule frequent, short sessions, which produce better learning.
6. Categorize the material, or ask the patient to structure it.
7. Refresh the learning to aid long-term retention.
8. Use cues to prompt recall.
9. Improve learning and recall by teaching in a range of settings.

The material taught should be meaningful and relevant to the patient, who may have preferences with regard to learning style.

A neglected technique in the clinical literature is expanded retrieval practice (see Moffatt, 1992), which is based upon the finding that the longer the interval between first and second successful recall of a piece of information, the higher the probability of subsequent successful recall (Bjork, 1988). Moffatt (1989) employed this strategy in rehabilitating problems of memory, dysgraphia, and naming, using a gradual expansion of the interval between first and second recall. This concept is very similar to that of spaced retrieval (Camp & Schaller, 1989), a method in which associations are recalled repeatedly with an increasing retention interval. The technique has been used successfully to improve naming in degenerative dementia (Abrahams & Camp, 1993; McKitrick & Camp, 1993). Evidence of generalization beyond the training task was observed, and this approach appears particularly relevant to memory deficits in older stroke patients.

There has been relatively little research on patients' own compensatory mechanisms for their memory impairment. Backman and Dixon (1992) addressed this issue, providing a theoretical framework for its consideration. Following from this paper, Wilson and Watson (1996) offered a practical approach to understanding patients' compensatory behavior. Both papers are essential reading. Wilson and Hughes (1997) provided a detailed description of a patient's compensatory processes for dealing with memory deficits after an aneurysm hemorrhage.

An area of the literature that is not fully exploited by clinicians is research on normal aging. In a review of nonpharmacological treatments for memory loss in old age, Yesavage (1985) discussed a number of strategies that have been utilized, including group mnemonic training, categorization, visual mediators, spatial loci, and visual imagery. The studies he reviewed suggested that the method of spatial loci, in which persons name a number of locations within a familiar setting (e.g., their home) and then associate a visual image of the thing to be remembered with each of these loci, is very effective in improving recall. Verbal elaboration, too, appears to be a successful strategy when, for example, older people are attempting to remember faces. Yesavage indicated that anxiety often adversely affects the attentional capacity of older adults, and a number of studies have shown the recall benefits of training elderly subjects in relaxation techniques.

In a subsequent study involving 40 elderly people, Yesavage, Sheikh, Tanke, and Hill (1988) investigated variability in individual response to memory retraining. These authors found that higher WAIS Vocabulary scale scores correlated with better use of a combined mnemonics and verbal elaboration retraining strategy, and that higher state anxiety scores were associated with better recall performance after relaxation training (see also Hayslip, 1989).

A key issue is generalization to objective neuropsychological tests and to real life. Panza et al. (1997) dealt with it by offering most of their rehabilitation program for memory deficits in patients' own homes, with a minority of the retraining procedures employing a PC in the rehabilitation center. Their results showed significant improvements in memory on objective tests.

When reviewing the use of PCs in memory remediation, Glisky (1995) cautioned against the assumption that a retraining procedure is helpful merely because it is delivered via a PC. She predicted PCs will make a larger contribution to rehabilitation in the future, so it is important that we fully test and critically evaluate their programs in terms of their basis in psychological models and their relevance to treatment goals. As indicated in the next section, home use of PCs should offer greater independence to patients.

Language Dysfunction

Detailed consideration of language dysfunction rehabilitation in older stroke patients is beyond the scope of this chapter, although a few illustrations of the research findings will be offered. The cognitive neuropsychology strategic approach is most popular in this field.

Excellent reviews of language remediation are available (e.g., Holland, Fromm, DeRuyter, & Stein, 1996). The general field of speech therapy for aphasia following stroke has received a mixed press, some studies providing little support for its use. For example, Lincoln et al. (1984) randomly allocated 191 stroke patients to either speech therapy (two sessions per week for 24 weeks) or a no-treatment control group. No significant differences were observed between the two groups at the start of therapy, at 12 weeks into therapy, and at end of therapy. Similarly, Hartman and Landau (1987) failed to observe significant effects in their study of 60 stroke patients randomly assigned to 6 months of speech therapy or of emotionally supportive counseling.

Studies focusing upon specific aspects of language disorder have sometimes produced significant results. For example, Helm-Estabrooks, Emery, and Albert (1987) successfully remediated perseverative speech errors in three case studies of stroke. In a large study of 281 aphasic patients, 85% of whom had suffered a stroke; Basso, Capitani, and Vignolo (1979) noted significant gains in their treatment group, though a number of difficulties exist in this study: Over 200 patients were excluded, as they dropped out before completing treatment, and the control group comprised 119 patients unable to attend for rehabilitation. In their review of the literature on rehabilitation of naming disorders, Nickels and Best (1996) concluded that therapeutic gains can be expected. Davis and Pring (1991) obtained significant improvement in their study of seven patients with word-finding deficits, though they also observed generalization to unrelated, nontarget items in the therapy material.

Following the cognitive neuropsychology strategy, Ellis, Franklin, and Crerar (1994), recommended the use of a large number of case studies, covering a range of language disorders, each of which would have detailed profiling prior to receiving replicable treatment interventions. In this way, therapeutic outcome can be related to pretreatment characterization of patients. Patterson (1994) provided an excellent review of the cognitive neuropsychology approach applied to disorders of reading and writing. She concluded that this approach is proving helpful, although the field is still young, while noting the mixed evidence on the generalization of gains beyond the training task.

Chute and Bliss (1994) advocated the use of PCs as prostheses in cognitive rehabilitation following stroke, presenting SpeechWare, a prosthesis developed for people with expressive language impairment and physical disability; the program seeks to compensate for the deficit by offering augmented assistance in the person's particular environment. In order to be effective, it needs to be ecologically valid for that individual. SpeechWare provides both digitized and synthesized speech and can handle programmable events and word processing. In addition, video clips or photographs of the user offer the most realistic reminders to ensure that ADLs are carried out. Thus, customization and empowerment of the user are maximized; interfacing with telephones, faxes, and so on is facilitated. Weaknesses of the approach include the necessity for expensive hardware to gain good environmental control (the SpeechWare software itself costs only $50), the sophisticated programming skills required for customization, and the potential additional medicolegal risks associated with its inappropriate use.

Other Cognitive Functions

The most difficult cognitive impairment to rehabilitate is dysexecutive syndrome, involving poor planning, inappropriate social behavior, and so on. Von Cramon and Matthes-von Cramon (1994) used the cognitive neuropsychology model of Norman and Shallice (1986), centered on the concept of a supervisory attentional system (SAS) to reduce the dysexecutive difficulties of a medical practitioner. The patient (GL) had sustained a closed head injury, rather than vascular damage, but is presented here because of the scarcity of relevant studies. An MRI of GL approximately 9 years after the head injury, indicated bilateral frontal lobe damage. The authors found most cognitive abilities to be intact (GL had managed to complete his medical degree 6 months after the injury), including an IQ of 130+, though GL was relatively poor on tests sensitive to frontal lobe dysfunction. Complaints relating to his behavior included making sexual jokes in front of his boss at a social function, interrupting work colleagues in their rooms without warning, and being unable to organize coherent autopsy/biopsy reports in the lab where he worked. Von Cramon and Matthes-von Cramon (1994) concentrated upon improving GL's monitoring of his own behavior in the work environment; this case provided an excellent opportunity to assess generalization of cognitive retraining directly, although evaluation of outcome in such a subtle behavioral area was difficult. Using goal attainment scaling, the authors used observable work performance, such as accuracy, structure, and relevance of pathology reports. Feedback, offered via graphs, proved useful in increasing GL's motivation. Von Cramon and Matthes-von Cramon reported significant gains in work performance within a few weeks of retraining commencing. Therapy consisted of 2–3 hours per week over 12 months, and the authors found Norman and Shallice's model (SAS) helpful in both formulating the intervention and in discussing their treatment findings.

Crepeau, Scherzer, Belleville, and Desmarais (1997) provided a useful analysis of central executive (CE) deficits in a number of workplace tasks, correlating these with cognitive test scores, which should assist therapists plan rehabilitation routines to meet occupational requirements. Alderman (1996) advanced the hypothesis that SAS or CE deficits are associated with a poorer response to retraining procedures that are based on behavioral methods.

Practical assistance for those attempting to treat executive disorders has also been provided by Sohlberg and Mateer (1989), who discussed a clinical model for assessment and intervention comprising the selection and execution of cognitive plans, time management, and self-regulation. They gave a range of activities to help with this difficult area of retraining.

Other Aspects of Strategy

Depression

The adverse effects of coexisting depression upon cognitive functioning has often been suggested by significant correlations between mood state and neuropsychological test scores (e.g., Morris, Raphael, & Robinson, 1992; Downhill & Robinson, 1994). However, few studies have attempted to assess the benefits for cognitive recovery of treating depression following stroke. An exception is the research of Gonzalez-Torrecillas, Mendlewicz, and Lobo (1995). These authors compared the Mini-Mental State Examination (MMSE) scores, over a 6-week treatment period (starting 3–4 weeks poststroke), of 37 patients receiving antidepressant medication, 11 depressed patients who were not treated, and 82 patients who were not depressed. Initially, the nondepressed group had a higher MMSE score than the depressed groups, though differences between that group and the "treated depression" group, disappeared over the course of treatment. However, the untreated group showed little improvement in MMSE score, and by Week 5, significant differences were noted from the "treated depression" group. These findings are potentially very important in determining stroke rehabilitation strategies, and a replication study is needed. The Gonzalez-Torrecillas et al. (1995) investigation does not seem to have included active cognitive rehabilitation ("just" natural cognitive recovery), and it would be even more interesting to examine the effects of antidepressant medication on patients undergoing cognitive retraining.

The Contribution of "Normal" Aging

Reviewing the field of cognitive retraining with elderly people, Hayslip (1989) considered the factors important to efficacy and utility and pointed up the deleterious effects of anxiety *about* performance *on* performance. Hayslip was concerned about the durability and generalizability of any gains achieved, advocating that these aspects receive more attention in future research. When discussing individual differences, Hayslip suggested that low self-esteem, lower intellectual competence, and an external locus of control can mediate for a better training outcome, and that individuals showing these features are more likely to find the training procedures credible and effective. Amount of practice with the training material also seems important for training efficacy.

Psychosocial Aspects

The research literature on cognitive remediation after acquired brain damage is mainly concerned with formal, targeted attempts by therapists to improve functioning (usually in the rehabilitation ward or unit). The literature fails to recognize the informal potential contribution of family and friends of the patient to the remediation process. In addition, the stress of the cognitive deficits exhibited by the stroke patient falls heavily upon family and friends. One way of addressing the needs of both patient and family is via self-help groups. Wearing (1992) outlined the case for such groups and their additional possible purpose as a vehicle for "training" family and friends to act as informal cognitive rehabilitation assistants.

Discussion

Basic cognitive rehabilitation strategies exist, the most popular to date being based upon drills and exercises. Wilson and Hughes (1997) criticized this approach, as evidence for its effectiveness is mixed. Choice of area of cognitive impairment for retraining and method of implementation (PC or otherwise) are important factors when weighing the available support for the approach. There is sufficient evidence for the use of PC-based exercise rehabilitation for visuospatial and attention/information-processing deficits. Results are very variable in relation to retraining in the face of memory deficits by means of PCs (e.g., Bradley et al., 1993). The exercise approach can also be criticized, as it lacks theoretical infrastructure, and it does not address the psychosocial aspects of stroke.

A refinement of cognitive rehabilitation strategies is the cognitive neuropsychological strategy. This is grounded in theory, and it is argued that identification of the underlying deficit by means of an appropriate cognitive model allows greater specificity of retraining elements: The treatment is tailored to fit the model's view of the functional impairment. Wilson and Hughes (1997) argued that description of the *impairment* does not necessarily lead to treatment of the *disability* (World Health Organization, 1980). The cognitive neuropsychology approach is best suited to patients with pure deficits, who can be characterized by means of their models. Like exercise retraining, this strategy does not incorporate psychosocial elements, and usually its studies are not concerned with generalization to ADLs.

The combined strategy (cognitive psychology, neuropsychology, and learning theory) is popular with researchers and practitioners who are trained as clinical psychologists. Its strengths include careful monitoring and the evaluation of outcome. It might be argued that while it is wide-ranging, this approach still fails to encompass the emotional sequelae of stroke, although this lack is debatable. From an ethical viewpoint, it is very difficult to argue against the holistic approach (Prigatano, 1995, 1997), because it takes the widest possible psychological view of patients' problems poststroke. There is a resource issue here, and in many countries, there would not be enough adequately trained psychotherapists to meet the needs of the number of people suffering stroke. Psychological therapies that are relatively brief may be preferred, and the continued success and development of cognitive therapy offer a proven, cost-effective method of intervention for a range of problems and settings (Padesky & Greenberger, 1995). The routine extension of cognitive therapy to the psychological sequelae of acquired brain damage seems only a matter of time.

Most reviewers and researchers remain optimistic about cognitive retraining following acquired brain damage. This is a young field, and there is need for well-controlled studies to test the validity of the various proposed approaches to cognitive rehabilitation. These studies should prioritize the evaluation of generalization from training-task gains to ADLs and other real-life activities. Careful and detailed pretraining assessment data should also be gathered to allow adequate investigation of the "matching" of retraining strategy to specific patient characteristics.

Summary

Cognitive deficits following stroke are not important only because they are an essential part of a person's identity and his or her ability to function satisfactorily in the world. These deficits are also significant predictors of a person's ability to benefit from the general rehabilitation process. This chapter outlined the available strategies for cognitive retraining and provided some example applications across a range of cognitive areas. The evidence remains mixed with regard to efficacy, although many studies are able to demonstrate robust improvements in the retraining tasks themselves. The critical test is generalization of retraining effects from the training tasks to objective neuropsychological tests and to the patient's real-world environment.

The use of PCs in the retraining process has sometimes been criticized, but as long as their employment is not regarded de facto as a guarantee of good-quality cognitive retraining, they appear to have a part to play (particularly when the rehabilitation process becomes sophisticated enough to routinely utilize the patient's own environment).

Even the most complex cognitive areas, including executive functioning, are now being researched, and we are increasingly aware of confounding factors in the retraining program, such as mood state. Until recently, the available literature from research on "normal" cognitive aging and compensatory strategies was largely ignored, but we are now beginning to use this source.

The recommendation of Ellis, Franklin, and Crerar (1994) is a good one to adopt: Future research needs to include a large number of case studies in each of the cognitive areas we wish to rehabilitate. Each case will require extensive and detailed pretraining assessment to yield a profile to act as the basis for undertaking replication studies on treatment efficacy. In this way, specific patient characteristics may be investigated.

References

Abrahams, J. P. & Camp, C. J. (1993). Maintenance and generalization of object naming training associated with degenerative dementia. *Clinical Gerontology, 12*(3), 57–72.

Alderman, N. (1996). Central executive deficit and response to operant conditioning methods. *Neuropsychological Rehabilitation, 6*(3), 161–186.

Ansley, J., & Erber, J. T. (1988). Computer interaction: Effects on attitudes and performance in older adults. *Educational Gerontology, 14*(2), 107–119.

Bäckman, L., & Dixon, R. A. (1992). Psychological compensation: A theoretical framework. *Psychological Bulletin, 112*, 259–283.

Basso, A., Capitani, E., & Vignolo, L. A. (1979). Influence of rehabilitation on language skills in aphasic patients: A controlled study. *Archives of Neurology, 36*, 190–196.

Bjork, R. A. (1988). Retrieval practice and the maintenance of knowledge. In M. M. Gruneberg, P. E. Morris, & R. N. Sykes (Eds.), *Practical aspects of memory: Current research and issues.* Chichester, UK: Wiley.

Bracy, O. D. (1982). Cognitive rehabilitation programs for brain-impaired and stroke patients: Visuo-spatial program. *Psychological Software Services.*

Bradley, V. A., Welch, J. L., & Skilbeck, C. E. (1993). *Cognitive retraining using microcomputers.* Hove: LEA.

Calvanio, R., Levine, D., & Petrone, P. (1993). Elements of cognitive rehabilitation after right hemisphere stroke. *Behavioural Neurology, 11*(1), 25–56.

Camp, C. J., & Schaller, J. R. (1989). Epilogue: Spaced-retrieval memory training in an adult day care center. Special issue: Cognitive aging: Issues in research and application. *Educational Gerontology, 15*(6), 641–648.

Carter, L. T., Oliveira, D. O., Duponte, J., & Lynch, S. V. (1988). The relationship of cognitive skills performance to activities of daily living in stroke patients. *American Journal of Occupational Therapy, 42*(7), 449–455.

Chute, D. L. (1994). ProsthesisWare: Concepts and Caveats for microcomputer-based aids to everyday living. *Experimental Aging Research, 20*, 229–238.

Crepeau, F., Scherzer, B. P., Belleville, S., & Desmarais, G. (1997). A quantitative analysis of central executive disorders in a real-life work situation. *Neuropsychological Rehabilitation, 7*(2), 147–165.

Davis, A., & Pring, T. (1991). Therapy for word-finding deficits: More on the effects of semantic and phonological approaches to treatment with dysphasic patients. *Neuropsychological Rehabilitation, 1*(2), 135–145.

Diller, L., & Riley, E. (1993). The behavioural management of neglect. In I. H. Robertson & J. C. Marshall (Eds.), *Unilateral Neglect: Clinical and Experimental Studies.* Hove, UK: LEA.

Downes, J. J., Kalla, T., Davies, A. D. M., Flynn, A., et al. (1997). The preexposure technique: A novel method for enhancing the effects of imagery in face-name association learning. *Neuropsychological Rehabilitation, 7*(3), 195–214.

Downhill, J. E., & Robinson, R. G. (1994). Longitudinal assessment of depression and cognitive impairment following stroke. *Journal of Nervous and Mental Disease, 182*(8), 425–431.

Egelko, S., Simon, D., Riley, E., et al. (1989). First year after stroke: Tracking cognitive and affective deficits. *Archives of Physical Medicine and Rehabilitation, 70*, 297–302.

Ellis, A., Franklin, S., & Crerar, A. (1994). Cognitive neuropsychology and the remediation of disorders of spoken language. In M. J. Riddoch & G. W. Humphreys (Eds.), *Cognitive neuropsychology and cognitive rehabilitation.* Hove, UK: LEA.

Finkel, S. I., & Yesavage, J. A. (1990). Learning mnemonics: A preliminary evaluation of a computer-aided instruction package for the elderly. *Experimental Aging Research, 15*(4), 199–201.

Galski, T. G., Bruno, R. L., Zorowitz, R., & Walker, J. (1993). Predicting length of stay, functional outcome, and aftercare in the rehabilitation of stroke patients. *Stroke, 24*(12), 1794–1800.

Glasgow, R. E., Zeiss, R. A., Barrera, M., & Lewinsohn, P. M. (1977). Case studies on remediating memory deficits in brain damaged individuals. *Journal of Clinical Psychology, 33,* 1049–1054.

Glisky, E. L. (1995). Computers in memory rehabilitation. In A. D. Baddeley, B. A. Wilson, & F. N. Watts (Eds.), *Handbook of memory disorders.* Chichester, UK: Wiley.

Glisky, E. L., & Schacter, D. L. (1987). Acquisition of domain-specific knowledge in organic amnesia: Training for computer-related work. *Neuropsychologia, 25,* 893–906.

Glisky, E. L., Schacter, D. L., & Butters, M. A. (1994). Domain specific learning and remediation of memory disorders. In M. J. Riddoch & G. W. Humphreys (Eds.), *Cognitive neuropsychology and cognitive rehabilitation.* Hove, UK: LEA.

Gonzalez-Torrecillas, J. L., Mendlewicz, J., & Lobo, A. (1995). Effects of early treatment of poststroke depression on neuropsychological rehabilitation. *Int Psychogeriatrics, 7*(4), 547–560.

Gordon, W. A., Hibberd, M. R., Egelko, S., et al. (1985). Perceptual remediation in patients with right brain damage: A comprehensive program. *Archives of Physical Medicine and Rehabilitation, 66,* 353–360.

Hajek, V. E., Kates, M. H., Donnelly, R., & McGree, S. (1993). The effect of visuo-spatial training in patients with right hemisphere stroke. *Canadian Journal of Rehabilitation, 6*(3), 175–186.

Harris, J. W. (1992). Ways to help memory. In B. A. Wilson & N. Moffat (Eds.), *Clinical management of memory problems* (2nd ed.). London: Chapman & Hall.

Hartman, J., & Landau, W. M. (1987). Comparison of formal language therapy with supportive counselling for aphasia due to acute vascular accident. *Archives of Neurology, 44,* 646–649.

Hayslip, B. (1989). Fluid ability training with aged people: A past with a future? *Educational Gerontology, 15,* 573–595.

Helm-Estabrooks, N., Emery, P., & Albert, M. L. (1987). The treatment of aphasic perseveration (TAP) program: A new approach to aphasia therapy. *Archives of Neurology, 44,* 1253–1255.

Holland, A. L., Fromm, D. S., DeRuyter, F., & Stein, M. (1996). Treatment efficacy: Aphasia. *Journal of Speech and Hearing Research, 39*(5), s27–s36.

Joanett, Y., Brouchon, M., Gauthier, L., & Samson, M. (1986). Pointing with left versus right hand in left visual field neglect. *Neuropsychologia, 24,* 391–396.

Kapur, N. (1995). Memory aids in the rehabilitation of memory-disordered patients. In A. D. Baddeley, B. A. Wilson, & F. N. Watts (Eds.), *Handbook of memory disorders.* Chichester, UK: Wiley.

Kelly, T. P., Skilbeck, C. E., Welch, J. L., Bradley, V. A., & Britton, P. G. (1993). Long-term follow-up of microcomputer-based cognitive retraining: 15th European Conference, INS. *Journal of Clinical and Experimental Neuropsychology, 15*(3), 396.

Klavora, P., Gaskovski, K. M., Forsyth, R. D., et al. (1995). The effects of dynavision rehabilitation on behind-the-wheel driving ability and selected psychomotor abilities of persons after stroke. *American Journal of Occupational Therapy, 49,* 534–542.

Kurlychek, R. T., & Levin, W. (1987). Computers in the cognitive rehabilitation of brain-injured persons. *CRC Critical Reviews in Medical Informatics, 1,* 241–257.

Ladavas, E., Menghini, G., & Umilta, C. (1994). A rehabilitation study of hemispatial neglect. *Cognitive Neuropsychology, 11*(1), 75–95.

Lezak, M. D. (1995). *Neuropsychological assessment* (3rd ed.). New York: Oxford University Press.

Lincoln, N. B., Mulley, G. P., Jones, A. C., et al. (1984). Effectiveness of speech therapy for aphasic stroke patients. *Lancet,* 1197–1200.

McClure, J. (1997). The iconic memory skills of brain injury survivors before and after iconic memory skills training. *Cognitive Rehabilitation, 15*(3), 20–23.

McKitrick, L. A., & Camp, C. J. (1993). Relearning the names of things: The spaced-retrieval intervention implemented by a caregiver. *Clinical Gerontology, 14*(2), 60–62.

Moffat, N. (1989). Home based cognitive rehabilitation with the elderly. In L. W. Poon, D. C. Rubin, & B. A. Wilson (Eds.), *Everyday cognition in adulthood and later life.* Cambridge, UK: Cambridge University Press.

Moffat, N. (1992). Strategies of memory therapy. In B. A. Wilson & N. Moffat (Eds.), *Clinical management of memory problems* (2nd ed.). London: Chapman & Hall.

Moroney, J. T., & Desmond, D. W. (1996). Cognitve impairment and risk of stroke in the older population: Comment. *Journal of the American Geriatrics Society, 44*(11), 1410–1411.

Morris, P. L., Raphael, B., & Robinson, R. G. (1992). Clinical depression is associated with impaired recovery from stroke. *Medical Journal Australia, 157*(4), 239–242.

Nickels, L., & Best, W. (1996). Therapy for naming disorders: (Part 1). Principles, puzzles and progress. *Aphasiology, 10*(1), 21–47.

Norman, D. A., & Shallice, T. (1986). Attention to action: Willed and automatic control of behaviour. In R. J. Davidson, G. E. Swartz, & D. Shapiro (Eds.), *Consciousness and self-regulation: Advances in research.* New York: Plenum Press.

Padesky, C. A., & Greenberger, D. (1995). *Clinician's guide to mind over mood.* New York: Guilford Press.

Panza, F., Solfrizzi, V., Mastroianni, F., et al. (1997). A rehabilitation program for mild memory impairments. *Archives of Gerontology and Geriatrics, Suppl. 5,* 51–55.

Patterson, K. (1994). Reading, writing and rehabilitation: A reckoning. In M. J. Riddoch & G. W. Humphreys (Eds.), *Cognitive neuropsychology and cognitive rehabilitation.* Hove, UK: LEA.

Prigatano, G. P. (1995). Personality and social aspects of memory rehabilitation. In A. D. Baddeley, B. A. Wilson, & F. N. Watts (Eds.), *Handbook of memory disorders.* Chichester, UK: Wiley.

Prigatano, G. P. (1997). Learning from our successes and failures: Reflections and comments on "cognitive rehabilitation: How it is and how it might be." *Journal of the International Neuropsychological Society, 3*(5), 497–499.

Riddoch, M. J., & Humphreys, G. W. (Eds). (1994). *Cognitive neuropsychology and cognitive rehabilitation.* Hove, UK: LEA.

Rizzolatti, G., & Camarda, R. (1987). Neural circuits for spatial attention and unilateral neglect. In M. Jeannerod (Ed.), *Neurophysiological and neuropsychological aspects of neglect.* Amsterdam: North-Holland.

Robertson, I. H., Halligan, P. W., & Marshall, J. C. (1993). In I. H. Robertson & J. C. Marshall (Eds.), *Unilateral neglect: Clinical and experimental studies.* Hove, UK: LEA.

Robertson, I. H., & North, N. (1992). Spatio-motor cueing in unilateral neglect: The role of hemispace, hand and motor activation. *Neuropsychologia, 30,* 553–563.

Rossi, P. W., Kheyfets, S., & Reding, M. J. (1990). Fresnel prisms improve visual perception in stroke patients with homonymous hemianopia or unilateral visual neglect. *Neurology, 40,* 1597–1599.

Seron, X., Deloche, G., & Coyette, F. (1989). A retrospective analysis of a single case neglect therapy: A point of theory. In X. Seron & G. Deloche (Eds.), *Cognitive approaches to neuropsychological rehabilitation.* Hillsdale, NJ: LEA.

Skilbeck, C. E. (1991). Microcomputer-based cognitive rehabilitation. In A. Ager (Ed.), *Microcomputers and clinical psychology: Issues, applications and future developments.* Chichester, UK: Wiley.

Skilbeck, C. E., & Robertson, I. H. (1992). Computer assistance in the management of memory and cognitive impairment. In B. A. Wilson & N. Moffat (Eds.), *Clinical management of memory problems* (2nd ed.). London: Chapman & Hall.

Sohlberg, M. M., & Mateer, C. A. (1989). *Introduction to cognitive rehabilitation.* New York: Guilford.

Sturm, W. & Willmes, K. (1991). Efficacy of a reaction training on various attentional and cognitive functions in stroke patients. *Neuropsychological Rehabilitation, 1*(4), 259–280.

Sturm, S. W., Willmes, K., Orgass, B., & Hartje, W. (1997). Do specific attention deficits need specific training? *Neuropsychological Rehabilitation, 7*(2), 81–103.

Von Cramon, D. Y., & Matthes-von Cramon, G. (1994). Back to work with a chronic dysexecutive syndrome? (A case report). *Neuropsychological Rehabilitation, 4*(4), 399–417.

Wade, D. T., Skilbeck, C., & Langton-Hewer, R. (1983). Predicting Barthel ADL scores at 6 months after stroke. *Archives of Physical Medicine and Rehabilitation, 64,* 24–28.

Wagenaar, R. C., Van Wieringen, P. C. W., Netelenbos, J. B., et al. (1992). The transfer of scanning training effects in visual attention after stroke: Five single cases. *Disability & Rehabilitation, 14*(1), 51–60.

Walker, R., Young, A. W., & Lincoln, N. B. (1996). Eye patching and the rehabilitation of visual neglect. *Neuropsychological Rehabilitation, 6*(3), 219–231.

Wearing, D. (1992). The need for self-help groups. In B. A. Wilson & N. Moffat (Eds.), *Clinical management of memory problems* (2nd ed.). London: Chapman & Hall.

Wienberg, J., Diller, L., Gordon, W. A., et al. (1977). Visual scanning training effect on reading-related tasks in acquired right brain damage. *Archives of Physical Medicine and Rehabilitation, 58,* 479–486.

Wienberg, J., Diller, L., Gordon, W. A., et al. (1979). Training sensory awareness and spatial organisation in people with right brain damage. *Archives of Physical Medicine and Rehabilitation, 60,* 491–496.

Wilson, B. A. (1987). *Rehabilitation of memory.* London: Guilford Press.

Wilson, B. A. (1992). Memory therapy in practice. In B. A. Wilson & N. Moffat (Eds.), *Clinical management of memory problems* (2nd ed.). London: Chapman & Hall.

Wilson, B. A., Evans, J. C., Emslie, H., & Malinek, V. (1997). Evaluation of Neuropage: A new memory aid. *Journal of Neurology, Neurosurgery & Psychiatry, 63,* 113–115.

Wilson, B. A., & Hughes, E. (1997). Coping with amnesia: The natural history of a compensatory memory system. *Neuropsychological Rehabilitation, 7*(1), 43–56.

Wilson, B. A., & Watson, P. C. (1996). A practical framework for understanding compensatory behaviour in people with memory impairment. *Memory, 4,* 465–486.

Woods, R. T. (1996). Psychological "therapies" in dementia. In R. T. Woods (Ed.), *Handbook of the clinical psychology of ageing.* Chichester, UK: Wiley.

World Health Organization. (1980). *International classification of impairments, disabilities and handicaps: A manual of classification relating to the consequences of disease.* Geneva: World Health Organization.

Yesavage, J. A. (1985). Nonpharmocologic treatments for memory losses with normal ageing. *American Journal of Psychiatry, 142*(5), 600–605.

Yesavage, J. A., Sheikh, J., Tanke, E. D., & Hill, R. (1988). Response to memory training and individual differences in verbal intelligence and state anxiety. *American Journal of Psychiatry, 145*(5), 636–639.

Index

abilities, 166
  basic, 18
  fluid *vs.* crystallized, 45–46
acquisition. *See also* learning; skill acquisition
  of information, 24–25, 50. *See also* encoding
acquisition assistance, and use of cues, 231–34
activities of daily living (ADLs), 212–13, 251, 270, 275, 276
ADEPT (Adult Development and Enrichment) program, 4, 5, 17
age
  and memory training outcome, 31
  processing resources and, 48–49
age-associated memory impairment (AAMI), 23
age-related loss, control, and motivation
  conceptual model of, 112–13
aging
  cognitive changes associated with normal, 45–50, 124, 208–10, 280–81, 284. *See also* memory aging
  and skill usage and acquisition, 42–43

stereotypes regarding, 170
  "usual" and "successful," 209
Alderman, N., 283
Allen, C., 26
Alzheimer's disease (AD), 29, 240–41. *See also* Dementia of the Alzheimer's Type
  depression in, 178
  exercise and, 133–34
  interventions and, 227, 235, 238
  case studies, 258–63
  smoking and, 148, 150–51
amnesia, source, 236
anger management, 168
anxiety, 90, 110–11, 116. *See also* relaxation training
apathetic clients, 169
apolipoprotein E (ApoE), 177–78
assessment, 182–85, 214. *See also* psychometric test performance
  determining the cause of impairment, 215–18
  interpretation of test results, 209
  of mood, 181
  of suspected cognitive decline, 207–8, 210–15